Monument to Failure

Monument to Failure

COMPANION PIECE TO

So Much Pleasure,
So Little Pain

NICKOLAS VASSILI

authorHOUSE™

1663 LIBERTY DRIVE, SUITE 200
BLOOMINGTON, INDIANA 47403
(800) 839-8640
WWW.AUTHORHOUSE.COM

AuthorHouse™
1663 Liberty Drive, Suite 200
Bloomington, IN 47403
www.authorhouse.com
Phone: 1-800-839-8640

AuthorHouse™ UK Ltd.
500 Avebury Boulevard
Central Milton Keynes, MK9 2BE
www.authorhouse.co.uk
Phone: 08001974150

First published by AuthorHouse 1/29/2007
(This printer's revision date is irrelevant of the actual publication date of May 2007.)

ISBN: 978-1-4259-8587-5 (sc)

Printed in the United States of America
Bloomington, Indiana

This book is printed on acid-free paper.

Library of Congress Control Number: 2006911179

In dedication to life, which is for living and love—not death.

Acknowledgements

I dedicate this book to my wife Nan, who has endured much above and beyond the call of duty and without whom I would never have experienced so many joyous years; and to my four brilliant children, Billy, Jenny, Julie, and Ellie, whose very existence has enriched my life beyond words.

To my dear friends, Neil and Lee Selden, whose loyalty, love, and support has meant so much to my entire family for almost 40 years; Brent and Peg Gushowaty, whose matchless personalities give me what little hope I hold out for the future of humanity; to Randall Nozawa, who brought the gift of friendship, and a smile for the rest of my life; and to Maurice and Rose Foley, who stood by me at the worst of times and whose humor I shall always cherish.

To Edmund Spencer, a man of great dignity, charm, and conceptual awareness, who taught us a lifetime of things we could never have learned otherwise; to Ray Hauserman, who taught me to meditate and appreciate the teachings of Sree Sree Thakur Anukul Chandra; to Father John Pallas, who inspired my awakening and never lost sight of what was important; and to James Germano, who pointed me in a direction that taught me how to help others.

To Harry Bovain, my first teacher and mentor, who set an example for me that I will never forget; to Joe Ray and Nate Resch, two mensches of the first order, who gave me my first legitimate job; and to Eddie Cohen, my first true friend and fellow Scout.

Regarding my editor, Mi Ae Lipe ... What can I say that would possibly cover the extent of my gratitude for your labor of love? You took what I hoped would be readable and turned it into something I can be proud of, giving me the freedom to expand the book to heights that I never dreamt of. You not only edited the book but also took on a myriad of other responsibilities, all above and beyond the call of duty. So how can I ever thank you? I don't know—but I'll try.

Contents

Preface

For those of you who have not (or do not plan to) read *So Much Pleasure, So Little Pain,* which is the autobiographical precursor to *Monument To Failure,* there are some vital missing links related to obesity and dieting that I must fill you in on, or else you will more than likely be left in the dark about certain aspects of this healthcare book.

I started out more than 30 years ago to write a book about my experience with obesity and dieting. I have been plagued with obesity from early childhood, and had spent 23 years excessively dieting, fasting, exercising, and trying every sane or cockeyed method of dealing with the problem. In the process, I became a professional dieter.

Over the decades of constant struggle with my weight problem, I pursued two careers, one in show business, the other as a group therapist. During both of these periods, I involved myself in numerous alternative health dynamics, ranging from emotional and sense-memory exercises to hypnotism, bodybuilding and weight-lifting, Eastern philosophies, and a succession of therapies and nondrug-related approaches to building a healthy lifestyle. As a result, I accumulated a wealth of knowledge and personal experience about healthcare in general—not just dieting—and decided to expand my writing to include a large chapter titled "Monument To Failure" in the book.

However, I did not recognize just how much material I had amassed, and with the help of an editor who wanted to see the mission completed to the fullest, I embarked on what was to become the book adventure of a lifetime.

Initially thinking that the entire work would total no more than 600 pages, we soon discovered that it could not be contained in 650, 700, or even 800 pages! And when the page count reached 840—we had no choice but to accept the fact that we would have to publish this opus as a two-part book.

Having arrived at this decision, we realized that many people might not initially be interested in reading my autobiography (I'm not a famous Hollywood star or a well-known personality), but that they might opt for reading *Monument To Failure* because of their personal medical issues. With that in mind, we knew that it was necessary for the healthcare work to stand on its own.

To fill you in on all of the essential text that is contained in the autobiography, we extracted the story material dealing with obesity and dieting and made it a chapter titled "Roman Emperors of Old." With this addition, you should have no problems understanding and bridging the two volumes.

Not that this is to say that you needn't read *So Much Pleasure, So Little Pain.*

Although you will be able to access all of the vital healthcare material in *Monument To Failure,* there is much you can learn from the autobiography. For instance, you will determine what drove me to be such an extremist and consequently arrive at the viewpoints presented in *Monument To Failure.* Above and beyond that, you will get to know me in a very personal way ... which should ensure that you will hopefully have a clear sense of where I'm coming from at every turn of the page.

I would also like to express my deep gratitude to Dr. Barbara Starfield for her prompt and gracious willingness to read *Monument To Failure* and to offer her positive comments and suggestions. All those who are concerned about our deplorable healthcare system can be thankful to Dr. Starfield for many years of service not only as America's foremost healthcare advocate, but also for her courage and determination in the face of insurmountable odds and opposition. She is a shining example of how people can support others in common cause, and I am beholden to her for her affirmation and enthusiasm.

In marked contrast to Dr. Starfield's readiness to read and proffer her opinion and endorsement, I must—in the spirit of this book—confront those healthcare advocates and organizations who were unwilling to as much as review it, even though doing so might advance the overall cause of healthcare. The very people and organizations that should join together in solidarity and in my effort to inform and enlighten the American public have shown that we must all be aware of the enemy within—who refuse to get down in the trenches with comrades-at-arms.

I take special exception to HealthGrades, the leading healthcare ratings company, whose executive staff "declined the opportunity," and CodeBlueNow!, The National Coalition on Healthcare and the Center for Public Policy, whose founder and CEO Kathleen O'Conner would not as much as read even this book's four-page introduction, much less offer any comments.

Throughout my professional life, one of the most disturbing realities that I constantly faced was that so many individuals and organizations that supposedly supported progressive human causes would not—under any circumstances—show a united front in advancing the very cause to which they were committed to.

This has been the case with prison reform movements, drug prevention programs, and environmental organizations. They all talk the talk—but fail to walk the walk with others dedicated to the same objectives. That's one of the main reasons that so little progress has been made in dealing with the most serious issues of our time.

Ultimately, we must come together ... or we shall all fail....

Be safe on your journey. Joy Guru!

Nickolas Vassili
Seattle, November 2006

Part I.
Monument to Failure

Monument to Failure

I must warn the reader that this book is not for the faint-hearted. It won't mince words. It will be brutally frank, forcing you to either put it out of sight because you are unwilling to examine what it represents on a personal level, or else to read it in its entirety and face a reality that is truly terrifying.

The American public has grown accustomed to a way of life that involves drugs, surgeries, unhealthy eating that results in excess weight and obesity, lack of proper exercise, self-destructive lifestyles, mental and emotional unhealthiness, declining healthcare standards (we are ranked 37th among industrialized nations), a meek tolerance for a political system that no longer serves the needs of the people, and a paralyzing indifference to the fact that we are, through ignorance and greed, aiding and abetting the willful demolition of our environment and our planet.

Before embarking on this potentially hazardous journey of lies, manipulations, deceit, bureaucratic corruption on an unimaginable scale, and the threatening postures of a corporate and political mentality immune to decency and truth, I must ask one thing of the reader: Understand from the beginning that this book is meant to confront the powers that be within the entire industry of healthcare in America, and to unearth and expose those individuals, groups, corporations, non-profits, and governmental agencies directly responsible for the horrendously inadequate healthcare conditions in America, **ones that cause the needless deaths of 500,000 people every year.**

This will not be a pretty story, nor will it indulge in seeking moderate and less confrontational ways of revealing the full extent of the enormous human tragedy and disaster that engulfs our nation's healthcare system. This book will meet the truth head-on, with no apologies for profane language or what might be regarded as assault tactics.

We must regard our journey as a war zone, and we can ill-afford the luxury of politeness or inane respect for people and organizations merely because they have titled positions and control the workings of our derelict healthcare system, or our government for that matter. As such, I will not give in to some false notion of supposed respectability and reverence for institutions merely to appease those at the helm of these deficient organizations. (When I was in the Air Force, I never bought into the regulation "Respect the uniform, not the man," because I witnessed untold abuse of this sacrosanct command. It's simply too easy to hide behind titles, and commit all manner of crimes. Just examine President Bush's misuse and outright abuse of office, which has wreaked havoc on our healthcare and environment; caused war, death, and destruction; and threatens the future of civilization itself.)

Neither should you look for a balanced opinion, nor complain that this section of my book is overly negative in its views and does not give equal time and space to the more positive aspects of our healthcare structure. **It is not meant for these purposes.** It is meant to create a tidal wave of action against the entire heartless healthcare system that is deservedly ranked as the worst in the industrialized world.

On the same serious note, for those who immediately challenge my claim that the American healthcare system is a monument to failure, and attempt to detract from this overall truth by pointing out positive aspects (which certainly exist for those who can afford a superior brand of healthcare), I must further clarify my position:

One of the biggest reasons that Americans are insulated from the overwhelming dimensions of our healthcare problems is that the issue is fed to us piecemeal; from A to Z, we read, listen, and watch the various elements presented as individual and separate parts, but never internalize them as a whole.

The pharmaceutical industry, drug marketing, hospitals, surgery, insurance companies, care providers, doctors, dentists, psychiatrists, social workers, nurses, emergency treatment, foster care, smoking, cancer research, drug prevention, environmental protection, the Federal Drug Administration, Katrina victims, a thousand and one studies, and the media—to hell and back. The components of the American healthcare system are always fragmented into convenient sound bites and then parceled out as separate and unique stories.

It's as if the dropping of the first atomic bomb on Hiroshima was a series of distinct and individual accounts: a B-29 named the *Enola Gay* flying toward its destination, the bomb bay door of the plane opening, the bomb dropping, the mushroom cloud, a small section of the bombed area, individual bodies buried beneath rubble, stunned bomb victims walking about, radiation burns on people's backs, the *Enola Gay* returning to base. **Everything but the total devastation of an entire city, leaving more than 100,000 dead civilians.**

Likewise, we bear witness to these apparently disconnected problems and catastrophes related to our healthcare, and as these separate events circle about our everyday existence, we focus our attention on them only one at a time. We are never completely deluged by the entire range of deadly events at their destructive worst.

We never see the full tsunami, the total Hurricane Katrina, the greater backdrop of horror and destruction. It's easier to accept the carnage when it is presented one bloody account at a time, one frightening occurrence on a given day, one shocking eyewitness revelation, without losing sleep over any of it.

Even if it's 9/11, which brings the full story closer to home, it's still not close enough to make us stop in our tracks and realize that a full-scale war is taking place—and we're not yet actively involved in it. Although we *feel* involved, we keep relatively clear of all the issues that do not personally impact our lives, simply leaving all the conflict areas in the hands of the very individuals and organizations that are ill-equipped or unwilling (as many of them are) to deal with them. It's as if we were hoping that our lame government would painlessly and effortlessly cure the problems, allowing us to reap the benefits without taking on any of the responsibilities.

In case you're still wondering what the point of my popping off about our limited understanding and acceptance of our total healthcare disaster is all about, let me illustrate it in another way: There are numerous accounts, reports, books, articles, studies, websites, blogs, and documentaries about various parts of the healthcare system of America. But they all focus on separate issues. At best, they sometimes overlap in one or two other near-related areas. But by and large, they are fragmented stories, not the complete picture—**which is what we must see if we are ever going to realize the full extent of what must be dealt with.**

We are also unmindful of the political ramifications of our disastrous healthcare system, naïve enough to think that solutions to the myriad of problems, conflicts, and deficiencies within the wide range of healthcare systems can be enacted on a selective basis. Nothing could be further from the truth. Without an overhaul of our present political situation as it directly affects healthcare, meaningful improvement is, on all practical levels, improbable, if not impossible.

As an example: An estimated 103,000 people died in 2005 as a result of infections, including staph, contracted in American hospitals. These people died needlessly because our hospitals fail to maintain proper hygienic standards. It's that basic. And it would be relatively elementary to solve that problem—as many nations have. But it cannot happen because the White House controls the regulatory agencies—such as the Center for Disease Control (CDC)—and that agency has refused to respond to the crying need for improvement in the hygiene standards within American hospitals. In fact, the CDC will not even provide the public with the vital information and statistics related to the names and locations of the worst of these hospitals, so that people could at least avoid going to these places.

So it's as much a political problem as it is a healthcare issue. Don't think you can separate one from the other. Not in America.

And if you still want to hold on to some vestige of hope that the powers that be can bring about meaningful change and improvement in our healthcare without political mending and restoration, remember what happened when President and Mrs. Clinton attempted to reconstruct the healthcare system in 1993—and the insurance industry made mincemeat of their attempt. It was "No contest!"

※ ※ ※

To the very best of my knowledge, this book titled "Monument to Failure" is the most comprehensive study and critique of the American healthcare system that has ever been made. And I am uniquely qualified to be making it. Why? Because, whereas all the other written accounts about the American healthcare system have been written by specialists in one field or another, I bring a much broader range of skills and experiences to the table.

If you doubt that I possess this range of skills necessary for such a comprehensive accounting of our healthcare system, then I don't think you've read *So Much Pleasure, So Little Pain,* the precursor to this book—in which case you should read that first before tackling this volume.

And once you've read and examined my in-depth involvement with such issues as drug use, abuse, prevention, and treatment; a broad spectrum of therapies; hypnosis; dieting; health-related issues; medical experiences; exercise; and writing, reporting, and publishing, you'll understand that these credentials, although not an M.D. or Ph.D, have equipped me to accomplish what very few people might be able to do in terms of presenting this comprehensive study.

I am also uniquely qualified to solve the wide range of problems associated with the healthcare system. Why? Because I ran more than 4,000 therapy groups over a period of 15 years, and my objective was to become the best problem-solver in the world. And pardon me for tooting my own horn—but I did it!

I should also mention that I initiated and created training programs specifically related to the behavioral therapies in America (confrontation, encounter, reality therapy) during the 1960s and '70s that became the model for all such training that followed. In essence, I wrote the modern-day manual on the subject of problem solving. (It's an everlasting shame that my study, research, and experiences were vandalized and bastardized by individuals and organizations that were interested only in profits. It's also amazing—agonizing—to realize that so many nonprofits aligned themselves with insurance racketeers to peddle these watered-down versions of genuine therapeutic tools and programs to the unsuspecting masses.)

So if I'm challenged to come up with answers to all the horrendous things I'm about to outline, I have them! Starting with the all-important proviso of first identifying the problem—not in legal, bureaucratic, or economic terms—which only results in watered-down compromises and failure—but in human and conceptual terms, and concluding with a commitment to change, this is the way to go!

If we start from that point, we have a much greater chance of getting on the road to recovery and good health.

And don't forget that doctors, lawyers, legislators, and the so-called elite of the healthcare world have been at it for many decades, and look at the results! Failure upon failure, and absolute resistance to change. That's all the more reason why any effective change in the system must begin on a political level.

I am telling this "elite" group to move over already and give someone else a shot at solving the problem; that's what this is about. And I will take it off the ground by speaking the ugly truth, confronting those responsible for the debacle, awakening the public to the true dimensions of this cataclysmic healthcare tragedy, and moving on to face the monumental political measures that must be grappled with and adopted. Fair enough?

In that regard, I must herein quote Winston Churchill's beseeching statement to President Roosevelt in 1941: "We shall not fail or falter. We shall not weaken or tire. Give us the tools, and we will finish the job."

Above all, please believe that as highly confrontational as it is, **this book is meant to inspire vast change.** But if we are to recreate and move forward, we must first acknowledge and then tear away the obstacles that stand in the way of progress. Then we must redefine the healthcare system—from top to bottom—and begin anew. That's what we need—a fresh start.

Author's note: Large parts of this book will be written in a question-and-answer format to anticipate the reader's curiosity. It also uses and reviews factual information from original sources to illustrate premises and concepts, criticism (denoted by shaded boxes with the header "NF" for "NICKFACT"), and other commentary on the subject matter.

✳ ✳ ✳

What is life all about? Is it just hard work and a struggle to have some money in the bank, a pension, health plan, and a good primary care physician, so that the rest is gravy? Is that what you've been up to all your life? When you get right down to it, this general matter of security, for whatever it's worth, does seem to be our purpose for existence.

"Not so," you say. "It's more about living, loving, feeling self-esteem, and dealing with life's challenges." Yeah, that sounds like the real McCoy to me, too. But for most of us, this is a pretense because by the time you reach 40, the ideals and images of a supposedly greater meaning in life begin to fade into the background, and you become increasingly attached to other ambitions, security, and sustenance, not to mention the provisions of your medical insurance.

With this growing awareness, the older you get, the more frightening this aging becomes, and for one simple reason: You have only so many more years to live, and you want them to be "quality" years. But will they be? Will the security measures you've taken through the decades really be worth all the hard work and struggle you put into them? Or will they just be eaten up by doctors, drug costs, insurance and hospital bills, leaving you with little reward for all those years of planning ahead?

If you think I'm exaggerating, talk to some middle-class senior citizens and find out what they're going through. You'll learn that the overall picture of their preparations for a quality existence in their senior years is becoming more muddled, depressing, and insecure with each passing year. They can do little about it.

And it's safe to say that times are going to get a hell of a lot worse for upcoming generations. If everything is left to the corporate scheme of things, the insurance companies, our present administration in Washington, D.C., and the next feckless breed of political leaders lying in wait, your future pensions[1] and Social Security payments won't be worth the price of admission to a cheap movie. And God only knows what shape America's healthcare system will be like in the future. (Don't be naïve enough to think it can't get much worse.)

As reported in the *Boston Herald:*

HEALTH-CARE EXPENSES KEEP RISING
FOR PEOPLE IN RETIREMENT

Jay Fitzgerald, *Boston Herald***—March 7, 2006**

Retiring elderly couples will need $200,000 in savings just to pay for the most basic medical coverage during their golden years, according to new estimates by Boston's Fidelity Investments.

The latest figure is up 5.3 percent from last year's $190,000 estimate. Cost estimates have been rising at an average 5.8 percent clip a year since 2002, Fidelity said.

"Health-care costs have the potential to significantly erode an individual's retirement savings," said Brad Kilmer, a vice president who oversaw the study at Fidelity.

The survey notes that fewer companies are offering health-care benefits for retirees—increasing the financial burden on the elderly after they stop working.

The survey is based on the assumption that a couple 65 years old or older relies heavily on Medicare.

---

[1] Currently, company pension plans are underfunded by an estimated $450 billion, and The Pension Benefit Guaranty Corp.—the federal agency that insures private pension plans much like the Federal Deposit Insurance Corp. insures bank accounts—estimates that $100 billion of that is with companies with serious funding problems. Without drastic change, which Congress has failed to achieve, the entire system could implode in much the same way as the late 1980s savings and loan crisis, which resulted in a $130 billion taxpayer bailout.

*Taking into account premium costs, deductibles, pay-per-visits
and supplemental insurance, a couple's health-care bills can run
into big bucks, Kilmer said.*

*"This is the part of retirement people frequently forget," he
said.*

I'll let you in on a secret: You were wrong from the beginning to think that you could guard against all the possible eventualities of old age by building your nest egg and surrounding it with all the medical provisions outlined in your retirement plans. You were equally wrong to think that you would not only have the necessary resources but that you would also know how to carry out the crowning plan of your older years.

How could you have made such huge mistakes?

It's simple—you were led down the golden path by an organized, systematic, nearly foolproof scheme that you bought into when you were very young and never really considered thereafter because it made all the sense in the world. And why should you have had second thoughts about your long-range security program, when all the other smart people you know also bought into it? Could so many intelligent people be wrong?

I compare it to living in Los Angeles, where much of the white middle class lead lives seemingly devoid of basic human virtues, touting such ostentatious materialism, lack of respect, and severe insecurity made apparent by extreme denial that it's hard to believe. Imagine shouting out and confronting the lot of them to say, "You know—you're all nuts!" They would look at you, and with one collective expression, make it clear that you're the one who's insane.

It's the same thing with your health provisions—because it takes a different dimension of thinking to accept the fact that **so many people could be wrong. But they are! And you're most likely caught in the trap of believing otherwise.**

I suggest that you put your ego aside to examine what I am about to outline as if your life depends on it—because it really does. That is, **if** you're concerned with having a quality life instead of mere existence. Even if you think that you're okay with things as they are, I implore you to consider all the implications and consequences. **People of all ages—listen up!**

What is this "scheme" that you have bought into?

It's a national plot, a conspiracy of unbelievable dimensions to destroy your health and well-being and empty your wallet and bank accounts, leaving only enough for your burial.

Whether you like it or not, you have been hijacked from the time your mom and dad conceived you and been suckered ever since by this **conglomerate** of greedy, self-serving, vainglorious, power-hungry megalomaniacs and thieves.

Who makes up this conglomerate?

- Government leaders who turn a deaf ear to healthcare issues and align themselves with the highest bidder.

- Politicians who are lobbied, bribed, and remain at the beck and call of the conglomerate.

- Lobbyists who crank up all the illicit schemes for the various sectors of the conglomerate.

- The media that advertise and promote this conglomerate's killing fields, lending unholy credence to the mindless, heartless, ongoing ecumenical genocide.

- Pharmaceutical companies.

- Medical insurance agencies.

- Managed-care facilities and operators.

- Medical schools.

- Medical publications.

- Doctors (including psychiatrists, psychologists, and dentists).

- Lawyers.

Following close behind the conglomerate, although not quite charter members of this sick fraternity, are the regulatory agencies that are pro-business rather than pro-people: the Federal Drug Administration (FDA), the Centers for Disease Control and Prevention (CDC), and the Environmental Protection Agency (EPA).

In support of these administrative lapdogs, we have the prominent and highly influential professional associations: the American Medical Association (AMA), the American Dental Association (ADA), and the American Psychiatric Association (APA).

For good measure, we must also include the National Cancer Institute (NCI), which all but ignores cancer prevention in favor of aiding and abetting the pharmaceutical industry's stockpiling of more and more drugs—which, by and large, do not cure cancer.

I might be hard-pressed to prove beyond a shadow of a doubt that the different heads of this conglomerate dragon hold regular meetings to arrange for the deadly tools of their trades to be brought to bear against the population, but denying its existence is like denying the existence of organized crime, the military-industrial complex, the ozone layer, global warming, and the Holocaust. I mean, "Do big brown bears live and shit in the woods?"

This is not to question whether the conglomerate's leaders and corporate heads meet to discuss the ways of maintaining complete control over our bodies and minds. However, unlike criminal organizations like the Mafia, whose Appalachian-style meetings have been recorded, documented, and used as evidence to convict mob bosses of everything from criminal conspiracy to extortion and murder, the conglomerate's purveyors of drugs, disease, and death follow the "gentlemen's agreement."

And, of course, they employ a thriving community of underlings who knowingly carry out the dirty work for the conglomerate heads-of-state. This is why the big shots themselves are rarely prosecuted for crimes, much less spend a day behind bars.

Coupled with this supporting network **AND** the ignorant public—who are nothing more than fodder for these werewolves and their clan of demons—the conglomerate is, for all intents and purposes, untouchable and immune to prosecution, **above the law.** All the more so because they have the complete and undying support of the administration in Washington, as well as most elected officials in both political parties.

Yes, I most assuredly demonize and condemn this entire alliance of conspirators and killers because it has robbed our people of the will to resist this daily encroachment on their lives, has destroyed the nation's health and sanity, and rendered obsolete our minds and immune systems.

How does the conglomerate
get a foothold on our lives?

It begins at conception, when expectant mothers (and usually in the background, fathers) visit their doctors and are given their walking papers. Here's where the deceit that will last a lifetime begins: The doctors don't necessarily say anything that is outwardly negative, or forcefully insist that their instructions be followed. No, they don't have to do it that way because they know beyond a shadow of a doubt that when push comes to shove, their patients will obey their commands at fear of death. Better believe it!

Their scare tactics and manipulations, like their superficial smiles and hand-shakes, are precise tools of their trade, honed and polished in much the same way car salesmen or telemarketers craft their business pitches. Patients are left with the threat of loss ("I can't guarantee that the procedure will be effective unless. ... ") should they fail to heed the warnings of their physicians.

That's why hundreds of thousands of pregnant women, who have researched their childbearing needs and determined well in advance that they will not be given a drug to induce labor, fall by the wayside at the last minute, agreeing to the doctor's bedside warnings to submit to the needle. They're afraid of what might happen to their children if they don't do what they're told. And, just like a child who doesn't want to be punished, they will obey the command of the authority figure—who society tells us "knows better and is doing it for our good."

To induce labor, the drug (Pitocin or misoprostol) enters the mother's AND the baby's system. **With this, the lifelong game of drugs and medical fraud has begun.** Although you haven't officially signed up for life, your chances of escaping the all-encompassing network of deception and carnage are now next to nil because you'll want to play it safe and stick with the ruling institution's directive.

Look at it this way: My wife Nan and I were initially dumb enough to be thankful to a jerk doctor who almost killed her and our son during his delivery. We felt grateful because they survived the ordeal, but we didn't stop to think about what had actually happened. In fact, the average person will probably go a lifetime without thinking about what has happened for the same reason. You're alive, apparently well, and afraid to question or confront the doctor, even when s/he is obviously guilty of malfeasance (unless a clever lawyer convinces you to sue).

We are shackled to our fears, addicted as such, and will go to our deaths that way. In fact, **if**, at the moment of our passing, a voice were to cry out, "You didn't think—you could have been healthy and lived a quality life for many more years had you used your mind—instead of drugs—and not followed your doctor's advice," I'll bet you dollars to donuts that you'd look up and call out, "No—don't tell me that! I did what was right!"

Wanna bet?

I find it uncanny that seemingly intelligent people are so willing to accept the advice of physicians merely because they have the title and license to administer supposed healing. I find it equally mysterious that the average individual can be so cowed by authority figures that they accept the smile and handshake of the doctor as proof positive that they are in good hands. We never consider the possibility that the physician in question may be greedy, uncaring, and incompetent. In fact, even when we see signs of fault, laziness, or indifference, we are still obedient to the doctor. Nothing else seems to filter into our general landscape of thought and awareness.

Would we employ such blind faith in the case of a bus driver? Just because he works for an established company, obviously has a license to drive a bus, and smiles politely doesn't necessarily mean he's a conscientious driver, much less an excellent one. He may be a terror behind the wheel.

The same holds true for most professions; when we bring our cars in for repair, we don't automatically believe that our means of transportation (and safety) is being cared for by a good mechanic. We expect the job to be done correctly, the car to operate efficiently, and the bill to be fair payment for a job well-done. If it's not—we generally raise hell.

So how is it that we treat doctors as someone above the human and professional standard of almost all others? Why do we follow "blind faith," failing to react and respond intelligently with common sense and natural defenses against potential harm, even death, as a result of serious medical misgivings? Why are we so damn blind, deaf, and dumb to the obvious and to the need of caution?

Try to remember that the doctor is no less and no more human and professional than the next person. He is capable of all things. And that includes ineptitude, callousness, apathetic behavior, even criminality. If we go into our medical situations with this rational and objective understanding, we have a much better chance of coming out of them with confidence and well-being. This clear-minded approach will also level the field, so to speak, and persuade the healer to mind his sworn oath to "First, do no harm" instead of giving him carte blanche.

The next stage of "obedience training" happens during the child's early years, when s/he is required—by law—to be vaccinated or immunized. This is a social doctrine supported by all areas of the unaware public, including the school system and all public health organizations.

Don't jump to the conclusion that I'm going to assail the entire system of vaccinations that has been devised over many decades of trial and has all but eradicated numerous diseases throughout the world. That's not necessarily the case, because I can't vouchsafe for whether or not my four children would have been better off had they not been vaccinated. But I should have known vaccination's pros and cons before allowing it to happen. We should all know what is happening to us before we agree to any vaccination or injection. **We should all be informed citizens, not obedient cattle.**

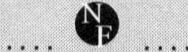

The federal advisory committee on immunization practices has recommended that the vaccine that protects against a sexually transmitted virus that causes cervical cancer be among the routine immunizations for 11- and 12-year-old girls. The committee recommends that the shots be available to girls as young as nine, in order to safeguard future generations.

Based on the way vaccinations are customarily school-mandated, chances are good that these shots will be accepted by most parents without careful evaluation and scrutiny. Therein lies the problem: No public forum on this issue will be held and no one will debate the pros and cons; and future generations of women who were vaccinated could possibly be at risk because of the lack of thorough and long-range studies of the vaccine's effectiveness and safety.

Simply put, the public will rubber-stamp its approval for this vaccine—as it does with so many other vital healthcare questions and issues.

I must address another point regarding vaccinations that has puzzled me for many years. Since almost all forms of vaccinations (including flu shots) are made from killed virus, which is derived using a homeopathic procedure, why does the medical profession deny the efficacy of homeopathic treatment, which was quite popular in the early part of the 20th century? (It reminds me of how American politics persecutes socialism while simultaneously supporting social security.) This mystery is shrouded in medical opinions that have little to do with the true reasons for keeping homeopathy out of the mainstream of medical care: namely money (from the sale of drugs) and power, which are always at the root of all these debatable and unsolved medical Catch-22s.

Likewise, the American Dental Association has been pussyfooting the issue of using amalgams as a filling material for over 150 years! The same arguments for and against the use of amalgam have not been resolved. As the battle rages, the public, as well as dentists throughout America, are caught in this vortex of contention. Of course, the only winners are those with financial interests, and the public be damned.

※ ※ ※

The third stage in the domination of our minds and bodies happens without notice or scheduling, and at any given time that we get sick or suffer an injury that is treated by a doctor or clinic. By this time in our lives, we are fully indoctrinated and programmed to obey doctors' commands, following the rules laid down by the ever-forceful medical fraternity and its subcultures. In the process, we are made to feel thankful and privileged to be receiving treatment in the first place—that is, if we are among those who are insured.

And if you do ask why a particular procedure or drug is necessary, don't over-extend the concession and show any signs of doubting the word of the "healer." That wouldn't be good form—at least not according to these clockwatching specialists.

As you leave the office or clinic bandaged up and with prescription in hand, once again you feel secure and healthy, totally relieved of any potential loss, because everything's okay. Right? Wrong. Let me tell you why.

We can rightfully be thankful for many natural gifts, and I seriously doubt if anyone would deny that the two most vital and treasured of these endowments are the mind and the immune system. Without these, we would not survive for more than a few hours beyond birth.

Bearing this in mind, we must ask ourselves, *why do we allow the conglomerate to control and ultimately destroy these two wonderful gifts from nature?*

※ ※ ※

Let's first take a good look at what happens to our minds. According to numerous scientific studies, we use only a small fraction of our brain power. Why is that? For one thing, we have been trained to not ask questions. And without asking questions, we cannot learn very much and we cannot stimulate our brain cells.

This underuse of our minds usually begins in public school, where we are forced to memorize dates and facts and to follow a prescribed course of learning, which is merely absorbing details, not asking questions or using our imaginations.

Case in point: When I entered my freshman year at James Madison High School in Brooklyn, New York, one of my classes was social studies. During the first two weeks of the term, the teacher focused on the three branches of our government. Much to her credit, she kept it interesting and even strangely exciting, making me want to learn more.

When the third week began, she discussed lobbies, explaining how high-priced lobbyists corner congressmen and senators in the halls of Congress to use their means of persuasion (including political contributions) to enact or defeat laws that will affect the corporations that pay them the big bucks.

Listening to her describe the way that lobbying went on with nothing short of outright bribery and conflict of interest touched something in me. Perhaps it had to do with being the son of poor immigrants who had to break their asses to make a go of it in America. In any case, I deeply resented the richer classes who had it easy and got their way with everything their money and power brought them.

The thought of bringing attention to myself in a classroom was scary, and I normally kept my views quiet, so I could not be embarrassed. But I felt compelled to be heard. My hand shot up in the air so that I could ask a question.

The teacher saw my hand in the air, and with a polite smile on her face, asked, "Yes, do you have a question?"

I couldn't have known it, but I was about to begin my rabble-rousing career at that moment. I stood up and blurted out, "I don't understand something; for the first two weeks of this class, you told us how the three branches of our government work. You also pointed out several times that there is a system of checks and balances that protects the way our democracy operates. But now you're telling us about lobbyists that just walk into Congress and sidestep this system and are given special treatment because they represent powerful interests. That seems unfair to me. My mother or father can't do that. Why do these people have such a privilege?"

The teacher's civil expression immediately changed to that of someone on the defensive, and she answered in a way that made me feel personally attacked.

"I don't think you quite understand what it's all about—and it's best that you stay within the bounds of what I'm trying to teach you."

She might just as well have said, "Mind your own business."

As I sat down to nurse my feelings, I cautiously looked about the room to see if the other students were staring at me. What I saw was frightening. The entire class of 30-odd students was looking down at their books, *hiding*. I instinctively realized that the teacher's cold message had, in fact, a stifling effect on everyone's minds. I knew that these students would now think twice before daring to ask a question, and that they would hold back their views for fear of being attacked the way I had been.

That painful classroom experience has stayed with me throughout my life. Along with numerous other put-downs at the hands of teachers and authority figures, by the age of 16, I decided that I would never allow my own children to be *confined* in the public education system. Without knowing it then, my kids would all be home-schooled.

* * *

The imagination is usually the next victim along the path of being trained to not operate at full throttle. Eventually (a lot sooner than you realize), we lose this precious talent. In that regard, the world can be thankful for the fact that Albert Einstein's schoolteachers treated him so poorly. Instead of being like the other students, he retreated into a fantasy world of his early childhood, nurturing his ability to imagine and create. (Einstein believed that the imagination was more important than knowledge.) That's what so many of us miss out on—we become like many unthinking and unimaginative others.

Because we have fallen into line, we are easily manipulated and coerced into doing exactly what we are told—for our own good, of course. That gives authority figures almost absolute power over our underused, underexposed, cornered minds.

The worst offenders are doctors and lawyers, followed closely by religious leaders, educators (yes!), corporate heads, our military, the media, and of course politicians, all of whom have a huge stake in keeping your brainpower in check. Thinking people pose a great threat. Better believe it!

The net results of this brain deprivation are predictable: fewer and fewer Einsteins, Eleanor Roosevelts, Gandhis, Thakurs, Schweitzers, Mother Theresas, Martin Luther Kings, Churchills, and Mandelas, and more illiterates and despots in positions of leadership. This leaves our depleted civilization on the brink of self-extermination through wars, poverty, malnutrition,[2] disease, and the destruction of our environment.

So, it's not just a question of the conglomerate controlling the destiny of your health. The conglomerate's plan subjugates your mind and your actions, leaving you unable to use the immense talents you might actually possess. We can't see it happening because we're aligned with the masses of ignorant people whose minds have become *damaged goods.*

I must hereby state for the record that the American public suffers from massive ignorance. Otherwise, why would we subscribe to inane drug advertisements, accept gas price gouging, support deceit and corruption in government, go along with Bush's personal war in Iraq, ignore the gulag at Guantanamo Bay, rationalize torture, and pretend we're unaware of the suffering of tens of thousands of people being dumped on 21st-century Hoovervilles in America (cultural genocide). Suggestion: Instead of acting insulted by this aggressive confrontation, take a good look at yourself and what you stand for.

---

[2] According to the U.N. Children's Fund (UNICEF), poor nutrition contributes to the deaths of some 5.6 million children every year.

And because we're so damned defensive (and unwilling to admit to any fault—another trademark of our system of noneducation), we can only identify with all the other dummies who think they're really much smarter than they are. We go along our merry ways and DON'T "GET IT."

Right up to the very end, we don't get it. In fact, we stray even further from reality as we approach our final years, becoming thankful just to be breathing. *Like slaves.*

✳ ✳ ✳

As for our immune systems, the conglomerate has laid waste to what is easily one of the universe's greatest success stories as we know it. We have become willing victims of this arch-treachery and madness, surrendering ourselves to inane advertisements, needles, drugs, and medical procedures.

> *What makes you such an expert in all this?*

I'm not a doctor, chemist, or research scientist, so I can't address technical questions about our immune systems. I do know what I have learned through personal experience and observation, and what I have to say makes perfect sense to most people who examine it. So, I ask you to start by considering my health résumé.

During my childhood, I was overweight and in poor physical condition, suffering from headaches, backaches, stomachaches, and the inability to coordinate my mind or body. As an adolescent, I became obese, smoked, and started having migraine headaches. As I reached adulthood, I suffered from severe migraine attacks and asthma, had gallstones, ranged from overweight to obese, smoked up to four packs of cigarettes a day, and regularly came down with colds and the flu. And until the age of 35, I could characterize my overall physical health as problematic, typical in the sense of the average person who follows conventional medical advice and uses prescribed drugs.

As a result of various medical experiences (including severe migraines), my lifelong weight issues, decades of focus on problem-solving, our children's births (three of them home births), enormous reading and personal research into a wide range of medical subjects, and my observation of people under medical treatment for everything from sports injuries to menopause, **I have adopted a strict policy of avoiding doctors and hospitals.** And I allow my body to do its own healing without the standard use of medication.

These are the net results of this rebellious thinking and behavior:

1. Although I was given a disability benefit for my asthma, I haven't suffered from the slightest trace of it in 40 years.

2. Since September of 1959, I have never had another migraine headache, nor have I had a single ordinary type of headache. Not one headache in 46 years! Not even a stress-oriented headache—and my work in show business and as a group therapist has been very stressful. Do you know anyone else who hasn't had a headache in 46 years?

3. Except for my appendicitis, I have not had a stomachache in 35 years. Not even a tiny one.

4. I have not had a cold in 10 years.

5. I can't remember when I last had the flu—and I do not take flu shots.

6. If you examine my medicine cabinet, you won't find even an aspirin, which is something I haven't used in 20 years.

7. At the age of 70, I am in remarkable physical condition, work out strenuously four to six times a week, and feel as if I'm a healthy 30 years of age. And I look damn good, too!

If everyone were like me—the conglomerate would go out of business!

How did I go from being a dismal physical schnook to a perfect specimen of good health? Is it some kind of medical miracle or simply the power of positive thinking?

In 1983, while traveling back to my Greek island paradise and the waiting arms of my family, I reached over to my carrying case for a book and felt a strong pain in my right shoulder. At first I thought that I had accidentally pulled something out of place, but the pain persisted throughout the trip, and by the time I got home it was excruciating. The next morning, I could not raise my arm more than a few inches without causing even greater strain and ache.

Over a period of weeks, I waited for the pain to subside, but it didn't. As I had to carry bundles of our *Journey To Greece* newspaper aboard ferry boats, I found it increasingly difficult to carry out my work responsibilities.

I finally took the plunge, visiting a doctor who had been recommended by my publisher friend John Chapple. After a thorough examination, X-rays, and questioning, he told me that I was suffering from arthritis. He advised me to stop doing any lifting with my right hand and to give my shoulder as much rest and rehabilitation as possible for up to six months. The doctor also recommended that I begin a prescribed program of pain medication.

I left his office growling under my breath because I had no intention of dumping my work responsibilities, nor did I intend to start taking any form of medication stronger than aspirin.

At Nan's urging, I visited two more physicians, one of whom was a sports injury specialist. Both of them concurred with the first diagnosis of arthritis and pointed me in the same treatment direction as John Chapple's physician. I felt that none of these doctors held out any hope that I might return to normal physical activity in the very near future, or at all for that matter; *arthritis was not curable.*

Several days later, while walking along Syntagma Square in Athens, I came upon a brand-new store, the first of its kind in Greece, which sold professional bodybuilding equipment, including everything connected with the art of pumping iron, which I hadn't done for years.

As I walked through the store, aware that my shoulder might really fall apart if I dared to try lifting a weight above my head, I remembered some advice given to me years earlier by my bodybuilding guru, Kimon Voyages.[3] Kimon told me that one of the wisest things I might do for any son of mine would be to get him into weightlifting and bodybuilding at an early age. (This is quite contrary to the preachings of most sports advisors and experts.)

At that very moment, I knew exactly what I would have to do for my 10-year-old son Billy and myself.

The Greek dockworkers whom I paid to load the dumbbells, free weights, bars, and benches into the hold of the ferryboat were incredulous at the thought of a middle-aged man—much less a 10-year-old boy—lifting weights. They thought that nothing could be more ridiculous. According to their great wisdom, it was as much a waste of time and energy as jogging, which made the native population of Naoussa throw up their hands and exclaim, *"Ti na kanoume!"* ("Dear God—what's going on?!") every time they saw Nan jogging along the road.

Nonetheless, I managed to transport my newly purchased equipment to the port of Paros, to Naoussa, and then on to my home, where I was greeted by my astonished family, who laughed at my latest attempt to introduce something new to the island of Paros.

Billy did most of the setup, and we put together a small gym in the middle room of the adjacent house that we had recently rented to accommodate our fami-

---

[3]   Kimon Voyages placed second in the 1945 Mr. America Contest in the Most Muscular category.

ly's growing needs. I began to instruct Billy on the basics as they had been taught to me by Kimon and our mutual friend and wrestling champion Chris Tolos. As Billy began to learn them, I decided to deal with my arthritis in a way that would show it who was boss.

When I lay down on the bench and extended my arms for that first attempt to lift just the 40-pound bar, with Billy spotting behind me, I knew it would hurt a great deal—but I wasn't going to back down unless my shoulder fell off!

The pain was horrific, as would have been expected, and I could barely lift the bar before returning it to the rack. Then I sat up and felt the rush of pain continue through the entire region of my right shoulder and down my arm, followed by a burning sensation that lasted some 20 to 30 seconds before dissipating.

Billy looked at me and said, "Does it hurt bad? What are you going to do?" My face must have been flushed at that moment, and I could feel sweat beading on my forehead as I thought about my next step, which was to lower myself back on the bench and get ready to lift the bar again.

As unbearable as it felt, I slowly lifted the bar above my head and held it up, furiously determined to keep it there as long as humanly possible, no matter how painful it was, all the while cautioning Billy to be ready to help me lower it back into the cradle position.

I could feel the sweat on my forehead dripping into my eyes and the strain on my right shoulder was almost unbearable. But I kept holding out for another few seconds at a time, remembering how I had done the same kind of thing at Boy Scout camp so many years before. When I felt my lungs would burst, I refused to give up until I was sure I had set the underwater record. With that sensory memory working for me, I held out another 10 seconds before telling Billy to help me lower the bar.

Billy waited until I took a few deep breaths and lifted myself into a sitting position before asking how I felt. As I answered the question, I knew that I would win this fucking battle. "It hurts a lot ... but it's no worse than when I tried the first time. So, let's go again. ... "

The third lift was just as agonizing as the previous two, but nonetheless more manageable because my mind was now focused. I was able to call upon a reserve of energy and strength that was there since the long years of migraine attacks, when I had to find a way to resist the terrible pain.

Within three weeks from the time I started to lift weights again, the pain in my shoulder began to lessen. In less than another two months, by which time I was bench-pressing **165 pounds,** no sign of any "arthritis" remained.

Had I been cured? You're damn right! My immune system, in consort with my mind, worked it all out. How can I be so sure? Well, as I write this story, it's the year 2006, I'm 70 years old, still bench-press my own weight (and then some), do 50 pushups at a time, been boxing for the past two years, and haven't had a bout with arthritis since that initial experience back in 1983. Which begs the question—what happened to the arthritis? Where did it go? You tell me!

✳ ✳ ✳

Let's go again. In 1986, while selling *Journey to Greece* on a ferryboat in Piraeus one morning, the departure announcement was made, and I headed for the ship's ramp to leave the boat before it sailed. I had left hundreds of boats hurriedly over many years, and except for a few near-skirmishes with last-minute travelers coming up the ramp on foot, I had never had a problem, but this time was different.

As I tramped down the 40-foot-long ramp, which angled down at about 45 degrees, a large truck began to back into the boat. Without warning, the driver stepped on the gas and the truck came barreling up at me. As I was about halfway down the ramp, I couldn't possibly turn back in time. Even if I tucked myself right against the hull of the ship, I might still be crushed by the truck.

With no time to do anything else, I made an instant decision and jumped overboard!

Some 20 feet down, I landed on the boat's heavy towlines and immediately felt my right ankle give way. When I got back up, I writhed in pain, unable to stand and holding my ankle, which I was sure had been broken by the fall.

With the help of the port police, I was placed in a taxi and taken to a doctor's office, where I was examined and X-rayed. I had a slight break, and my ankle would have to be immobilized for a long time. As the break did not require a cast, the ankle was wrapped tightly and I was told to get in a cab, go home, and stay off the leg for six weeks.

Sounds like good advice, right? But not for me! I couldn't afford a six-week vacation from work, and I had long since decided to tough it out, not because I wanted to prove something—but because *I believe that my body will repair itself if given the chance, because the mind and the immune system are the strongest medicines in the universe.*

I got into a taxi, returned to Piraeus, and went right back to work!

By now, my ankle had swollen to twice its normal size and I was still in a great deal of pain. As I hobbled around, I wondered if I could actually climb stairs and move around the boat. A practitioner of self-hypnosis, I meditated as I walked around, and knowing how little time I had on each deck, I acted as if there were no pain or swelling. My brain got the message: It released endorphins that acted as natural painkillers, and I continued to do my job.

Without any pain reliever and with no other medical consultation, I continued to work each day.

Within three days the swelling diminished considerably, as did the pain.
By the end of the second week, my ankle was back to normal.

Most medically minded pundits (professionals and laymen) would challenge my assertion that the immune system could have anything to do with healing my ankle injury or curing my arthritis. This narrow view of the overall scope of the immune system's capability makes no sense because it limits it to nothing more than a textbook definition of the body's dealing with pathogenic organisms. It ignores the universal truths of the interaction, interdependency, and integration of every particle of existence, failing to recognize the medical and scientific correlations between body, mind, and spirit.

Apropos of this philosophy:

SCIENTISTS FIND REGENERATING HEART CELLS
Research raises hopes of new ways to treat cardiac disease
Gareth Cook, *The Boston Globe*—February 10, 2005

Scientists announced yesterday the discovery of cells in the heart that can create new muscle cells, raising hopes that doctors may find dramatic new ways to treat heart disease, the nation's leading cause of death.

The team, led by Dr. Kenneth Chien at the University of California-San Diego, showed that the cells, which are similar to stem cells, can be expanded from just a few hundred in a laboratory dish to more than a million, and these cells can be guided into becoming the pulsing muscle cells that power the heart.

The finding, published in today's issue of the journal Nature, *may yield new insights into the heart's development and might further the quest to regenerate damaged heart tissue—an idea once thought impossible....*

PLANT MAY HAVE BACKUP OF ITS GENOME
Offspring possessed corrected copy of defective gene
Nicholas Wade, *The New York Times*—March 23, 2005

In a startling discovery, geneticists at Purdue University say they have found plants that possess a corrected version of a defective gene inherited from both their parents, as if some handy backup copy with the right version had been made in the grandparents' generation or earlier.

The finding implies that some organisms may contain a cryptic backup copy of their genome that bypasses the usual mechanisms of heredity. If confirmed, it would represent an unprecedented exception to the laws of inheritance discovered by Gregor Mendel in the 19th century.

Equally surprising, the cryptic genome appears not to be made of DNA, the standard hereditary material. ... But there are hints that the same mechanism may occur in people, according to a commentary by Detlef Weigel of the Max-Planck Institute of Developmental Biology in Tuebingen, Germany. Weigel describes the Purdue work as "a spectacular discovery."...

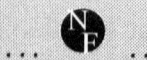

· · · ·　· · · ·

As these two articles point out, a lot of ideas once thought impossible may one day be a natural part of our existence, which proves the point that **there is so much we don't know.**

This is where quantum physics and the mind both play an enormous role. This is also where you place your trust in your immune system, which not only prevents illness and protects you from disease but also repairs bodily damage and **GROWS!!!**

I'll bet you never thought of that. **Your immune system actually grows**—just like the rest of your cells and muscles. Its genius lies in the fact that its overall capabilities are vast, ongoing, and unfathomable to our limited understanding. But how can you possibly begin to understand its range and capacity when you're so busy defeating its purpose with drugs?

Here's one more example of the immune system at work. I was a smoker for 18 years, and when I quit, I was smoking four packs a day. Coupled with my asthma, my lungs and respiratory system were in bad shape.

One year after I quit smoking, I went to a clinic in Astoria (Long Island, New York) for my then regular yearly checkup. When I finished the examination, which included chest X-rays, I sat down with the attending physician. He gave me a great report card on all counts, going out of his way to tell me that my lungs and respiratory system were in perfect condition.

When I told him that I had smoked for 18 years, had quit only one year earlier, and had suffered from disabling asthma, he shook his head and said that I was either making it up or that a miracle had occurred, because the scar tissue from smoking all those years would be evident in the X-rays. He insisted that there had to be some other explanation.

At the time, I didn't know what it was, but I certainly do now. I had started my physical recovery when I quit smoking, detoxified myself in Greece, rebuilt my respiratory system as well as my lungs with bodybuilding, refrained from the use of drugs, and left the rest to my immune system, which thanked me profusely and swore allegiance to my health for the rest of my long life. Ever since—it's never let me down.

Again, I must stress that any medical definition that limits our immune system to dealing with pathogenic organisms and the like is fundamentally flawed and ridiculous. It has only been devised to aid and abet the conglomerate's profiteering schemes. **If you don't believe in your immune system—you'll buy into drugs!** That's the conglomerate's game plan.

Under the conglomerate's disfiguring guidance, our drugged society has presumed that its magical pharmaceutical potions—**manufactured by the rat pack of drug companies that are responsible for more drug addiction and death than all the opium and heroin growers, methamphetamine labs, and street dealers in the world**—are the cure for whatever ails you. Your foolish need to solve your medical problems with drugs reduces your immune system to nothing more than a second-rate backup plan.

And just as AIDS destroys the body's immune system, overuse of drugs does the same in that you not only lose the ability to neutralize pathogenic organisms and substances, but you also drastically alter the body's natural defense against illness. **That's why most people get sick on a fairly regular basis.** And they're dumb enough to think it's normal!

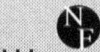

A comparison between the United States and England shows that white, middle-aged Americans have higher rates of hypertension, heart disease, diabetes (twice as prevalent as in England), cancer, lung disease, myocardial infarction, and stroke as their cousins across the Atlantic. This is all in spite of the fact that we spend more than twice as much for healthcare than the Brits.

What's even more revealing is that those in the upper education and income level in America had similar rates of diabetes and heart disease as those in the bottom level in England.

The survey stated that the varying levels of health could not be attributed to such factors as smoking, obesity, alcohol abuse, or the differences between the nations' healthcare systems.

So what does that leave us to conclude? If you need to think twice, you're blind to the overwhelming reality of drug use, abuse, and addiction in America. Nowhere in the world is there anything like it. The results are plain to see: OUR COLLECTIVE IMMUNE SYSTEMS ARE SHOT! And no manner of healthcare expense will change this.

In effect, you have told your body that Eli Lilly, Pfizer, Merck, Johnson & Johnson, and all the other drug giants are better than its own natural gift of immunity.

"Sorry old boy—but we've got drugs to cure all your ills," says the doctor as s/he scribbles a prescription. And you know what? You got just what you ordered and probably deserve—an immune system that is weakened, no longer growing, and barely a facsimile of what it once was.

This is exactly what the conglomerate has masterminded. It's been its brain-child since the day you were born and will be until you die. **Our society's poor health is the conglomerate's success story.** Our immune system has been sacrificed for its gain. What patsies we are!

If you think I'm misguided, then tell me why (and pardon the redundancy—but I must reemphasize this to shake you awake)—at the age of 70—I no longer have asthma, arthritis, headaches, stomachaches, and colds; why my knees and back are sound (not a creak or strain anywhere); why I move down the street with speed, agility, and stamina; have no pains anywhere in my body; can do 50 pushups and 600 situps at a time; attend boxing classes and handle myself as well as men and women 40 years younger; and still bench-press more than my own weight? And I never feel sick or under the weather!

Ask your doctor how many pushups he can do! Chances are, he can't do five! No surprise. These medical experts, who advise, guide, and prescribe for you, neglect balance in their lives and put themselves and their patients at risk. That's one reason why they have the highest rate of drug use, divorce, and suicide of any profession.[4] Did you know that? Does it matter?

---

[4]   A 2005 Harvard Medical School study concluded that male doctors committed suicide at a rate 41 percent higher than that of other men and women. The more startling finding was that female doctors take their lives at a rate more than twice (2.27 times) that of the general public.

Furthermore, the medical experts, including your personal physicians and sports doctors who advise "rest and drugs" for your illnesses and injuries, might just as well be charter members of the conglomerate. They are guilty of doing great harm to your mental acumen and untold permanent damage to your immune system and body.

Under the guise of protecting you from further pain or injury, and with some carefully placed "strokes," they aid and abet your weaknesses (your acceptance of drugs and your willingness to submit to a long rehab instead of building up your body through good nutrition and exercise). They severely limit your will to fight the good fight and trust your body to recover without self-indulgence and drugs. By the time they're through, you're thinking and behaving like a helpless child—which is exactly where they want you.

Like the dumb schnook that you've become, you'll return for more of the same "treatment" because, having accepted the premise that rest and drugs are the correct one-two punch, you become addicted to it. And as this solution has dissuaded you from trusting the greater powers you were born with, you abuse your mind and immune system to the extent that they are no longer even dormant. For all intents and purposes, they no longer exist. They're buried!

And what are you left with? The conglomerate, whose representatives are wolves in sheep's clothing, treating you as nothing more than an annuity to be banked and preserved as a cash cow for as long as possible before being dumped into the heap of bodies long abandoned for the sake of greed and vainglory.

Providing that you have the adequate means and insurance, the various conglomerate members guide you through your middle and senior years, making you feel relatively comfortable along the way with rest and drugs. That's why you will go to your grave thinking that the warlords of the conglomerate really had your interests at heart. All the while, they feast on your body and bank account, like a swarm of charlatans and vultures.

To better serve the public interest—which is why I'm going to such an extreme in confronting the **scumfucks**[5] of the unholy conglomerate—I'm going to open myself up to questions raised by people who hear me talk about the overall issue of health in America.

---

[5] Just as we denounce tyrants and terrorists, I will never apologize for using foul language to describe and characterize these evil people, because we must see them for what they actually are. Furthermore, many people will undoubtedly take exception to my use of the worst language I can think of, but I ask you to consider this: If you were to suddenly receive a 9/11-type wake-up call one morning telling you the inconceivable news that all life on the planet will cease to exist in three months because we destroyed the environment and subsequently our health—will you wish I had cursed even more? Think about it.

> *Are all doctors and healthcare officials*
> *greedy and uncaring monsters?*

No, there are quite a few decent and concerned physicians and healthcare workers out there, many of whom are not consumed by greed or the need to control our minds and lives. However, their numbers pale in proportion to the professionals who have long since positioned themselves in the conglomerate's camp.

These mindless people number in the millions, representing the body politic of the healthcare industry, along with a legion of weak-minded bureaucrats who are too lazy or unwilling to stand up against the powerbrokers, and the subordinate workers and officials who don't stand a chance of getting their concerns aired. They constitute the heart of the conglomerate, leaving us shackled—mind and soul—to a healthcare system that is a disgrace, a disaster—**A MONUMENT TO FAILURE.**

And it will only get worse. If you doubt that for a moment, just look at the spiraling costs for all types of healthcare: a 73-percent increase in the last five years; the growing numbers of underinsured or uninsured (more than 83 million Americans in 2006); the huge number of yearly deaths (**half a million!**) as a result of medical malfeasance and prescription drug use and abuse; and the profiteering of the entrenched conglomerate, which is calculated in the hundreds of billions.

✳ ✳ ✳

On another level, the catastrophic disaster caused by Hurricane Katrina proved beyond a doubt that a caste system exists in America when it comes to healthcare. Hundreds of thousands of people (mostly poor and black) were abandoned by the Federal Emergency Management Agency (FEMA) and our administration's leaders, including our weak-kneed president, who would only view the catastrophe from a distance, because the Katrina victims didn't count as being important enough people.

. . . .

Our president wasn't the only important figure to keep his hands unsoiled; the leaders of the Democratic Party were equally at fault when it came to showing humanitarian concern for the victims of Hurricane Katrina.

You didn't see any ranking member of that once-proud political party walking among the casualties, or manning the crumbling levees. In fact, all of America's national figures were conspicuously absent from the catastrophic scene, having chosen to keep away from New Orleans and other heavily damaged areas. Where were they?

To add insult to injury, the press manhandled the situation by labeling those who had lost their homes and loved ones as "refugees."

Only when President Bush and his henchmen began to get bad press throughout the world did they finally come to the aid of those who had been left behind to fend for themselves or die. And that was only temporary help—a Band-Aid in place of true relief.

> *How would you generally characterize*
> *the state of our health?*

Too often we spend our lives eating the wrong foods, breathing in and surrounding ourselves with toxins, taking drugs, and engaging in lifestyles that fail to truly nourish us physically, mentally, and spiritually. In our quick-fix mentality, we would sooner swallow some pills to relieve the symptoms of pain than to do what is necessary to solve the root causes of that pain.

Over many years, the consequence of all these combined unhealthy practices is that our bodies' natural immune systems simply cannot bear the strain of this accumulated poison in our systems. This manifests itself in the form of cancer or other serious, chronic conditions.

By the time cancer is diagnosed, toxins in the body have reached critical levels, and only drastic measures will cleanse or reverse this scenario. This usually means starting all over from ground zero, completely changing one's diet, lifestyle, and mental outlook.

Finally motivated by the threat of death, millions of people who have completely and faithfully followed this level of change have successfully overcome their cancer and survived to be healthy again.

The same analogy can be made for the state of the American healthcare system. The conglomerate, in its ruthless greed for profits and power, has infused our healthcare system with similar poisons that slowly but surely have accumulated to the point where not only Americans as individuals are flooded with misleading, dangerous, and expensive medical information and practices, but to where our very economy is being crippled by the spreading cancer of soaring employer medical coverage.

Political tumors of a sort also influence our decisions about international healthcare realities; we would treat the underdeveloped nations as an incubator for our own destructive healthcare policies (just as we export cancer-causing tobacco), especially when it comes to helping nations deal with the scourge of AIDS and other deadly diseases.

How did things get so bad? Well, the American healthcare system's roots are deeply embedded in our corrupt political system, which freely takes contributions and payoffs from the conglomerate on many levels. And the self-absorbed American public has generally turned a blind eye to the goings-on of politics in this country, naïvely believing that somehow they are going to be taken care of or that things are not really as bad as they seem.

However, the conglomerate's corruption has become so ubiquitous and deeply rooted that it will take a catclysmic event to turn the nation's undivided attention and energy to actually solving the problem, not just ignoring it or masking its symptoms with Band-Aid legislative measures or half-baked bills that will be reversed when the next lobbying group raises its ugly head.

✳ ✳ ✳

In the meantime, with all the supposed research, new medical breakthroughs, and scientific discoveries, **we are not a healthy society.** Far from it. In a July 2000 article in the *Journal of the American Medical Association,* Dr. Barbara Starfield of the Johns Hopkins School of Medicine studied the overall health of the American people and compared our conditions to those in other industrialized countries. This is what she found:

- Of 13 countries in a recent comparison, the United States ranks an average of 12th (second from the bottom) for 16 available health indicators.

- The United States places 13th, dead last, for low birth weight percentages; 13th for neonatal mortality and overall infant mortality; 13th for years of potential life lost (excluding external causes); 11th for life expectancy at the age of 1 for females and 12th for males; and 10th for life expectancy at the age of 15 for females and 12th for males.

- Children in the U.S. are particularly disadvantaged, but even the relatively advantaged position of elderly people is slipping. The U.S. relative position for life expectancy in the oldest age group was better in the 1980s than in the 1990s.

"The fact is that the U.S. population does not have anywhere near the best health in the world," Dr. Starfield wrote.

In 2004, she was asked by *The New York Times* op-ed columnist Bob Herbert whether the situation had improved over the past four years.

> ... *"It's getting worse," she said, noting, "We've done a lot more studies in terms of the international comparisons. We've done them a million different ways. The findings are so robust that I think they're probably incontrovertible."*
>
> *The U.S. has the most expensive health care system on the planet, but millions of Americans without access to care die from illnesses that could have been successfully treated if diagnosed in time. Poor people line up at emergency rooms for care that should be provided in a doctor's office or clinic. Each year tens of thousands of men, women and children die from medical errors and many more are maimed.*
>
> *But when you look for leadership on these issues, you find yourself staring into the void. If you want to get physicians' representatives excited, ask them about tort reform, not patient care. Elected officials give lip service to health care issues, but at the end of the campaign day their allegiance goes to the highest bidders, and they are never the people who put patients first.*
>
> *To get a sense of just how backward we're becoming on these matters, consider that in places as Texas, Florida and Mississippi the politicians are dreaming up new ways to remove the protective cloak of health coverage from children, the elderly and the poor. Texas and Florida have been pulling the plug on coverage for low-income kids. And Mississippi recently approved the deepest cut in Medicaid eligibility for senior citizens and the disabled that has ever been approved anywhere in the U.S.*
>
> *Even the affluent are finding it more difficult to obtain access to care. For patients with insurance the route to treatment is often a confusing maze of gatekeepers and maddening regulations. The costs of insurance are shifting from employers to employees, and important health decisions are increasingly being made by*

bureaucrats and pitchmen interested solely in profits.

In the maddening din that passes for a national conversation in this country, distinguished voices like Dr. Starfield's are not easily heard.

Echoing so many other patient advocates, she continues to call for movement on two crucial needs: coverage for the many millions who currently do not have access to care, and the development of a first-rate primary care system, which would bring a sense of coherence to a health care environment that is both chaotic and wildly expensive.

... "We don't have any national health policy at all in this country," said Dr. Starfield.

And there is no sign of that changing anytime soon.

This statement was made by an internationally respected physician, professor, and researcher, and it clearly echoes many issues I will hammer away at in this book. If you are among the conglomerate supporters who claim that the medical statements made herein are strictly the opinion of the author of this book—take another look!

Although I'm in complete agreement with Dr. Starfield, what she fails to mention is that the movement she speaks of cannot happen without radically changing the political structure that controls healthcare in America.

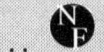

····   ····

According to the 2005 July/August Kaiser Health Poll Report tracking survey, Americans rank healthcare (22%) behind only war and foreign policy issues (28%).

However, we are firmly entrenched in a political status quo, do nothing but "wait and see what's going to happen" mode of thinking and behavior about healthcare—which won't get the job done.

Here's another statement about our healthcare, made by Kathleen O'Connor, founder and CEO of CodeBlueNow! America's Health Care Voice, a national grassroots advocacy group for U.S. healthcare:

... Our healthcare system is fundamentally flawed. There's no vision

for what the system should do, much less the outcomes we want. Not only is it fundamentally flawed, it is outright harmful:

- *More than 200,000 people die every year because of medical mistakes. That's more than the deaths by guns, drunk driving and airline crashes combined.*

- *More than 50 percent to 60 percent of the care we get is probably wrong or inappropriate, according to a RAND study.*

- *New, really expensive drugs like Vioxx or Celebrex may cure one condition but may also cause deaths.*

- *We won't invest in health promotion but we'll cover the cost of last-ditch ER efforts.*

- *Meaningful competition on quality and cost are elusive when the insurers tell us which providers we can and cannot see.*

All past reform attempts have held the American public at arm's length. We must change that. We need a healthcare revolution not by the industry but by the public. We need a revolution founded on the belief that the system should support the health of all people and the communities in which we live, with health promotion and wellness as the cornerstone, not the stepchild....

I'm all in favor of such a revolution, but it won't happen until the public wakes up from its drug-fix mentality and takes back its national life from the conglomerate. *And that would call for a revolution on many levels—including the political sphere.*

＊ ＊ ＊

Another deploring reality about our healthcare is that we treat foster children as if we wished they would go away. That's proven time and again by the fact that we refuse to provide the financial resources needed to improve the system of foster care. Instead, we bounce these children around foster homes without adequate services. Nationwide, it produces thousands of horror stories, and there is little that can be done about this enormous human tragedy because it's the old axiom of "It's either guns or butter." And the world of George W. Bush will always go for the guns. That's where the big profits are. The health of our people is not even on the same chart with the importance of enshrining the military-industrial complex in the hearts and bank accounts of America's chosen elite and powerful.

To understand how easy it is for the big shots to ignore the plight of disadvantaged and homeless children, you must first accept the fact that these wealthy and titled people do not in any manner, shape, or form identify with the lesser classes. They breathe rarified air, look down upon the masses, and only pretend to be part of what they disdainfully refer to as "society." And should they or any member of their elitist crowd have need for medical attention, they have access to the best doctors in every field of medicine—and no worries about costs or insurance. They want for naught. That's one of many reasons that healthcare reformation cannot be accomplished without appropriate political change. In this specific case, millionaire senators and congressmen need to be replaced with some common folk that understand what it's like to be left out in the cold.

Speaking of children's horror stories, do you have any idea of the number of children reported lost, runaway, or kidnapped annually? It's staggering. In 2005 there were 662,196 reported by police to state and federal authorities. Think about that: Where are they? What's being done to them? How will they end up? Does anyone care?

The same general standards and conditions that apply to the care of foster children also apply to the way we treat the developmentally disabled. They're at the bottom of the list of healthcare priorities, and they will remain in that neglected zone as long as America continues on its current destructive path.

The plight of the homeless in America is another national health disgrace. The vast majority of these millions of neglected people never even register on the radar screen as a healthcare priority, and the fact that not they're not ever factored in spells out more guns for the ruling class.

Although community healthcare organizations for the homeless do exist, no national safety net is provided by the government, and lawmakers hardly count the homeless as constituents.

Here's another important indicator of America's poor healthcare:

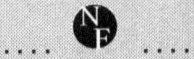

Did you know that the United States is one of only two industrialized countries (the other is Australia) that doesn't provide paid leave for new mothers nationally? The U.S. Family and Medical Leave Act provides for only 12 weeks of job-protected leave—but that's only for workers in large companies.

What's even more revealing: Out of 168 nations in a 2004 Harvard University study, 163 had some form of paid maternity leave, while the U.S. stands with **Lesotho, Papua New Guinea, and Swaziland.**

Can you imagine?

And where are the feminists? You would think that they'd be at the forefront to get paid time off and long-term job protection for new moms. But they couldn't get the Equal Rights Amendment passed, and they've long since stayed in the background on important national issues. They are as much to blame for this backward condition as U.S. employers and our legislators. Where's the fight in them?

> *Are most Americans affected equally*
> *by healthcare problems?*

A survey reported in the *New England Journal of Medicine* in 2006 showed that **all Americans get equally mediocre care.** It doesn't matter whether you're white, black, or Hispanic, nor does it matter if you're insured or uninsured. Overall, we receive only 55 percent of recommended care, and the quality of that American medical care falls short of expectations.

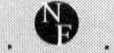

Upper and middle-class Americans pay little attention to the plight of the lower classes, especially their poor level of healthcare, thinking that it's not their problem, but the aforementioned survey points out that **ALL AMERICANS—rich or poor—ARE BAMBOOZLED BY THE CONGLOMERATE!**

Speaking of how the conglomerate bamboozles all people, don't for a minute think that our veterans are not included in this horrific reality. Did you know that hundreds of thousands of U.S. veterans have been denied healthcare from the Veterans Administration system?

Here we are, putting out the flags for our servicemen and women, urging Americans to support our troops in Iraq, but when they return home to civilian life, they're in for a painful dose of reality—the government and the people they fought and risked their lives for turn a deaf ear to them when it comes to VA healthcare benefits.

And in the case of Gulf War veterans, we're still denying that our government knowingly exposed our fighting men and women to various chemical and biological agents that caused widespread illness and premature death.

We've covered up the deadly truth and will go down in history for crimes against our own servicemen and women.

Even with the support of the American Legion, the Disabled American Veterans, and the Veterans of Foreign Wars (who represent over seven million military veterans), as well as ranking members of Congress, we continue to turn our back on our veterans. If they haven't earned the right to quality healthcare—who has?

While I'm speaking of how our government treats returning veterans, I was recently appalled to read an account of a wounded soldier in Iraq being forced to pay his Uncle Sam $632 for body armor that was destroyed by medics because it was soaked with the soldier's blood. How low can you get?

Speaking of body armor, did you know that our leaders in Washington and the Pentagon aren't providing our troops in Iraq with appropriate military helmets? In fact, private citizens and organizations are raising money to purchase better headgear for our fighting servicemen. While that goes on, our congressmen just gave themselves another raise. Wouldn't you believe it!

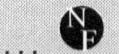

To make this point sink in: I just read the account of an American staff sergeant who was paralyzed from the waist down after being shot by a sniper in Iraq in 2005, and like thousands of other veterans, this man, his wife, and four children ended up staying in seedy hotels, living on credit cards and the kindness of strangers.

Where is his Uncle Sam? He's sitting in the White House, playing palsy-walsy with his oil-rich friends and cronies, keeping clear of such human problems—just as he did after Hurricane Katrina.

It goes without saying that our veterans should be treated with greater respect and consideration, and one way to do it would be to enact a new GI Bill of Rights for the 21st century. It would improve veterans' services, healthcare, and education, and boost the morale of servicemen returning home from active military duty.

If that weren't bad enough, take a look at this:

WOUNDED SOLDIERS LEFT IN DEBT

The Associated Press—April 28, 2006

After suffering paralysis, brain damage, lost limbs and other wounds in war, nearly 900 Army soldiers ran up $1.2 million in debt because of the military's "complex, cumbersome" pay system, congressional investigators said Thursday.

The report from the Government Accountability Office said another 400 who died in the wars had $300,000 in debt but that the Defense Department doesn't pursue collection of people killed in combat.

"We found that hundreds of separated battle-injured Soldiers were pursued for collection of military debts incurred through no fault of their own," said the report. . . .

For those of you who have felt the wrath of bill collectors pursuing you for health-care-related debts (and there are millions of you, many forced into bankruptcy), you can certainly appreciate the fact that you are not alone in your grievous circumstances. Even our battle-injured soldiers are caught in the same type of predicament—chased down by the very government of the people they fought and sacrificed for. And that includes both Democrats and Republicans.

Before moving on, I feel a deep personal need to clarify something to readers who may be under the illusion that America has, by and large, been kind and just to our veterans. Although there have been periods following wars, both declared or otherwise, when veterans were given their due, many stains remain on our nation's conscience that are difficult for the average American to believe.

One in particular stands out: In June 1932, 20,000 hungry, harassed, and ridiculed veterans of the "Bonus Army" marched on Washington, D.C. to demand immediate payment of a bonus that a grateful Congress had voted on in 1924 to give World War I veterans. As it stood, the payment would not be made until 1945, but as the nation had entered the Depression, the unemployed veterans needed their money immediately.

However, on June 17, 1932, the Senate, voting on a bill already passed by the House to immediately give the vets their bonus money, defeated the bill by a vote of 62 to 18.

A month later, on July 28, Attorney General Mitchell ordered the veterans, 10,000 of whom were living with their wives and children in shanty towns built from materials dragged out of nearby junk piles across the river from the Capitol, to evacuate the area.

Entrusted with the job of clearing out the veterans, the Washington police met resistance, shots were fired, and two marchers were killed. President Hoover then ordered the army to go in.

Led by General Douglas MacArthur and his aide Major Dwight D. Eisenhower, with Major George Patton leading the cavalry supported by six tanks, and with thousands of Civil Service employees lining the streets to watch, the veterans, assuming the military display was in their honor, cheered.

Suddenly Patton's troopers, with fixed bayonets, turned and charged, hurling tear gas into the crowd, while spectators cried "Shame! Shame!"

When it was over, the 10,000 inhabitants were routed and the camp was on fire. Two babies perished and nearby hospitals were overwhelmed with casualties. Eisenhower later wrote, "The whole scene was pitiful. The veterans were ragged, ill-fed, and felt themselves badly abused. To suddenly see the whole encampment going up in flames just added to the pity."

You may read this brief account of the Bonus Army and weep—but also remember that it can happen again.

On that note, I want to warn all veterans—regardless of your political persuasions—that you are once again being used by the government in its typical underhanded fashion. President Bush claims that America is at war, but in truth **it is our President who is at war,** and he doesn't care how many young American men and women, as well as innocent civilians, die on HIS behalf. He has managed to get away with this illegal war because there is not one single politician in America who is willing to put his or her political future at risk.

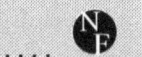

As a nation, we have not voiced our true feelings and concern for those thousands of dead servicemen and women because, unlike the Vietnam era, there has been no military draft, so the majority of Americans haven't had personal reason to become antiwar activists. In other words, the Iraq war isn't worth every citizen's involvement.

President Bush and his cabinet are also aware of how easy it is to distract Americans, including millions of veterans, with patriotic slogans and an array of political tactics. And during the months leading up to the November 7, 2006 congressional elections, with so much at stake for both political parties, the administration—once again—unfurled its Constitutional amendment to ban flag desecration. Supporters (including Democratic Senator Hillary Clinton!) claimed that "this is a chance for Congress to salute veterans."

What absolute cock and bull! If Congress and the American people truly want to salute its veterans, then give them a new GI Bill of Rights, provide them with all the benefits that they deserve, and declassify all the information about the true causes of Gulf War illnesses suffered by hundreds of thousands of servicemen.

Veterans—WAKE UP! Don't buy into flag burning as the enemy. That amendment won't get you respect from the political hooligans who run this country.

What about our government's role in our healthcare crisis?

The most glaring reality about our government's role in the American healthcare crisis today is the consensus of healthcare agencies and officials throughout the country that transforming the entire system is impossible. In other words, the best we can hope for are small, incremental changes—and you can bet your bottom dollar that none of them will include such vital areas as the lack of preventative medicine, providing healthcare insurance to all Americans, dealing with our national drug-fix mentality, or curbing the control of the ruling conglomerate—and that certainly includes the present administration in Washington. In fact, George W. Bush, aided and abetted by the Democratic Party, is the lynchpin who holds this status quo in place the way he would guard one of his oil holdings.

Anything of a more progressive nature will automatically be called *too ambitious,* which dooms any possible transformation of our healthcare system even before anyone dares to venture forth with a greater goal in mind. So let the word go forth—*aim low*. Very low. That's what our leaders tell us.

This defeatist philosophy of nicking at the edges of a problem—instead of going to the heart of the matter and applying all the necessary means to solve it—is really the crux of the conflict that exists within the various structures of the American healthcare system. It mandates low-level expectations, compromise, and the certainty of continuing the downward spiral of America's health and well-being. And almost everyone buys into the philosophy that it's the reasonable and responsible way to go. We've actually been trained to believe this nonsense.

✳ ✳ ✳

A major share of the responsibility for the narrow view of change and progress belongs to apologists who keep pointing out the good things about various healthcare programs. For instance, CEOs of healthcare organizations will tell you about the few possible alternatives open to uninsured people, such as Health Savings Accounts (HAS), or Health Reimbursement Accounts (HRA). While I understand and to a limited extent accept that these plans have something to offer, they do not help solve the existing root causes of our healthcare dysfunctionality. In many ways they contribute to its greater problems because they ultimately serve the conglomerate's purpose.

As long as lesser healthcare services can be dangled before the poorer classes of Americans, the powers that be will continue to neglect those most in need. These patchwork healthcare programs will be offered in place of the comprehensive national healthcare that is desperately needed. In effect, maintaining these meager attempts is making it impossible to move in the direction of a universal healthcare program, and this paralysis only benefits the conglomerate.

This point must be made about those CEOs and agency heads who support minimalist efforts at healthcare improvement: By supporting minor advances, they help perpetuate their positions as well as the status quo that is strangling the entire healthcare system in America. These supposedly well-meaning officials are in fact protecting themselves from being swept away by any meaningful change. These people and their small ideas must be cleared from the playing field before any march toward quality healthcare for the masses can advance.

On a governmental level, we must also realize that healthcare progress can never be made unless our Congress is willing to make an all-out effort to deal with the overall issue—and that takes time, as well as energy and innovative thinking. But our Congress does not have the time for such an effort. In fact, the 2006 congressional schedule called for Congress to be in session for the fewest number of days in 60 years. That's because our elected officials have to spend the bulk of their time raising money for reelection. That's what they're really up to most of the time, because that's what counts for them.

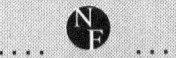

Not only does our Congress fail to devote adequate time and energy to healthcare matters, the subject is barely on its horizon because the various lobbies (primarily those working on behalf of pharmaceutical companies, HMOs, the medical profession, and the insurance industries) do everything in their considerable power to prevent movement on the healthcare front.

If you doubt this, just think back (once again) to President and Mrs. Clinton's proposed healthcare reform act of 1993. It quickly died in its tracks—as it always will unless there is significant political reform.

Besides being the biggest obstacle to change, "thinking small" is also a complete blunder of horrific proportions. In reality, the exact opposite would serve us well. As an example:

I grew up during the Great Depression. In spite of the idealistic intentions of Franklin D. Roosevelt's administration and numerous national programs (including the New Deal and the advent of Social Security), there was no coming out of the ruinous times. Progress was at a standstill, and hope waned. And then we were plunged into World War II.

So there we were, still mired in the Depression, at war on two major fronts—and unprepared for the strength of action that would be needed to save our very existence as a nation. At that crucial time, something magnificent happened in America: We became a nation again. Then we turned on our imagination, rolled up our sleeves, abandoned our isolationist course, and accepted the responsibility of leading the free world against the totalitarian forces that would otherwise rule the world. With that, we pushed aside all our doubts and fears and geared up for the job ahead.

And when the three major American car manufacturers (Ford, Chrysler, and General Motors) were challenged to retool their assembly lines and go from producing recreational vehicles to delivering several million military vehicles, as well as some 75 essential military items (most of them unrelated to the motor vehicle), they were up to the task. These materials had a total value of $29 billion, one-fifth of the nation's war production.

To kick it up a notch, with our backs still to the wall, we undertook the seemingly inconceivable objective of designing and building an atomic bomb—which eventually brought about the end of the war.

And guess what? Not only did we win the war, we knocked off the Depression as well. That's American resourcefulness!

If you need another example of how successful America can be when it accepts an unreachable challenge—and refuses to compromise—think about the fact that **WE GOT TO THE MOON!** Because we decided to. It took one decision!

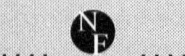

If you think we're not capable of doing the same thing with the American healthcare system as we did to build the atomic bomb, win World War II, come out of the Depression, and land Americans on the moon—you're dead wrong!

The same innovative thinking and decision making would work today. Not only would we create a new and successful healthcare system—for all people—but we would also create millions of new jobs. But the effort would require a war footing—not pussyfooting.

That's what's needed today! **And don't tell me it can't be done,** or that we should compromise, aim low, not be too ambitious.

As an example of what could be done, America's three largest car manufacturers could retool their assembly lines to turn out millions of electric cars. Not hybrids, but fully electric cars. These cars would reshape the automobile industry, decrease pollution, greatly reduce the oil and gasoline consumed in America, cut back on environmentally produced diseases, create hundreds of thousands of new jobs, and once again show what we can do when we put our minds to it.

But General Motors, Chrysler, and Ford would rather have you believe that they are not capable of so much change and advancement. They represent corporate mentality at its worst—nothing more than weakness and the need to maintain stock options without daring to go out on the limb for the good of all people.

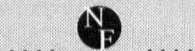

The technology for the success of the electric car IS available. Don't think otherwise. Were it not for the lack of vision and dedication on the part of the environmentalists, we would today be witnessing the appearance of millions of these vehicles on our streets and highways. By the way, the problems associated with electric car battery units have also been solved.

Although most liberal-minded people blame the demise of the electric-car potential on America's three auto giants, as well as the world's oil companies, nothing could be further from the truth. The automakers and oil companies would have yielded on the issue because there was just as much for them to gain (the sales of millions of electric cars, and there are thousands of other uses for oil) and it was almost in the cards for the emergence of the electric car in America. Who derailed it? *The environmentalists!*

Across the boards, they refused to join together to get the job done. They caved in—not to the auto and oil industries—but to their own undisciplined, vainglory needs. That I can attest to. I was in the thick of that battle for many years and witnessed a constant pattern of sabotage against the electric car carried out by the environmentalists.

> *Aren't individual states enacting measures*
> *to improve their healthcare systems?*

I would love to report some positive movements in particular states, but very little of that is happening, for the same reasons that prevent advancement nationally.

First and foremost, on every conceivable level, it's a matter of money. If some legislator manages to propose meaningful healthcare bills and get them enacted, that doesn't necessarily mean that funds will actually be appropriated and eventually used to fulfill those healthcare programs. The process just doesn't work that easily.

Just as massive cost overruns often delay or derail vital building projects, the same goes for healthcare spending. By the time a bill is passed, funded, and given over to those officials, organizations, and otherwise involved people and agencies, the original budgets are no longer viable.

Even if some elements of the new healthcare provisions seemingly remain intact, what usually happens is that **the original focus ends up getting lost on the process rather than the outcome.** Bureaucracy replaces imagination, and it's back to business as usual.

There's also the matter of cutting up the healthcare dollar to satisfy everyone's needs. And you can bet that by the time the money gets spent, **very little actual new healthcare service is made available to those most in need.** In this regard, meaningful oversight is alarmingly scarce.

The big exception to the rule of the process being more important than the outcome is in the area of pharmaceutical drugs. **No matter what happens, drugs will be made available to the masses.** That's because the big shots know where their bread is buttered and will pass all manner of legislation to ensure the steady flow of their junk into the hands and veins of our drug-oriented culture. That's the deadly given, and it supplants almost all of the positive steps that are attempted on a state-to-state level. So much for healthcare progress.

> *Are all drugs dangerous? And do you advocate*
> *a no-tolerance level for all of them?*

Before getting into specifics, I want to make a general statement about drugs that ought to be drummed into everyone's head: Our society is abysmally ignorant about what's really going on with "medication" (the polite, soft-sell word that lessens the true meaning of the *junk)*.

No one, but no one—including all the doctors, chemists, and pill salesmen in the world—can accurately predict what will always happen when any drug enters your body. No one can fully establish how safe or unsafe a given drug may be, or what regulatory agencies (primarily the FDA) will do to protect the public against unproven or questionable drugs.

Why not? Here are the reasons:

1. **To begin with, all chemicals produce side effects,** which makes their use a crap shoot, not always by design, but nonetheless just as risky. As one of thousands of examples, risks of blood clots in legs and lungs are twice as high for women using the birth-control patch instead of the Pill. Even ordinary aspirin has side effects, and Tylenol may hurt the liver. And don't think for a moment that the questionnaires you fill out in the doctor's office cover all contingencies and possibilities. That's hardly the case, as the statistics bear out.

2. **Harmful reactions to some of the most widely used medicines—from insulin to a common antibiotic—send more than 700,000 Americans to emergency rooms each year.** This reinforces the fact that there are substantial risks involved with using drugs.

3. **More than a fifth of drug prescriptions written by office-based doctors in America are for medical problems that have not been included in the FDA's approval of the drug, and fewer than a third of these prescriptions were backed by evidence of effectiveness.** Nonetheless, this usage, known as "off-label prescribing," is legal and considered ethical (though God knows why!) by the medical profession. Likewise, an ever-growing number of American children are being prescribed antipsychotic drugs for attention deficit disorder or other behavioral problems for which these medications have not been proven to work.

4. **Just as each person's DNA is uniquely different, the same holds true for each individual's chemistry.** This helps to explain why at least 200,000 drug-related deaths and more than two million serious drug reactions occur in the United States every year. Also, more than half the population is believed to have detectable genetic variations that affect the 8 to 10 liver enzymes that are responsible for breaking down most drugs.

5. **Drug tolerance levels vary from person to person.** As such, drug users throughout the world have no way to know if they can tolerate a particular dose of their drug of choice, which is clearly illustrated when people overdose and die unexpectedly.

6. **Besides causing death from overdose, drugs are often factors in suicide, automobile accidents,[6] and murder.** When these statistics are factored in, the body count for drug use in general goes way over the top of any available chart.

7. **There is no way on earth that we can ever know exactly what goes into the drug manufacturing process from one day to the next, and from one lab to the next.[7]** In other words, one batch can be significantly different than another. And just as the purity of heroin varies from city to city, the strains of materials used for various pharmaceutical drugs and vaccines are subject to the same vagaries and inconsistencies.

There is also the ever-present danger of contamination, as occurred in the winter of 2004–2005 to a large amount of flu vaccine.

Speaking of contamination, on November 10, 2006, it was reported that 11 million bottles of the widely-used pain reliever acetaminophen were being recalled because the pills may contain metal fragments. The pills are made by Perrigo Company, which has carried out at least 32 other product recalls since 1993, according to FDA records.

It should be noted that the FDA—like the unaware American public—is more than likely kept in the dark about hundreds of other serious cases of pharmaceutical contamination, because the conglomerate is not in the business of snitching on itself, regardless of how many human beings suffer the consequences.

8. **By and large, drugs are first tested on animals or rodents, but not as extensively on humans.** At least not to my satisfaction, or that of thousands of people whose lives are destroyed by drugs of a dubious nature. In spite

---

[6] Ambien, the nation's best-selling prescription sleeping pill (26.5 million prescriptions in 2005) shows up regularly as a factor in traffic arrests. Often drivers have no memory of taking the wheel after taking the drug.

[7] On March 4, 2005, in a response to ongoing concerns about manufacturing quality, the FDA and the Department of Justice initiated seizures of Paxil CR and Avandamet tablets manufactured by GlaxoSmithKline. Manufacturing practices for the two drugs, approved to treat depression and panic disorder (Paxil CR) and Type II (Avandamet), failed to meet the standards set by the FDA that ensure product safety, strength, quality, and purity.

of regulations, controls, case histories, record retentions, progress reports, safety reports, and financial disclosures, clinical tests on human beings do not measure up as adequate protection against the drug companies that want to derive huge profits from their efforts. And needless to say, as much as a mouse may be able to survive a particular dose of a chemical and even show signs of health benefits from it, that doesn't necessarily mean that human beings will always respond in a similar way.

That's just one of many reasons why, after approving a drug for sale, the Food and Drug Administration (FDA) often pulls the plug when it discovers—sometimes many years later—that the drug is responsible for an elevated risk of stroke, liver damage, heart disease, cancer, or even suicide. It's happened hundreds of times, and in many cases the information and data are not adequately or accurately disseminated to the public, or the conglomerate pulls out its tried-and-true rationale that *its drug's benefits outweigh the risks.*

Another typical ploy is for the drug company to cover up the story or change the name of the drug—tactics that maintain lucrative sales. Likewise we will never know about thousands of other drugs that are causing negative, dangerous reactions because the data is insufficient, poorly analyzed, or kept under wraps. Remember Fen-Phen?

9. **Senior citizens pay billions of dollars for drugs made in the U.S., while Canadian pharmaceutical companies provide the same drugs at a much lower cost.** But American drug companies and their cohorts tell the public that Canadian drugs may be dangerous. A large percentage of Americans buy into this hearsay without realizing that, in most cases, it is the American drug that should be brought into question because of the lack of proper research into the drug's safety.

Compared to U.S. standards, Canada offers an environment that provides significant advantages for the conduct of clinical trials for new drugs. With high-quality research expertise, lower clinical costs, and overall savings as high as 45 percent, the positive results speak for themselves.

10. **Thousands of drugs exist that are next to useless.** As such, they may prove harmful because their user's condition can deteriorate while the person thinks they are receiving appropriate medication. Cough medicines are among the more obvious worthless drugs; except for a class of antihistamines, these medicines do not significantly help relieve coughs that are cold-related.

11. **There is no way to accurately predict the cumulative, long-range effects**

of any drug on your body. These effects mount up day by day, like grains of sand, until you wake up one day to find something is wrong—and you've had no way of preventing it from happening because you've had no way of monitoring what's happening to each of your vital organs over the course of years. All the computers in the world couldn't figure it out. When this happens, you will go back to your doctor and he will prescribe more junk!

12. **Many variables factor into a person's drug reaction, such as age, race, and overall physical condition.** For instance, a recent FDA report asserts that Asian-Americans who use the cholesterol-lowering drug Crestor had an increased chance of muscle damage, and someone suffering from high blood pressure will react differently to a particular drug than someone with low blood pressure.

    There's also the frequent case of an undiagnosed illness, which could severely alter the body's reaction to a chemical. Not to mention the coincidental use of alcohol, creating a hazardous double-jeopardy situation—which has killed untold numbers of people.

13. **Overuse of antibiotics are playing havoc with disease control** as more and more "super bugs" pop up around the country, striking healthy people and stunning their doctors. Until a few years ago, these drug-resistant infections were present only in hospital patients, prison inmates, and the chronically ill. Now, resistant strains are infecting healthy children, athletes, and others with no connections to a hospital.

14. **Doctors often prescribe drugs that they know practically nothing about.** Large numbers of physicians accept payments (bribes) by pharmaceutical companies to prescribe costly medications. In this regard, they are no different than heroin dealers on the street. *These scribblers are worse than common drug dealers.*

15. **To add to this mayhem, antidepressants and other drugs are often prescribed to as many as half of the college students seen at student health centers.** These students fake symptoms of depression or attention deficit disorder to get prescriptions for *recreational* use. To further add to the dangers, a recent study in *The Journal of American College Health* found that 14 percent of students at a Midwestern liberal arts college reported borrowing or buying prescription stimulants from each other. Like trading CDs!

    These amateur pharmacists also manage quite easily to locate doctors who are willing to prescribe antidepressants, sleeping pills, or other psychiatric medications. There are also doctors writing hundreds of fraudulent prescriptions and charging big bucks—like $2,000 for each one! Then we have illegal online pharmacies operating offshore that openly dispense drugs without prescriptions. Just like ordering sneakers. All of this creates more legions of drug zombies who will of course graduate to being full-time drug freaks, unable to function without some form of medication (junk).

16. **The FDA was the lone cop on the drug industry beat a quarter-century ago, but its enforcement powers over drug marketing have been severely curbed** since 1976 by a series of court rulings based mainly on the drug companies' free-speech rights. (Would you believe it!)

    This left a vacuum that the drug industry has exploited to its full advantage, with practically no check remaining on what it is allowed to do. And when you realize just how cozy the FDA has become with the pharmaceutical companies—well, it's no wonder that so many drugs fall through the cracks before the public learns of their untold damage and potential recall.

    Federal prosecutors, state attorney generals, and plaintiff lawyers have stepped into the void, but in most instances it takes many years to bring charges against drug companies that are guilty of fraudulent marketing practices. In the intervening years, companies often conveniently name a new CEO and announce that they are reforming their marketing programs, as well as strengthening their internal policing of sales practices.

    What phooey. The brains behind these PR ploys are the same characters who tell the public that tobacco companies have reformed and are no longer aiming their marketing strategy toward young children and adolescents.

17. **I can't stress this enough: drug manufacturers—like tobacco companies—will sit on evidence that shows high risks of illness, disease, and death from the use of a drug, and keep this data from the FDA and the public.** When this information finally leaks out, they deny any prior knowledge. In this regard, they are no different from a tire manufacturer that knowingly produces defective tires and allows millions of unsuspecting drivers to risk their lives—*knowing all the while that people will die.*

18. **The pharmaceutical industry spends twice as much to market its junk than to research its effects on the human body.** Just look at all those TV commercials—that's one of the main reasons Americans pay such exorbitant prices for drugs. This should tell you where the industry's heart is. A dedication to profit above safety is the general rule of thumb; the industry gets away with it because it employs a thousand ways to cover up or deny inherent

dangers from the use of a drug.

Here's one such example:

ABBOTT LABS TO PULL CONTROVERSIAL ADHD DRUG
Scout News LLC—2005

A day after the consumer group Public Citizen petitioned the U.S. Food and Drug Administration to ban the attention deficit hyperactivity disorder drug Cylert (Pemoline), maker Abbott Laboratories said Friday that it had already planned to discontinue the medication because of declining sales.

Public Citizen petitioned the FDA on Thursday, citing reported cases of liver failure among Cylert users. The drug had been used to treat the disorder for some 30 years, the Associated Press reported.

The consumer group cited 193 adverse reactions to the drug from its approval in 1975 to 1996, including 13 cases of acute liver failure.

The company said letters advising doctors of the drug's withdrawal will be mailed within two months, the wire service said. ...

You will note the following regarding the "mechanics" of the drug maker's response to the petition:

- Rather than address the nature of the consumer group's petition (which was triggered by 193 adverse drug reactions ascribed to pemoline, including 13 cases of acute liver failure), Abbott Laboratories said they were already planning to discontinue the drug because of declining sales. You might wonder what would have happened if the drug sales were not in decline.

- The drug manufacturer will take up to two months to notify physicians about the discontinuation. Why should it take that long? How many more people will suffer liver damage in the meantime?

To show you that you can't trust a word out of the mouths of the conglomerate:

FDA WITHDRAWS APPROVAL FOR ADD DRUG (PEMOLINE)
The Associated Press—October 24, 2005

The Food and Drug Administration has withdrawn approval for a drug used to treat attention deficit hyperactivity disorder because it has been associated with liver problems, including death, agency officials said Monday.

The move means drug manufacturers will no longer produce generic versions of pemoline, which was developed by Abbott Laboratories and sold under the name Cylert. Abbott discontinued the drug earlier this year, but generic versions have remained available.

FDA is not recalling the drug, instead allowing pharmacies to sell their remaining stock as doctors still using it switch patients to alternative treatments, the agency said in a statement. ...

What liars, thieves, and killers! And that includes the FDA, who will now allow pharmacies to keep selling a drug that can kill children. And God only knows how much of the junk (sold under various generic names—which were not revealed when the drug was discontinued seven months earlier) is stockpiled!

This is but one of the typical deadly game plans carried out by the whole roster of conglomerate operatives. Needless to say, my attitude about the FDA has now gone from bad to worse. It's no wonder that the Bush administration says that the FDA is doing a spectacular job. Indeed, there is honor among thieves.

Just when you think that it's as bad as it can get—it gets worse!

Here's what I mean:

DRUG COMPANIES FALLING THROUGH ON STUDY PROMISES
Andrew Bridges, The Associated Press—March 4, 2006

Drug companies sometimes are allowed to hurry medicines to market in exchange for a promise to continue studying their safety and effectiveness. Those studies haven't begun in two-thirds of cases, the government reported Friday.

The Food and Drug Administration said Friday that drug companies had pledged to conduct 1,231 drug studies. But as of Sept. 30, 797—or 65 percent—were still pending.

"That doesn't mean they will never be started," said Dr. John Jenkins, director of the FDA's Office of New Drugs. ...

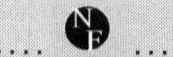

As difficult as it might be to believe, drug companies are allowed (given permission) to put their new poisons on the pharmacy shelves without proper safety studies, if they agree to do a study sometime (who knows when?) in the future. That's like giving airlines permission to fly fully loaded planes without having carried out proper flight tests, providing that the aircraft manufacturer promises to carry out the flight tests in the future. And our government does nothing about this deadly travesty!

This goes to show you that the American public will buy into anything. That's how lacking in self-respect we are. As a society, we're pathetic. It's no wonder we have elected officials the caliber of George W. Bush and company—we deserve as much.

For the record: Dr. John Jenkins should be forced to test all those drugs on himself and his family. That's what should be required of anyone who would dare to go along with such criminal behavior perpetrated against an entire society. If you think that this position is too harsh, then you are obviously aligned with all the drug traffickers in America—and I'm not talking about street peddlers.

To be redundant: Any official who says that 65 percent of anything of such a vital nature has not been completed but insists "That doesn't mean it won't be done" should be released from service and brought up on charges.

One last point on this healthcare deception: You'll notice that the report begins, "Drug companies sometimes. ..." *Sometimes?* We're talking about 1,231 instances (that we know of)—and that's called sometimes?!

America, these conglomerate goons are laughing in your face....

※ ※ ※

Generally speaking, drugs are *dangerous* because they drastically impact the immune system, frequently mask the root causes of the malady at hand, and their long-term effects are often unknown. They should be avoided whenever possible. You will never know if you might live longer and experience a much better quality of life over the years had you not taken them.

Having said that, I'm sure you've gathered by this point in my book that although I'm an extremist, I'm also pragmatic and believe in common sense. Ultimately, I am guided by one question, *"What upholds existence?"* That one question can serve all of us in remarkable fashion if we are honest and objective about the medical issues of our lives, especially the use of drugs.

Several years ago I went to the hospital for a hernia operation. As much as I'm a believer in the immune system and the power of the mind, I knew that the tear in the wall of my abdomen could not be repaired without a surgical procedure and that if I did not have it repaired, I could damage my overall health, just like my father did decades earlier.

But that didn't mean surrendering myself blindly to the will of the conglomerate. Every step along the way, I questioned and probed, making my needs known and respected. **This is not that difficult once you decide to stand up for yourself and refuse to allow anyone to abuse or bamboozle you.**

Among the questions I asked was whether hypnosis could be used instead of the usual anesthetic. (I have avoided using all drugs for many years and will continue to do so unless it is absolutely unavoidable.) I learned that Medicare did not provide for this (and the hospital would not consent to this surgery under hypnosis), so I could not do anything about that.

But when I came out of the operation and dressed to leave, I refused to take any painkillers they insisted I would need. I wasn't about to yield to anything else that was intrusive or unnecessary—no matter how highly recommended it was.

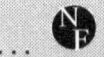

···· ····

This operation I described upheld my existence; taking painkillers would not have. This is where choice and common sense play huge roles. But in **99** percent of cases with the same general conditions, **a person will accept the painkillers without thinking twice.**

Doctors immediately prescribe painkillers and other medication as a means of protecting themselves from malpractice suits. In fact, they stand behind this defensive tactic as a matter of principle and financial practicality. That's why so many unnecessary biopsies and procedures are recommended and performed.

That doesn't necessarily mean that doctors do not want their patients to be comfortable following a medical procedure, or that patients' pain tolerance level is high enough to counterbalance their discomfort. It does mean that doctors' efforts are not always primarily focused on their patients' well-being or long-range recuperation—but on financial factors that impact their personal lives.

Had the medical fraternity been less interested in profit and its own comfort, it would never have surrendered patient care and treatment into the hands of the greedy insurance industry, the equally avaricious managed-care operators, and the pharmaceutical wizards. As a result of this restructuring of medicine, doctors have willingly become pawns in the sick game of healthcare in America.

If you have any doubts as to the degree of this medical racketeering, here's a report that should alert you to the truth:

DOCTORS ORDER NEEDLESS TESTS, SAY EXPERTS

Lee Bowman, Scripps Howard News Service—May 20, 2006

Needless medical tests are costing the U.S. healthcare system potentially billions of dollars a year and are adding unnecessarily to patient stress, according to a new study.

A review of data from more than 4,600 Americans older than 20 found that diagnostic tests not recommended under professional guidelines, or even advised against, were ordered for more than a third of the patients.

The researchers found that at least one of three common exams— urinalysis, electrocardiogram and X-rays—was inappropriately ordered for 43 percent to 46 percent of the patients. That would project to $194 million, the researchers said. ...

This report clearly indicates that these unnecessary tests are standard procedure, making it relatively easy for doctors driven by financial incentives (especially if their office includes a lab or links to a diagnostic facility) to take advantage of unknowing and trusting patients. As already mentioned—but worth repeating—doctors also carry out such unneeded tests to protect themselves from malpractice suits.

. . . .

One of their time-honored "padded-profit" schemes is to tell patients who are about to undergo a medical procedure that certain tests are necessary, including blood work. So the patient gives the okay and tests are made and appropriately billed. However, in an ever-growing number of these cases, the test results are not made known or available to patients unless they request them—and then they are charged for copies of the results. The charges can be as much as $20 for a page.

As if that weren't bad enough, in many cases, the doctors aren't even informed of or don't bother to review the test results themselves!

Needless to say, a myriad of reasons exist whereby the use of a drug will definitely uphold existence. Some obvious situations include people who are HIV-positive or suffering from AIDS, requiring various medical cocktails to control their disease; terminally ill patients who need painkillers; transplant patients who need drugs that will inhibit their bodies' attempts to reject organs; hemophilia sufferers who must have blood-clotting agents; and most people having operations who require anesthesia.

There is also some validity in using drugs for such maladies as toothaches, allergies, morning sickness, migraine attacks, and other debilitating illnesses, as well as major national and international immunization programs that apparently protect the public from deadly diseases.

But our society as a whole, guided by the conglomerate's thousands of tentacles, does not discern between those legitimate reasons and those motivated by nothing more than greed and stupidity.

As a direct result of this quick-fix insanity, we are the most medicated society in the world. And no amount of common sense or legislation will halt this because we have crossed over into a netherworld that feasts on tens of millions of drug-addicted bodies and minds, leaving no room for any discernment or wisdom in the use of drugs. We are addicted to our drug mentality.

When I was growing up, the hot dog was America's number-one food treat. It was replaced by the hamburger, and followed by pizza. Even *souvlaki* made a brief run at the top spot. But today, the number-one food of choice isn't tofu or whole grains—but DRUGS! If you think I'm exaggerating, just look at the big sign above Safeway's major grocery stores. It reads: FOOD and DRUGS. Yeah, what a team!

This mentality has escalated to the point that we are now openly addicting millions of children to drugs. (Even dogs are given psychotropic drugs, not to mention meds for racehorses!) These young people are destined to go the way of many drug abusers and addicts—with nothing in sight to stop the deadly cycle.

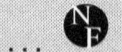

The conglomerate completely controls this genocide, raking in so many billions of dollars that dealing with any part of the overall problem and addiction is nearly impossible. The drug companies manufacture the junk, the FDA approves its use, the media advertises and promotes, the doctors prescribe unconscionably, the willing public buys, and adults and children swallow. And politicians in both the Republican and Democratic parties stand by and do nothing.

Meanwhile, no cure for cancer or AIDS is in sight, healthcare costs have escalated out of control, tens of millions of people have no health insurance, the average American medicine cabinet is stocked with a variety of prescription drugs (a different one for every ailment and problem), and a million people lie up in prisons because they are guilty of selling small amounts of illegal drugs such as marijuana.

On that note, on May 9, 2005, a federal judge sentenced former volunteer University of Washington team doctor William Scheyer to only 60 days of home confinement for indiscriminately dispensing a wide range of drugs (including narcotic painkillers) to athletes at the university. This is not even a mild slap on the wrist for such a crime! **Another example of the American caste system.**

At the same time, the real narcotics dealers—the charter members of the conglomerate—continue to operate their drug empire with total immunity from prosecution or public accountability. Just like the tobacco scions who are responsible for hundreds of millions of deaths worldwide, this conglomerate remains untouchable.

If any government agency should ever indict these people for crimes against humanity (which is bloody hell what it is), you can bet your bottom dollar that none of these mass killers will ever see the inside of a prison cell, and that, of the billions of dollars collected in fines, 99 percent of that money will go to lawyers who will see to it that it eventually makes its way right back into the conglomerate's pockets. That's the way of our society.

And only a revolution will change it.

> *You mention millions of child drug addicts;*
> *isn't it possible that a large percentage*
> *of these children are being helped?*
>
> *And don't you think that children's parents*
> *have their interests at heart?*

Pardon me if I sound sarcastic and sing, "And the farmer took another load away...." Never in my life have I witnessed such a dangerous lack of awareness as it pertains to the issue of children and drugs.

Let's put it in perspective:

Yes, there are cases where children require drugs—such as situations where no other possible hope exists for treating serious medical conditions. However, in a soaring number of cases, children are medicated as a matter of standard treatment. **That's because many ordinary problems and ailments are now labeled as diseases.**

Although drugs may provide short-term relief from individual ailments, these children face a future of increased drug use and dependency, with severe lifelong limitations and disabilities. And regardless of most parents' good intentions (and unfortunately there are those who are eager to transfer their parental responsibilities to the pharmacy), by resorting to drug regimens, parents contribute to the addiction and ultimate destruction of their children's lives while also supporting the conglomerate's growing need for power and profit.

Here's a typical example: Dr. James McGough, associate professor of clinical psychiatry at UCLA Neuropsychiatric Institute, said, "It's not necessarily a bad thing that these medicines are being used more." He goes on: "... kids on attention-deficit drugs tend to avoid substance abuse and other problems and do better in school."

What a crock! Of course the average parent will look at this guy's credentials and assume that he knows what he's talking about. **But nothing could be further from the truth.** Our nation's parents buy into this scheme at a frightening ratio: a 49-percent rise in the use of attention-deficit/hyperactivity disorder (ADHD) drugs by children *under five between 2000 and 2003* (we're not talking about adolescents with severe behavioral problems) and a corresponding 369-percent rise in spending on these drugs.

More on the same issue:

MORE KIDS GETTING ANTI-PSYCHOTIC DRUGS, STUDY FINDS
Little is known about medicines' effect on minors
Benedict Carey, *The New York Times*—June 6, 2006

The use of potent antipsychotic drugs to treat children and adolescents for problems such as aggression and mood swings increased more than fivefold from 1993 to 2002, researchers reported yesterday. ...

... "We are using these medications and don't know how they work, if they work, or at what cost," said Dr. John March, a professor of child and adolescent psychiatry at Duke University. "It amounts to a huge experiment with the lives of American kids, and what it tells us is that we've got to do something other than what we're doing now" to assess the drugs' overall impact." ...

... Dr. Mark Olfson, a professor of clinical psychiatry at Columbia University and the lead author of the study, financed in part by the National Institute of Mental Health, said the popularity of antipsychotic drugs might result in part from "the fact that psychiatrists have few other pharmacological options in certain patients." ...

Here we have psychiatrists telling us that one, we're knowingly experimenting with the lives of children and two, they have few other pharmacological options. Know what? These people should all have their licenses revoked and be charged with criminal behavior. They are part of the psychiatric wing of the conglomerate, guilty of crimes that are far more serious than those typically committed by common felons.

And the ignorant public—especially the parents of children being given these drugs and the teachers who often advise parents to have their children placed on them—should be brought to task.

This drug story is but another indication of how far the psychiatric profession has fallen; they've made a science out of dispensing drugs instead of mental and emotional health. And you can bet that they are the prized pets of the conglomerate.

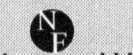

According to a federal survey cited by Dr. Andrew Mosholder, a medical officer in the Office of Drug Safety, about 2.5 million children between the ages of 4 and 17 take ADHD drugs. The survey also found that 9.3 percent of 12-year-old boys and 3.7 percent of 11-year-old girls use the drugs.

The use of other behavioral drugs has also increased dramatically in the past three years. Antidepressant use rose 21 percent, while drugs for autism and other conduct disorders jumped 71 percent, compared with a 4.3 percent rise in antibiotics, and the use of medicines for gastrointestinal problems jumped 28 percent.

Overall 5.3 percent of children took some type of behavioral medicine in 2003. It should also be noted that with the use of these drugs, more and more children are becoming prone to suicide.[8]

And that's only the beginning. Leave it to the conglomerate, and those percentages will more than double in the next few years. Be assured that the conglomerate will not be satisfied until all middle- and upper-class children are on its bandwagon.

The media's role in this children's drug insanity is unconscionable. Pick up any newspaper and you will find multiple advertisements that read "Does your child suffer from any of these symptoms?" while listing some of the most normal everyday problems that all children experience on one level or another, including anxiety, restlessness, lack of attention, etc.

For God's sake—if you accept these ridiculous criteria as proof positive that a child needs drugs to deal with this range of Mickey Mouse problems—then the entire human race should be medicated from birth!!!

This medieval attitude would be laughable (a classic Woody Allen scenario), were it not for the fact that the real sickies—the conglomerate—get away with this calculated genocide and do so with impunity. Even babies and toddlers are being given prescribed sedatives and powerful, mood-altering medications.

---

[8] In October 2003, the FDA issued a warning that children and teens who take antidepressants may face a higher suicide risk. And in February 2004, the FDA advisory panel recommended stronger warnings about the risk of suicide in kids who take antidepressant drugs.

EVEN BABIES GETTING TREATED AS MENTALLY ILL
Prescriptions on the rise even though they haven't been tested on children

Encarnacion Pyle, *The Columbus Dispatch*—April 25, 2005

Doctors prescribed sedatives and powerful, mood-altering medications for nearly 700 Ohio babies and toddlers on Medicaid last summer, according to a Dispatch *review of records.*

There's no doubt that mental health drugs can help troubled youngsters, whether they're on the government insurance program for the poor or not. But dozens of advocates, child-welfare workers and psychiatrists interviewed by the Dispatch *question the wisdom of prescribing potent medications, most of which have never been tested on kids, for so many young, vulnerable children.*

"It's shocking," said Dr. Ellen Bassuk, associate professor of psychiatry at Harvard Medical School. "Who's really being helped by these children being drugged? The babies? Or their caregivers?

"These medications are not benign; they can have dangerous side effects and have to be closely monitored." ...

Well spoken, Dr. Bassuk, but poor children on Medicaid are generally not monitored. That's one of the reasons they're being given drugs; the government won't spend the money to provide quality services to these youngsters. It's much easier and less expensive to drug them into submission. And of course it's more profit for the conglomerate.

By the way, Dr. Bassuk, there is a great deal of doubt as to whether mental health drugs really help troubled youngsters. I could write a separate book on that topic alone!

As for the possible side effects of these drugs, Stephanie Hall died after her daily dosage of Ritalin was doubled, and her parents blame the stimulant for her heart attack at age 11. Stephanie began taking medication for ADHD when she was six, after a teacher pressured her parents.

Read it and weep; thousands of well-meaning teachers have been duped or otherwise trained to follow psychiatric guidelines of the most dubious nature and recommend the use of drugs to trusting (or ignorant) parents.

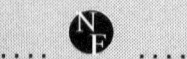

.... **N F** ....

It's no wonder that drug education within our school system has produced limited results ("Just say no to drugs" is a farce). For one thing, there's an obvious inherent hypocrisy in trying to warn children of the dangers of drug use while at the same time recommending that supposed problem children be given drugs. There's also the well-known reality that school children are aware of the fact that their own parents' medicine cabinets are fully stocked with prescription and over-the-counter drugs.

Also, many teachers themselves turn to prescription drugs for relief of their anxieties and other symptoms, so these teachers see nothing wrong with children being turned over to psychiatric counselors who will prescribe drugs rather than concern and counseling.

Here's another example of what the conglomerate is up to:

SLEEPING PILL USE BY YOUTHS SOARS, STUDY SAYS
Practice lacks FDA approval
Gardiner Harris, *The New York Times*—October 17, 2005

The use of sleeping pills among children and very young adults rose 85 percent between 2000 and 2004, in yet another sign that parents and physicians are increasingly turning to prescription medications to solve childhood health and behavioral problems.

And about 15 percent of people under age 20 who received sleeping pills were also being given drugs to treat attention deficit and hyperactivity disorder, according to the study by Medco Solutions, a managed-care company that makes estimates about medication use in the whole population based on extrapolations from its own data. Drugs used to treat attention disorders can cause insomnia.

Few of these prescriptions have the approval of the Food and Drug Administration, because no sleep medication has been approved for use in children under 18. Still, doctors commonly use medications for patients and disorders for which the drugs have never received formal approval, particularly when those patients are children. ...

Dr. Robert Epstein, Medco's chief medical officer, said, "It leads you to wonder whether these children are being treated for insomnia caused by hyperactivity or whether the medication itself causes the insomnia,"

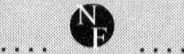

Medco officials would be wise to recognize that side effects from drugs are not only commonplace but built into the drug companies' marketing programs: Drugs approved by the FDA for specific use are then advertised and prescribed for other uses. For instance, cardiac drugs and anticonvulsants are prescribed "off-label" 46 percent of the time, allergy therapies 34 percent, and psychiatric medicines 31 percent.

Although this off-label promotion doesn't sit well with the FDA (it's actually illegal), and for that matter, the FCC, it's business as usual, unless federal prosecutors intervene.

Also be aware of the reality that, if a drug used for ADHD causes insomnia—that gives the conglomerate the added benefit of treating the insomnia with more drugs!

I call that the "MGM" procedure. Metro-Goldwyn-Mayer's medical people supplied Judy Garland (and dozens of other young performing artists) with uppers, downers, and in-betweeners so she could keep cranking out those fabulous musicals. That is—until the pills took their lasting toll.

They murdered her. By "they," I mean the doctors (pill-pushers) employed by the studio. These loathsome bastards never gave her a chance, even at the age of 14! And the evidence to support this fact is incontrovertible. Every actor, writer, director, grip, cameraman, right down to background players knew what was going on. Personally, I've known at least 30 people who worked on the MGM lot in those years, and every one of them openly spoke of this daily drug scene. Some of them were even subjected to it themselves.

Either way you look at it, doctors dispense the nonapproved script to children, creating more future American junkies. And the FDA does nothing about it.

✳ ✳ ✳

And this problem is not limited by any means to children:

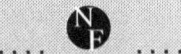

A study conducted by Medco Health Solutions, a managed care company, found that sleeping pill use among adults 20 to 44 years old has doubled in the past four years, while spending on them has almost doubled.

Concurrent with this increase, drug companies spent $2.1 billion advertising them in 2004. As for senior citizens, they are still the largest users of prescription sleeping pills. Also, use of prescription drugs for ADHD is growing at a faster rate among adults than children. Between March 2002 and June 2005, adult use of these drugs grew by 90 percent!

I must point my finger directly at the psychiatrists and psychologists who are guilty of neglecting their patients and of gross malfeasance. *These Ph.D characters have abandoned their chosen professions and become nothing more than legal drug dealers.*

Thinking about the issue of psychiatry in America is enough to make my blood boil. We're sending young people to noted universities to learn how to scribble prescriptions! *We'd be better off hiring ex-convicts to act as psychiatrists.* Someone who's done hard time in prison knows a hell of a lot more about human problems, probably has more compassion than the degenerates with Ph.Ds, and sure as hell knows more about the junk he would prescribe than the quack psychiatrist does.

Part of the problem is that **so many of these shrinks do not know how to deal with human problems**—so they resort to the use of drugs. That's what they do best! Once these quacks start dispensing the script, it becomes routine. They not only swear by it but they also advise commissions and hospitals (and teachers and parents) to follow this method of treatment, making drugs the acceptable form of treatment on a national level.

To quote Dr. Douglas Jacobs, associate clinical professor of psychiatry at Harvard Medical School, "The general evidence is that the best treatment for depression is a combination of medication and psychotherapy."

Sure, doctor, but by the time you have finished medicating your patients—especially the younger ones—they're in no shape for psychotherapy. Many of them are zombies! You can see them walking city streets without the mind to know what they're doing with their ruined lives, left adrift in a world they cannot cope with.

Not that you psychiatric pill-pushers would even begin to know how to apply any meaningful therapeutic concepts to those you diagnose as suffering from depression or the wide assortment of problems you no longer treat—because it's much easier and a lot quicker to pull out your prescription pads.

It should also be pointed out that the drug mentality is now so ingrained within the framework of psychiatry (and psychology) that it has filtered into school curriculums and all but replaced the idea of psychotherapy as the cornerstone of treating mental illness. *Why even bother with the pretense of treatment?*

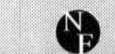

> During my tenure as executive director of Encounter, Inc. (America's first and foremost community-based drug prevention and treatment program) from 1965 to 1968, we successfully treated many methamphetamine users. Our counseling, conceptualizing, grouping, and concern did the job, and our methods and training became a model for other treatment programs.
>
> That was before the insurance industry, aided and abetted by the conglomerate, took control of treating drug users. Using the credentials of their psychiatric sidekicks, these meatheads (once again, I'm being polite) have turned what was a serious social problem **that could be dealt with on a therapeutic level** into a legalized drug den that ravages the minds and bodies of millions of people in desperate need of help.
>
> These professional psychiatrists-cum-drug dealers representing noted universities (as well as pharmaceutical companies) are now treating methamphetamine users with MORE DRUGS! The latest is something called The PROMETA Protocol (sounds like the title of a Robert Ludlum book), a combination of genetic drugs already on the market.

All these medical traitors and their associate allies (including the weak-minded leadership in both houses of Congress) are the loyal right hands of the pharmaceutical companies, directly responsible for the destruction of millions of human lives, including those of my friend Eddie Cohen and my ex-wife.

> *What do you think of President Bush's plan*
> *to subject all American schoolchildren*
> *to mental health screening?*

My immediate thought is that the infamous George W. Bush should be first in line for mental health screening himself, followed closely behind by his cabinet of psychotics, as well as the spineless elected officials in both parties who turn their backs on their constituents. Once that mindless group is taken away and put in the iron bar hotel, the next step will be to treat them the same way that millions of other Americans are treated for mental health problems—medicate the hell out of them.

Let each of these mentally and emotionally deformed lunatics experience what it's like to be in the hands of the psychiatric drug dealers. And as they go through their paces and slowly become zombie-like creatures, document the entire process on film—so that the world can see the overlords of madness finally get their just medicine and comeuppance.

Needless to say, the conglomerate should also be dealt with in similar fashion; we should give it the same medicine that it prescribes for America. I mean—let's be fair to it!

Now that I got that sarcastic—but accurate—thought out of my system, let's take a close look at this sick plan: Cunningly called "TeenScreen," this supposed suicide-prevention program is nothing less than a Nazi-style forced program of eugenics, to cleanse the race of all inferiors. Its agenda essentially calls for eliminating any future potential threat to the powers that be.

For those of you unfamiliar with the Nazi era in Germany, the leaders of the Third Reich were adept at creating model programs for national healthcare and the future welfare of the state. On the surface of things, they appeared to the populace as progressive and humanitarian achievements. It wasn't until it was much too late that the true nature of these activities was discovered.

Demigods and dictators throughout history have successfully persuaded their subjects to trust in their munificent intentions.

With untold power comes the unchallenged opportunity to make a stink bomb smell like a rose. And American leaders in both parties (including supposed "progressives") as well as our health-care institutions and industries are not exempt from such devious behavior. Just look at the conglomerate! They're turning millions of people—including children—into drug addicts.

I'm not going to waste lots of time or book space on this Nazi-styled program (which has already been adopted in Illinois), because it's so simple to analyze and outline that it's pathetic—providing you can see what's obvious to anyone with intelligence and common decency.

Here's a quick breakdown:

1. School officials hand conglomerate operatives (those prescription-pad whackos with Ph.D nameplates) permission to give mental health checkups to all those who are deemed to "not act normally."

2. Psychiatrists start kids on the meds that will turn them into future druggies.

3. Parents of children enrolled in this program will of course be given positive progress reports, and if necessary, be highly encouraged to acquiesce to other solutions, including boot camps, suspension centers, or psychiatric treatment.

4. This Orwellian-type program will succeed because the American public, already drug-infested, will regard it as a progressive form of treatment.

5. Nothing will stop it because the conglomerate, with strong personal support from the Republican administration and lack of opposition from the Democratic Party, will be allowed to circumvent all legal restraints and create another death-camp industry under the guise of dispensing beneficial drugs and treatment.

In other words, American children are really in for it. And if you think that we are already drug-fixated, just wait until you see what the next generation brings.

> *What can be done about*
> *the drug issue in America?*

Our most immediate need is for society to deal with the drug issue on all levels:

- **Prescription Drug Abuse:** The biggest and most destructive drug problem of the lot by far, this takes a greater toll on lives than all the other drug problems combined. As I've said previously—and it's worth repeating a hundred times!—the big-time dope peddlers are not the ones who sell the junk on the streets or back alleys and end up in prisons. The true demons of the drug world are the charter members of the conglomerate. *They are more deadly than any group of terrorists that the world has ever known.* Their prime medical operatives—doctors and psychiatrists— suffer from a disease called *severe trigger finger,* a malady that causes rigorous itching—to pull out the prescription pad.

    It must also be said that the American public, who is blind to its own drug dependence, ignorantly regards its drug use as a legitimate use of medication, which is the biggest crock of you-know-what ever perpetrated. Drugs are legitimate medications only when they are appropriately prescribed and used to treat ailments and diseases that cannot otherwise be treated, or after all other options (such as lifestyle and behavioral changes) have been exhausted. In all other instances—which safely encompasses at least 95 percent of all prescription drug use—these substances are not meds. They are "junk," the street term for drugs.

    And you, the buyer and user, are a junkie in every sense of the word. The fact that you are not hustling on the streets for your junk and that you're obtaining it legally doesn't change that reality. Nor does it alter the fact that you're contributing to the ongoing growth of the drug industry and culture, and in the process supporting unimaginable human suffering and destruction.

- **The War On Drugs:** This ineffective, costly, mindless, legislative nightmare must be put in the dumpster and trashed for all time. *We need nothing short of a complete revision of drug laws, starting from scratch. And we can begin by starting a war on prescription drugs!*

- **Recreational Drugs:** We must finally deal with the overall marijuana issue (recreational and medical use) and also develop effective educational programs to greatly reduce the use of methamphetamine and hallucinatory drugs. Merely following former First Lady Nancy Reagan's "Just Say No" to drugs hasn't moved us in a preventative direction. As for the various community organizations like The Anti-Drug, the Leadership to Keep Children Alcohol Free, The National African American Tobacco Prevention Network, the National Asian Pacific American Families Against Substance Abuse, and many others associated with the Office of National Drug Control Policy, I would urge them to check out some of their associated allies—who are guilty of supporting the very abuse these groups are confronting.

    For instance, the American Academy of Child and Adolescent Psychiatry should be evaluated for its psychopharmacology services. In fact, whenever any independent community group aligns itself with other groups dealing with drug prevention, it should avoid any association with medical organizations that foster prescription drug use as a general form of treatment. To do otherwise puts it into the enemy camp—without even knowing it! You can't play it both ways!

    When I was executive director of Encounter, Inc., I refused to accept proposed associations with organizations that sanctioned any manner, shape, or form of drug use within their own jurisdiction—even if it meant turning down large grants and contributions. I would take that same uncompromising position today.

- **Reefer Madness:** On June 6, 2005, the Supreme Court ruled that people who smoke marijuana because their doctors recommend it to ease pain and control nausea can be prosecuted for violating federal drug laws despite state laws that permit the medicinal use of marijuana. Although I am obviously opposed to drug use in an overall sense, here's a case that falls under the same category of legitimate use as insulin for diabetics, blood-clotting agents for hemophiliacs, painkillers for those who truly need them, and various drug cocktails for AIDS victims.

    The Supreme Court's ruling goes counter to what upholds existence for people whose only alternative to suffering and suicide is the medicinal use of marijuana. It's a cold-hearted ruling that keeps America's drug policy in the dark ages and supports the aims of the conglomerate, who feels the need to control the marketing and sales of all medication. Along with our war on drugs, this policy must be changed. But don't expect it to happen anymore than you can hope for changes in our archaic Constitution. The conglomerate will never allow such changes to take place, and it has the entire legal profession to back them. Note: The FDA will also stand against the medicinal use of marijuana, as ordered by the White House.

- **Drug Treatment and Prevention:** For the most part, there are disproportionately few effective treatment and prevention centers (as opposed to community support centers that do not have the means to treat drug-related problems) for the millions of people who are hooked on some kind of junk. Nowadays, there are few Daytops (America's foremost drug-treatment center) and no Encounters, leaving millions of otherwise helpless people with no avenue of approach to their drug problems and addictions.

As an example:

JUDGE BLASTS LACK OF DRUG-REHAB CENTERS

Rebecca Boone, The Associated Press—November 22, 2005

The lack of long-term residential drug-treatment in rural Idaho is leading to prison overcrowding and forcing some judges to send offenders out of state for treatment, a judge said.
"The need is incredible," 2nd District Court Justice John Bradberry said Monday. "Why are we giving the responsibility for mental-health treatment to the criminal-justice system? It's a disgrace." ...

You bet your life it's a disgrace. A national one. That's because the American people basically do not care about those they classify as addicts. So why should lawmakers provide drug-treatment centers? Of course, if your addiction is caused by legally dispensed prescription drugs, that's okay. You're deserving of costly treatment—just part and parcel of our foul caste system. I must also mention that places like the Betty Ford Clinic are nothing more than would-be detox houses for the rich and famous. They are abominations because they too aid and abet the conglomerate, failing to truly uphold existence for the masses of drug-suffering people in America.

- **Sports doping:** I'm going to go off on a tangent here because, unlike all the other drug issues in America, sports doping (even more than show business doping) is not just taken for granted by the public. Although our sports heroes are as vulnerable and confused as most others when it comes to drug use, they stand out as models to be watched, followed, and emulated on many levels, from clothing to behavior. So the drug issue in sports takes on a greater meaning and contributes disproportionately to our national cancer.

  Ken Caminiti, who won the 1996 National League Most Valued Player award, and who in May 2002 told *Sports Illustrated* that he used steroids during his MVP season, died at age 41 of a heart attack induced by years of drug use.

Steroid use by athletes is not limited to Ken Caminiti or Jose Canseco, to Mark McGuire, Sammy Sosa, Jason Giambi, Rafael Palmeiro, or Barry Bonds. Track stars, basketball players, bike racers, and football players also use them. Do you think that all those 350-pound guards and tackles get so big by merely eating more than others and putting extra time in the weight room?

Note: The average life expectancy of NFL players is 57.[9] That should make you think. And what's even worse, tens of thousands of high school athletes have turned to steroid use to satisfy the needs of school coaches who will accept nothing less than victory.

Overall, the hierarchy of sports on all levels—including school, amateur, semi-pro, and professional—have always reacted to drug problems in typical fashion. First, do nothing, to see if the problem won't go away. If someone blows the whistle, deny it. If tests prove that people are using drugs, immediately tell the public that the practice is not widespread. If that doesn't bury the issue, then refuse to comment. This battle plan won't change until the public, as well as Congress, forces a change.

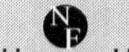

On November 15, 2005, baseball, spurred by the threat of legis-

---

[9] Twenty-eight percent of all pro football players born in the past century who qualified as obese died before their 50th birthday. Even more shocking, **19 percent died from homicides or suicides.**

lative action, finally agreed to tougher penalties for steroid use. Bravo! It only took countless deaths, insurmountable evidence of drug use, hundreds of thousands of young people getting hooked on steroid use, revelations and denial alike by major players, and God knows how much stupidity and avoidance on the part of the press, before concrete action was taken.

Needless to say, this is just the bare beginnings of what needs to be done. Hopefully it won't take another 30 years to deal with the use of other drugs such as amphetamines and human growth hormones.

The steroid problem has gotten enormous press coverage because of Jose Canseco's revealing book, *Juiced*. Besides fingering many star athletes as steroid users—in spite of their denials—Jose makes the following claims:

> *I have chemically restructured my body, giving myself one of the best physiques in the world and enabling myself to do things at 40 that most 22-year-old kids couldn't do. Best of all, I have prepared myself to maintain that body for years to come. My strength, vitality, and appearance are my best argument for what I'm saying.*
>
> *If I were exaggerating the effect that growth hormone and steroids can have when used properly and carefully as part of a program of weightlifting, fitness, careful nutrition, and clean living, then why would I look and feel as good as I do? The only answer is, I'm telling the truth.*

Jose goes on to say,

> *What I've learned is that there is a way to stop the aging process, or at least slow it down by 90 percent. I'm sure new chemicals will be developed in the coming years, which will open up new possibilities we can't even imagine at this point. As that happens, and other people experiment on themselves over time, I expect we'll see human beings commonly living to be a healthy 120 or 130 years old.*

· · · ·   · · · ·

Jose, you may be right on both counts—that you have enhanced

> your physical appearance and feel younger at 40 than most men at
> 20, and that the correct application of various chemicals may make
> it possible for people to live to be 130 years old. But what about
> the thousands of cases of people who don't know what the "correct
> application of various chemicals" is all about? And what about the
> quality of their drugged lives as they age? Will they end up like Ken
> Caminiti? How will *you* end up?
>   The jury is still out on that one.

And what about the millions of young people—including athletes, recreational drug users, and kids with absolutely no understanding of the proper use of drugs, weightlifting, fitness, careful nutrition, and clean living—who decide that they are as smart as Jose Canseco and start experimenting with steroids or growth hormones?

Have you thought about these people? How do you safeguard them? You can't! Like your fellow baseball players who want to be like you, these kids will want to be just as unique as you. They won't discern on any level, and many of them will suffer severe consequences, including death.

This compulsion to be as unique as the rich and famous extends to most areas of life and leads to hundreds of thousands (if not millions) of tragedies. For example, while President Kennedy and President Clinton were turning the White House into a whorehouse, millions of young, uneducated, and underprivileged teenagers decided they could be just as unique—resulting in high rates of sexually transmitted diseases and tens of thousands of unwanted births. (I know, because I treated many of these young people.)

The lesson, Jose, is that you must take direct responsibility for ballyhooing steroids and growth hormones and face up to the challenge of dealing with the potential results, which can be catastrophic. If you can do that—fine. Otherwise, take your money and run. And stop advising people to play it smart when you know they won't, especially if they don't know how to mix and match—not anymore than they do with prescription drugs or recreational drugs. Not any more than Ken Caminiti. No way, Jose!

I must also mention that the conglomerate will not allow private chemists like yourself to get a foothold on their marketplace, nor will the FDA sanction such private experimentation, even if the results are highly promising.

There is hope that in the future it will be possible for doctors to use DNA maps to predict and prevent illness and disease. If that happens, perhaps we can throw away all the drugs forever.

Ooops!—I take that back; by the time medical science has mapped the billions of pairs of genes that are the blueprint of the genetic code, chances are that the conglomerate will have positioned itself to control that aspect of healthcare as well. And no doubt our system will still be emphasizing reactive medicine instead of prevention. So all the scientific advancement will only result in more profits for the conglomerate—and the public [will still] be damned!)

A final thought on the steroid issue in baseball: The overlords of this great American pastime have covered up for their steroid-using superstars (as truthfully described by Jose Canseco, who undoubtedly will be blacklisted by the press and never be considered for the Hall of Fame). Meanwhile, they continue to bar Pete Rose and Shoeless Joe Jackson from the Hall of Fame for transgressions that jeopardize the integrity of the game. What hypocrisy—a double standard that damages baseball integrity more than all the drug issues combined. Shame.

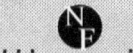

. . . .

In August 2005, Rafael Palmeiro was suspended for 10 days after testing positive for steroid use. He will remain eligible for the Hall of Fame. But Pete Rose, who bet on baseball many years ago, is still banned for life.

AND, in all fairness to those less-than-innocent players who have been penalized for various legal infractions, including Darryl Strawberry, Denny McClain, and Dwight Gooden (all of whom have served hard time), the real bummers have escaped all accusations, charges, and censorship, their reputations remaining clean and unscarred in spite of serious transgressions. Why? Because they are protected. Who are the protectors?

Here's a short list: Club owners who know where all the dirt lies but expose the lesser-known evils of the clubhouse only when it suits their purpose; the majority of players, trainers, coaches, and managers who are fully aware of who's doing drugs and pretend, lie, or cover up for all the bad examples; the players' union and representatives, who foolishly think that they are actually protecting the athletes; the commissioner's office in cahoots with club owners, who have lied about drug use in baseball for decades, preferring to protect the game's integrity by denial; and all the sports writers, commentators, and media analysts who turn a deaf ear to all the drug realities of which they are aware.

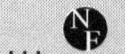

These media are quick to tear apart Mike Tyson every time he shoots himself in the foot (he is an immediate, easy target), but when it comes to the popular stars with clean reputations—the press follows a cowardly hands-off policy. In fact, it voted Gaylord Perry into the Hall of Fame in 1991, knowing he was a spitball pitcher, which is a violation of baseball laws.

All the aforementioned people are collectively responsible for doping in sports in that they have aided and abetted the worst examples that sports has to offer America's youth. Realize this: All those young people who get hooked on sports doping will graduate to more junk as they age. **That's why I'm focusing so much attention on it.**

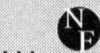

Baseball (and for that matter, most sports) is the mirror image of the true American pastime—drugs. In fact, it is perhaps the quintessential role model for the legal and illegal abuse of the junk. Athletes use steroids to enhance their performance, amphetamines for a quick pick-me-up, and a wide assortment of pills and injections while they're on the trainer's table or the disabled list. It's all accepted—by the general public—as the norm.

Once again, I must add another kicker to a vital question. In this case, this directly involves the steroid issue, as well as the related element of fairness and justice for all.

BALCO FOUNDER CONTE GETS EIGHT MONTHS

Maury Brown, The Associated Press—October 18, 2005

Victor Conte was sentenced to four months in prison and four months' home confinement Tuesday for his role as the mastermind in a scheme to provide pro athletes with undetectable banned drugs.

Conte, who negotiated a plea deal with federal prosecutors, started the Bay Area Laboratory Co-Operative. The lab, according to court records, counted dozens of prominent athletes among its clients, including Barry Bonds, Jason Giambi, Marion Jones and others.

James Valente, BALCO's vice president, was sentenced to probation after pleading guilty to reduced charges of steroid distribution. . ...

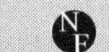

. . . .

It's no wonder that there is so little respect for the law. How can our citizens trust the court system when they see something like this? Hundreds of thousands of small-time drug dealers lie up in prison for years—while people who have developed and fostered a highly dangerous drug culture that affects hundreds of thousands—if not millions—of people throughout the country get off with a mild sentence that's laughable.

To put it in proper perspective, a man accused of supplying methamphetamine to the Billings, Montana area in 2003 was recently sentenced in federal court to 107 years in prison. Need I say more?

I'll go one up on that: A recently passed bill in the state of Washington makes lying on your résumé a class C felony, a crime of fraud that could land you in the can for five years, along with a $10,000 fine. Can you believe it?! If all the possible cases were tried, 40 million Americans would go to prison!!!

Not to mention what these inequities say to the Pete Rose situation and many others like it. Of course, the press won't make an issue of this injustice. They would have to go after the real big shots—and they will never do that. In fact, if Barry Bonds were to give the collective bunch of sports writers one hard stare—most of them would crap in their pants![10]

---

[10] It was widely accepted among sports writers that Barry Bonds used steroids because there was no other way of explaining the meteoric rise in his slugging statistics after the age of 30, any more than

In my final conclusion to this steroid issue, I must emphasize that the point of my lengthy discourse on the subject is that, although the public and the press view the steroid problem as unique to sports and distinctly different than the broader problem of illegal (street) drugs, nothing could be further from the truth. Whether we're addressing sports doping, illegal drugs, recreational drugs, or prescription drugs, **it's all one and the same problem**—a crippling disease that destroys millions of lives every year and feeds hundreds of billions of dollars into various conglomerates and drug cartels.

✳ ✳ ✳

While most of my comments and reports about drugs focus on conditions within America, we must also recognize that the conglomerate stretches its claws well beyond our shores, operating its wheels of drugs and death wherever it can get a foothold. As part of its outreach, it is of course aided and abetted by Big Brother George W. Bush and his henchmen.

Take a look:

U.S. TRADE REP HELPS POWERFUL DRUG INDUSTRY

Sherrod Brown, Member of Congress, *Seattle Post-Intelligencer*—June 28, 2005

When George W. Bush and the U.S. pharmaceutical industry team up in Washington, you know it's bad news for U.S. consumers. Now they are taking their show on the road—to Central America.

Guatemala—with an economy the size of Bismarck, N.D., and a population poorer than any U.S. community—seems to be the Chosen One. ...

... Last year, the Guatemalan Congress passed legislation to allow the sale of generic drugs to give its citizens more consumer choice and to bring down the price of name-brand drugs. Consumers in Guatemala cheered them on.

---

they could account for the added strength and muscularity of the man chasing Hank Aarons's home run record. But the press, along with baseball commissioner Bud Selig, chose to all but ignore the obvious fact that this mighty titan of baseball used performance-enhancing drugs. That changed in March 2006, when Barry Bonds was exposed in the 2006 book *Game of Shadows* by *San Francisco Chronicle* reporters Mark Fainaru-Wada and Lance Williams. These writers gave a detailed account of years of alleged heavy steroid use by the man who had consistently denied steroid involvement. So the book is still open on Bonds, and it will be played out for years to come—and the press will continue to treat him with kid gloves, even though he pretends that they're picking on him. Don't buy into that act.

Then the U.S. drug industry and its allies in the Bush administration moved in. Even though international trade law and World Trade Organization rules allow the sale of generics in member counties, the U.S. trade representative told Guatemalan leaders that there will be no Central American Free Trade Agreement unless the Guatemalan government gives the drug companies what they want. Not surprisingly, and against the vociferous opposition of millions of Guatemalans, the government repealed its own public health law.

This kind of strategy—presidents named Bush teaming up with the prescription drug industry—is not a new thing. In 1991, President George H. W. Bush told Canadians that, unless they repealed their compulsory license law that ensured significantly lower prescription drug prices for Canadians than Americans were paying, Canada would be excluded from the North American Free Trade Agreement. Ottawa repealed its law and soon Canada was included in the NAFTA agreement.

But this time, citizens of the victimized country took to the streets. In mid-March, 20,000 demonstrators assembled to protest the inclusion of Guatemala in the flawed CAFTA. Among their grievances? That CAFTA undercut their democratic rights and sold out their sovereignty. And that patent rules and the action of the Guatemalan legislation would limit the poor's access to life-saving medicine. The Bush-Pharmaceutical Alliance, they maintained, would make a poor country even poorer. ...

... Jessie Gruttadauria of the AIDS Healthcare Foundation, which operates three clinics in Honduras, said, "Poor Central Americans with AIDS will pay for CAFTA with their lives, since thousands of patients today rely on generics and CAFTA would cut off such access."

More than 150,000 protesters in 45 demonstrations in the six CAFTA countries expressed their opposition to this agreement. These demonstrators knew that CAFTA would not work for their country. They had seen that NAFTA failed Mexican workers, done little for Mexican consumers, and reduced the Mexican government's ability to deal with its national environment and health problems. And they figured that CAFTA, a dysfunctional cousin of NAFTA, could well be worse. ...

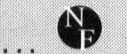

On July 28, 2005, the U.S. House of Representatives, by a vote of 217 to 215 approved the CAFTA agreement, a personal triumph for President Bush, who campaigned aggressively for the accord. Don't tell me you're proud to be an American after reading that.

Here's a kicker to U.S. foreign drug involvement:

On April 28, 2006, Mexico's Congress approved a bill to decriminalize possession of small quantities of drugs for personal use, including cocaine and heroin. All it would take for the bill to become law was the signature of President Vicente Fox. It never happened. American interests prevailed. After all, how could we explain Mexico's efforts to decriminalize illegal drugs to the million-odd Americans in prison for possessing or selling small amounts of drugs? And how could we appeal to the conglomerate to allow a neighboring country to control its own drug policy?

What about over-the-counter drugs?

That's a topic in and of itself. But, aside from the fact that over-the-counter drugs are typically less expensive than prescription medication, making them more affordable for those without insurance, these drugs are manufactured and marketed by the conglomerate, which equally manipulates their sale and distribution, just like the prescription stuff.

Whereas over-the-counter drug sales in other countries are less restrictive than in America (i.e., antibiotics are readily available in Greece without a prescription), **you must remember that we are the most medicated society in the world, which makes our over-the-counter drugstore purchases no less addictive or dangerous.** And pharmaceutical companies often attempt to switch the exact same drug from prescription to over-the-counter when their patents are about to expire, so they can avoid competition from generic brands.

As a result, you are no more protected from drugs of a dubious nature, regardless of whether you need a prescription or can purchase them over the counter.

As for "remedies" that treat such things as dandruff and athlete's foot—forget it! Nothing but worthless crap—in spite of all those TV commercials!

Some federal health advisors would like to see an in-between option, in which patients can buy certain drugs without prescription but only after speaking with a pharmacist. This option is currently available in Britain. But that would require U.S. federal laws to change, making such an option nationally available under FDA rules.

Anyway that you look at it, the drug scene (including the drugstore counter) is, on all levels, a rat race of such proportions that it makes organized crime and corporate scandal seem like child's play in comparison. And needless to say, this scene needs fixing in every conceivable way.

> *What are the general implications of*
> *supposedly "safe" drugs that are suddenly*
> *brought into question and recalled?*

In spite of the FDA's presence, drugs are constantly put on the market for use by millions of people without undergoing enough research to guarantee their safety. Even worse, studies sponsored by drug companies that clearly indicate serious (if not potentially deadly) side effects of a drug are often not published.

Here's a classic example.

DOZENS DIED, BUT DRUG WAS STILL KEPT ON MARKET

Gardiner Harris and Eric Koli, *The New York Times*—**June 10, 2005**

Dozens had died and more than 100 patients had suffered serious heart problems by March 1998 after taking Propulsid, a popular medicine for heartburn. ...

This was a drug for heartburn, given to children and babies for acid reflux, which caused heart problems and even death—and all the FDA did was add a watered-down label!

Because Propulsid had a good year (over $1 billion in sales), its manufacturer, Johnson & Johnson, continued to market its use for children. In fact, about 20 percent of babies in neonatal intensive care were given the drug in 1998.

Even though reports of heart injuries and deaths mounted, Johnson & Johnson maintained that Propulsid was safe for use. Only when a government hearing threatened to bring attention to the drug's long, mostly hidden record of problems did the drugmaker withdraw it from the market.

Corporate and government documents show that Johnson & Johnson did everything in its power to save a profitable drug, in spite of strong evidence of its harmful and deadly side effects.

Furthermore, documents from lawsuits against Johnson & Johnson showed that the company did not conduct the safety studies urged by federal regulators and their own consultants that could have revealed Propulsid's danger early on. Moreover, the FDA did not disclose Johnson & Johnson research that cast doubt on Propulsid's effectiveness against the very digestive disorders it was being used to treat, **since those studies are considered trade secrets.**

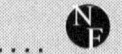

I find it amazing that while government officials are doing everything within and beyond their power to force reporters to reveal their sources of information, we obediently accept the illicit contract between the FDA and the conglomerate that allows for this trade secret conspiracy. Once again—there is honor among thieves!

The FDA later acquiesced to the "trade secrets" defense rather than take action to prevent human suffering and death. This is no different than the federal marshals of old allowing medicine men to peddle their magic elixirs to unsuspecting town folk. Only these days it's a hell of a lot more deadly!

In January 2000, the FDA scheduled a meeting to discuss its concerns with outside experts, but three weeks before the scheduled hearing, Johnson & Johnson announced it would stop selling Propulsid in the United States. The hearing was cancelled.

In reality, Johnson & Johnson, aided and abetted by the FDA, committed murder, then begged off a trial, and was allowed to go scot-free, but it will probably attempt to peddle its deadly junk in other countries.

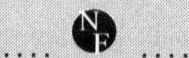

To conclude this report: Johnson & Johnson agreed in 2004 to pay up to $90 million to settle lawsuits that eventually involved claims that 300 people died and as many as 16,000 suffered significant side effects while taking Propulsid.

* * *

Along the same lines as the Propulsid sham and tragedy, here's news that might make you think about the conglomerate's direct involvement in a scam that is nothing short of life-threatening to millions:

On September 30, 2004, Merck & Co. announced it would withdraw Vioxx from the market after studies showed that long-term use of the product doubled the risk of heart attack and stroke. At the time of its withdrawal, about two million people were using Vioxx worldwide, mostly to treat arthritis.

When Vioxx first hit the market (in 1999) under a barrage of TV commercials, with celebrity endorsements from former athletes Dorothy Hamill and Bruce Jenner, it was hailed by Merck as a miracle drug. It became one of the most successful new drugs ever, racking up over $2.5 billion in sales in 2003, and 84 million prescriptions filed as of 2004.

Notwithstanding the drug's success, Merck was dogged for several years by research suggesting the drug increased risks of heart problems, but the company vehemently denied a connection until the drug was pulled from the market.

The FDA had said there were early signs of potential problems with Vioxx, and had monitored the situation since 2002. In addition, a Merck study led to warnings about heart risks being placed on the drug's label in 2002.

When the drug was finally withdrawn, experts advised patients to immediately stop taking Vioxx and talk to their doctors about alternatives. "Given the availability of alternative therapies, and the questions raised by the data, we concluded that a voluntary withdrawal is the responsible course to take," said Ray Gilmartin, chairman, president, and chief executive of Merck & Co.

"This is not a total surprise," said Dr. Steven Galson, acting director of the FDA's Center for Drug Evaluation and Research. In fact, Seattle-based Group Health Cooperative refused to approve Vioxx as part of its covered healthcare plans, citing the risks of increased heart attacks and other problems. "I think the concerns were very clear," said Jim Carlson, the director of pharmacy clinical services at Group Health.

Although I did not necessarily include the FDA as an original charter member of the conglomerate, let's look at some facts:

1.   The FDA said there were early signs of problems with Vioxx.

2.   A Merck study led to warnings—and the FDA had been monitoring problems since 2002.

3.   The acting director of the FDA's Center for Drug Evaluation and Research said, "This is not a total surprise."

4.   A regional managed-healthcare cooperative refused to approve Vioxx as part of its covered healthcare plans.

So what are we to assume about the FDA's actions over a period of five years? Should we call it complacency, stupidity, unwillingness to act quickly on behalf of the endangered public, or a sweetheart deal with the conglomerate that borders on criminal? The simple truth is that the FDA took five years to make a responsible move. And in that time, how many people needlessly died?

We're only talking about this one drug! How many other warning signs have the FDA ignored over the years? Must there be another Thalidomide tragedy[11] before we realize that the government agencies responsible for the public's safety are not doing their jobs effectively—no matter what they tell you? If they're not responsible for the nation's health mess—then who is?

I'll tell you who—the conglomerate—and all those who aid and abet it, knowingly or otherwise. And going back to the 1960s theme of "If you're not part of the solution, you're part of the problem," the FDA is certainly an integral part of the problem.

AFTER VIOXX, SAFETY DOUBTS RAISED ON CELEBREX, OTHER PAIN RELIEVERS

Marilynn Marchione, The Associated Press—October 7, 2004

... And researchers writing in the New England Journal of Medicine

---

[11] Thalidomide was first marketed in Europe in the late 1950s. It was used as a sleeping pill and to treat morning sickness during pregnancy. At that time no one knew Thalidomide caused birth defects. It was synthesized in West Germany in 1953 and marketed from 1957 to 1961, mainly in Germany and Britain. It was available in nearly 50 countries under at least 40 different names, although not in the United States (the FDA was on the verge of approving it when news of the disaster surfaced). It was later found to be teratogenic in fetal development, by interfering with the formation of blood vessels, especially if taken during the first 25 to 50 days of pregnancy. Around 15,000 fetuses were damaged by Thalidomide, of whom about 12,000 in 46 countries were born with birth defects, with only about 8,000 surviving past the first year of life. Most of these survivors are still alive, nearly all with disabilities caused by the drug. Researchers later discovered that the disabilities and deformities in many Thalidomide survivors are passed on to the survivor's own children through their DNA.

voiced their concerns as well with such drugs such as Pfizer's popular Celebrex and its newer drug, Bextra.

The medical journal published two reports on the issue yesterday on the Internet—more than two weeks ahead of their planned print publication—to help inform doctors and patients considering whether to stop using the drugs.

Studies done five years ago when Celebrex and Merck & Co.'s Vioxx were approved suggests that the same mechanism that inhibits inflammation and makes the drugs easier on the stomach than traditional painkillers also blocks a substance that prevents heart problems, according to Dr. Garret FitzGerald, a University of Pennsylvania cardiologist. FitzGerald led the studies, which were designed by him but funded by the drug companies.

"I believe this is a class effect," he said, meaning that the problem also applies to Celebrex and Bextra, which remain on the market. ...

... In a separate report also released by the medical journal, Dr. Eric Topol of the Cleveland Clinic chastised the FDA for not requiring Merck to do studies investigating heart problems with Vioxx when hints of them first appeared years ago, and for allowing the company to blitz consumers with TV ads touting the drug.

Vioxx was the largest prescription drug withdrawal in history, "but had the many warning signs along the way been heeded, such a debacle could have been prevented," Topol wrote. "Neither Merck nor the FDA fulfilled its responsibilities to the public... I believe there should be a full congressional review of this case." ...

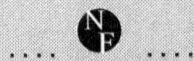

Know what fat chance is? Our dysfunctional Congress is not about to review the Vioxx travesty because our legislative troops (including newly elected ones in November 2006) are beholden to the drug companies themselves for contributing to their election campaigns.

Now get this:

PAINKILLER VIOXX MIGHT RETURN TO SALE
NewsMax.com Wires—February 18, 2005

The painkiller Vioxx, pulled from the market last fall because of reported heart problems and strokes in users, could come back on sale if federal regulators conclude it and similar drugs have benefits that balance the risks.

Dr. Peter S. Kim, president of Merck Research Laboratories, told a joint meeting of two Food and Drug Administration advisory committees on Thursday that new studies indicate the side effects aren't unique to the product. ...

FDA SCIENTIST DR. DAVID GRAHAM FORCED TO BLOW THE WHISTLE BY FDA NEGLIGENCE
NewsTarget.com—November 24, 2004

Dr. David Graham, a top FDA scientist, released information today that stated the FDA forced him to blow the whistle on Vioxx by neglecting to protect consumers. Dr. Graham felt that his hand had been forced after numerous studies showed that patients taking Vioxx were twice as likely to suffer a heart attack.

Dr. Graham feels that the FDA waited too long and should have banned the drug in 2000, when the studies were first released. Consumers would most likely agree with Dr. Graham, especially since more than 20 million people were prescribed Vioxx, not knowing the horrific consequences that could occur while taking the medication.

Here we have a classic case in which the FDA, the government, and the conglomerate work hand in hand to deceive the public. Not only will they try (and probably succeed) in eventually giving Vioxx a clean bill of health (or reinventing its use—as has been done with Thalidomide), they will attempt to shield the entire class of drugs from scrutiny, multiplying the hazards threefold. And if you are among those who will watch and see how this all plays out, odds are better than five to one that the result will favor the conglomerate. So much for truth, justice, and concern for the American public.

Guess what?

PAIN DRUGS' BENEFITS OFFSET RISKS, FDA PANEL DECIDES
Jeff Nesmith, Cox News Service—February 19, 2005

A government advisory panel recommended yesterday that the pain reliever Vioxx and two related drugs should be available to people with chronic pain, despite evidence that the drugs can cause heart damage. ...

... The panel also recommended a variety of measures meant to increase patient and physician awareness of the risks the drugs pose.

They suggested placing a prominent "black box" warning on the drugs' packaging, including more patient information, restricting which patients could get them, and possibly banning ads aimed directly at consumers. ...

... The action was condemned by consumer advocate Sidney Wolfe of Public Citizen.

"This was a very bad decision," Wolfe said, adding that alternative drugs are as effective as Bextra and Celebrex in relieving chronic pain and that the evidence of Vioxx's effectiveness "is swamped by the dangers."...

... Yesterday's votes caused a dramatic jump in the stock of Merck & Co., which voluntarily withdrew Vioxx from store shelves in September but now says it is considering putting the drug back on the market. ...

... Stock of Pfizer Inc. also rose. ...

If that's not enough to convince you that the conglomerate can get away with anything—including murder—try this on for size:

FDA PANELISTS HAVE TIES TO DRUG MAKERS
Ten members voted to keep marketing 3 popular medications
Gardiner Harris and Alex Berenson, *The New York Times*—February 25, 2005

Ten of the 32 government drug advisers who last week endorsed continued marketing of the huge-selling pain pills Celebrex, Bextra and Vioxx have consulted in recent years for the drugs' makers, according to disclosures in medical journals and other public records.

If the 10 advisers had not cast their votes, the committee would have voted 12–8 that Bextra should be withdrawn and 14–8 that

Vioxx should not return to the market. The 10 advisers with company ties voted 9–1 to keep Bextra on the market and 9–1 for Vioxx's return. ...

... Eight of the 10 members said in interviews that their past relationships with the drug companies did not influence their votes. The two others did not respond to phone calls or e-mails. ...

... An FDA spokeswoman said that no one at the agency would comment on specific panel member's industry ties. ...

... Ten members of the panel have worked in some capacity in recent years for Merck, the maker of Vioxx; Pfizer, the maker of Celebrex and Bextra; or Novartis, which is applying to sell Prexige, a very similar pill discussed by the panel, according to public disclosures. ...

... Of the 30 votes cast by the 10 panel members on whether Celebrex, Bextra and Vioxx should continue to be marketed, 28 favored the drugs. Among the 66 votes cast by the remaining 22 members of the panel, just 37 favored the drugs. The members with financial ties to the companies were 10 times more likely to favor the drugs as those without such ties.

When you deal with the conglomerate, the deck is always stacked against you.

❋ ❋ ❋

Again, not meaning to beat a dead horse, here's the kicker to this Vioxx scandal:

MERCK SOUGHT TO ALTER VIOXX
Document shows effort occurred while risk was downplayed
Theresa Agovino, The Associated Press—June 23, 2005

Merck & Co. researchers privately sought to reformulate Vioxx in 2000 to reduce its cardiovascular side effects, even as the drug maker was publicly playing down a study that highlighted the pain reliever's potential heart attack risk, an internal company document shows. ...

... That document, a communication between Merck researchers and the company's patent department, stated that the way Vioxx works to reduce pain might also increase cardiovascular problems. They suggested a patent be sought for a combination drug mixing Vioxx with another agent to lessen the risk. ...

... The document is potentially among the most damaging to emerge since the drug's sales were suspended because it calls into question the bedrock Merck defense that company officials were convinced of the drug's safety. The desire to reformulate the drug suggests a level of urgency that goes beyond previously disclosed internal e-mails that discussed safety risks. ...

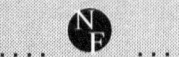

A week doesn't go by without a new report from one medical sector or another about other attempts by Vioxx maker Merck & Co. to cover up facts related to the scandal or of its failure to disclose a truth that was known as far back as 2000. I would need a separate volume to report on all of them!

Here's the kicker to the kicker.

MERCK LOSES VIOXX-RELATED LAWSUIT
$253.5 million awarded to widow of man who took the drug
Alex Berenson, *The New York Times*—August 20, 2005

In the first verdict of a Vioxx-related personal-injury lawsuit, a Texas jury found the drug's maker, Merck, liable and awarded $253.5 million to the widow of Robert Ernst, who died in 2001 after taking the painkiller and arthritis medicine. ...

... Under Texas law capping punitive damages, though, that part of the penalty will automatically be limited to $1.6 million, meaning the overall award would not exceed $26.1 million and could be reduced by Texas appellate courts.

But in interviews afterward, jurors said they had made the large punitive award to send a message to Merck and other pharmaceutical companies that drugmakers must disclose the risks of their medicines.

"Respect us, that's the message," said Derrick Chizer, one of the jurors. "Respect us."...

Respect? Are you kidding? That's the last thing in the world you will get from the conglomerate. And don't fool yourself into thinking large awards will force it to reform. If anything, this will motivate it to even further hide the truth about its drugs. That's standard operating procedure for this gang of outlaws.

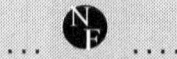

In passing, it should be noted that Merck will receive more favorable results from federal courts, who are generally more friendly to business than state courts. This will result in the Vioxx manufacturer getting off without paying damages in many instances. That was the case on February 17, 2006, when a federal jury in New Orleans cleared Merck of any responsibility in the death of a Florida man who had a heart attack after taking Vioxx for less than a month.

But no matter how you view the Vioxx scandal, it will continue to play out for a number of years, with juries handing out varied decisions throughout the country.

And you can be sure that the conglomerate will continue to receive complete support from the FDA, the Bush administration, both houses of Congress, and all the powers (bribed or otherwise) that be. In fact, the public will remain its biggest supporters—no matter how many Vioxx-type scandals there are.

There you have it! The beginning, middle, and end (more like the current status) of one conglomerate scheme that treats the American public like a bunch of chumps who can be deceived at every turn. The saddest part of it is, we *are* nothing but a bunch of chumps. We take it on the chin, the rascals laugh at us, and we have nowhere to turn. From start to finish, we're buffaloed and screwed over by the big shots that rule the roost.

And as bad as this scenario appears, it's really much worse than anyone can possibly imagine. Our health is declining and our environment is collapsing. We know terrorism of an unimaginable nature that, when coupled with wars and genocide in many parts of the world, poverty, and the spread of AIDS, will do the final job on this planet sooner than we can realize.

We'll go down for the count without even putting up a good fight. **That's because the anti-Christ is here in the person of Big Brother George W. Bush, and he's watching your every move.** And while he's lording it over the nation, both national political parties stand on the sidelines and look to taking care of their own "business as usual." Better believe it....

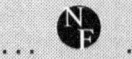

An anti-Christ figure usually conjures up visions of some strange and horrible-looking demon. Little did we expect it to arrive as an illiterate, psychotic despot with nothing in the way of intelligence or imagination. And little could we have expected our nation's leaders, on all levels, to have meekly bowed to his fiendish yet common ways. Note: Newly elected Democratic members of our Congress and Senate will continue to treat Demon Bush with undue respect.

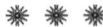

To add to the usual political spin generated by our present administration, on December 19, 2004 (barely six weeks after George W. Bush was reelected President), his White House chief of staff stated that the FDA was doing a "spectacular job" of protecting the public. A Senate critic then immediately charged that government oversight under the Bush administration has proved "a catastrophic failure."

Senator Edward Kennedy of Massachusetts added: "We need an FDA that looks out for the health of patients and not just the health of the pharmaceutical industry. Lives are at stake, and the president should put an FDA leadership team in place right away, with no ties to the industry it regulates, and that's committed to reform."

Bravo Senator Ted Kennedy, I'm all for it. Just as police departments need civilian review boards, the FDA needs watchdog procedures that will protect the public from the so-called regulators. But who would George W. Bush appoint? Which of his cronies? And what would you—or the Democratic Party—do to protest? Nothing.

Breaking news:

FDA ORDERS 'BLACK BOX' WARNING ON ANTI-DEPRESSANTS

Diedtra Henderson, The Associated Press—October 15, 2004

The Food and Drug Administration yesterday ordered that all anti-depressants carry "black box" warnings that they "increase the risk of suicidal thinking and behavior" in children who take them.

> *Patients and their parents will be given medication guides that include the warning with each new prescription or refill.*
> *Dr. Lester Crawford, acting FDA commissioner, said the agency based its decision on the "latest and best science."*
> *"We continue to believe, however, that these drugs provide significant benefits for pediatric patients when used appropriately," he told reporters. ...*

Even when the FDA finally makes the right move, it still acts as a shill for the conglomerate, giving it plenty of leeway needed to continue its nefarious practices. Note: One of the usual FDA manipulations (a classic end run) is to have black box warnings placed on these prescriptions. (A "black box" warning is the most serious type of warning placed on the labeling of a prescription medication, indicating that it may cause serious or even life-threatening adverse effects.)

For your information, *these supposed warnings are as effective as those on cigarette packs.* Warning labels rarely dissuade someone from using a product because people either ignore them or rationalize that "if the product has the approval of those that govern its availability to the general public, it must be okay." Call it naïveté—but it's true.

It's a horrific situation because we are fast approaching **the point of no return** in our drug-oriented culture. As it now stands, we cannot treat a fraction of those with serious drug problems (whether it be from prescription or nonprescription drugs, or illegal narcotics), so you can only imagine what the next decade of increased medication will bring to our drug-dependent society.

With the immense problem of a nonexistent national healthcare program, a growing population of people with no medical or dental insurance, the emergence of dangerous super-bugs that infect the healthy along with a growing resistance to antibiotics, a worsening obesity crisis, and a mentality of fear and hopelessness, we stand little chance of conquering our ills. Our destiny is to remain fodder for the conglomerate, with our children victimized at will. And we can expect nothing in the way of compassion or progressive movement from our idealistically impoverished government—and that includes both political parties.

> *In light of all of these medical inconsistencies, why aren't pharmaceutical and other studies complete enough to maximize safety standards and prevent these things from happening?*

You're naïve if you think that these studies can be improved, because they're not meant to be accurate and foolproof. **They're meant to mislead the regulatory agencies and the public to gain approval for the sale and successful marketing of a product or drug.**

It's all a big, fat, bogus manipulation of data, research, experiments, and interviews. We're led down the garden path hundreds of times a year by the sheer weight of these false studies. And the fact that it's criminal to knowingly endanger human life and conspire against the public's well-being doesn't stop these people from doing it.

Do you need a better example than the tobacco industry? How many studies were made that showed that smoking was not dangerous to health? Of course, every one of them was either paid for by the tobacco industry or an affiliate organization. Consequently, how many millions of lives have been lost? How many billions in profits have been pocketed? How many absolute falsifications have been sworn to publicly in front of Senate committees investigating the industry's deadly practices? And yet, not one of these genocidal maniacs (the CEOs of the tobacco companies) has ever been been sent to prison. Imagine—**these people have committed mass murder.**

Even when the tobacco industry's deadly game was finally recognized and in some cases even admitted to by tobacco CEOs (whose companies coughed up hundreds of billions of dollars in fines), who truly benefited from it? The public? You have to be crazy if you think the public, including the widows and widowers of the tens of millions of smoking victims, were the recipients of the bulk of the awards. Most of it went right back into the hands of the tobacco rulers, their lawyers and politicians, and their clan.

In the year of our Lord 2006, these same giants are still hard at their ghastly work of introducing tobacco into the lives of hundreds of millions of people around the world who will ultimately end up in cancer wards.

Note: **Current estimates indicate that over one billion people will die in the next 10 years of smoking-related diseases.**

Here's a recent report that sheds further light on the true nature of healthcare and the conglomerate in America:

REDUCED PENALTY IN TOBACCO TRIAL DECRIED
Hilary Roxe, The Associated Press—June 10, 2005

Federal prosecutors yesterday defended their decision to downsize dramatically a proposed penalty against Big Tobacco, saying they tried to put the focus on future smokers who might become hooked if

cigarette makers continue their alleged racketeering. ...
... Federal prosecutors this week told U.S. District Judge Gladys Kessler that they were seeking a $10 billion, five-year smoking cessation program as a penalty against the industry for a decades-long conspiracy to deceive the public about the health risks of smoking. That was a fraction of the $130 billion, 25-year program suggested by government witness Michael Fiore, a University of Wisconsin medical professor. ...

Here's more on the same gruesome story:

LAWYERS OPPOSED CUT IN TOBACCO PENALTIES
How senior Justice Department officials overrode objections

Eric Lichtblau, *The New York Times*—June 16, 2005

Senior Justice Department officials overrode the objections of career lawyers running the government's tobacco racketeering trial and ordered them to reduce the penalties sought at the close of a nine-month trial by $120 billion, internal documents and interviews show. The trial team argued that the move would be seen as politically motivated and legally groundless. ...
    Officials speaking on condition of anonymity said the decision to reduce the requested penalties provoked such strong objections from the trial team that some lawyers threatened to quit. ...

. . . .

The Justice Department lawyers spent five years preparing their case against the tobacco industry, only to have the Bush administration undermine the entire effort. And as we have grown fully accustomed to, the Democrats had little to say about the injustice and betrayal. That's because the two-party system has evaporated—even though the Democrats now have the voting edge in both houses of Congress.
    Big business as usual.

The kicker to the tobacco story:

COURT WON'T LET BUSH PUSH TOBACCO PENALTY
Gina Holland, The Associated Press—October 17, 2005

The Supreme Court refused Monday to let the government sue tobacco companies for $280 billion, a major victory for cigarette makers.

A federal judge presided over a nine-month trial and has not yet decided whether tobacco companies are guilty of wrongdoing.

The fight at the high court was over the amount of money the companies would have to pay if the judge rules that they violated a federal anti-racketeering law known as RICO by misleading the public about the dangers of smoking.

A lower court said that the government could not pursue the companies for profits that the government claims they earned illegally. ...

Gobbledygook upon gobbledygook—all meant to confuse the public and maintain the status quo of the tobacco industry. It just shows you how powerful the industry really is—**right up to the Supreme Court.** There's no justice.

On August 17, 2006, U.S. District Judge Gladys Kessler ruled that although the nation's top cigarette makers were "racketeers" who had deceived the public for five decades as to the hazards of smoking, she could not order them to pay the billions of dollars the government had sought. How's that for justice?

To continue answering the question of why studies don't maximize safety standards: If you think the conglomerate and all those who develop the drugs or conduct studies and research are any different from those in the tobacco industry—

you're dumber than dumb. From top to bottom, everyone tries to ride the gravy train and little else matters, no matter how many lies and distortions have to be covered up. The equation is quite simple: *If there are big bucks to be made, the studies and research will support the hypothesis.* As always, the American public be damned!

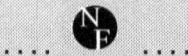

One of the conglomerate's basic tactics is to bait the public with success claims that are right out of the tobacco industry's textbooks. It does it with the sleekness of a sleight-of-hand artist, drawing your attention away from what's really going on.

As an example, a recent report claimed that high doses of a cholesterol drug, Crestor, offered a breakthrough in turning back heart disease, actually reversing it, not merely keeping it from getting worse. The claim was made by Dr. Steven Nissen, a Cleveland Clinic cardiologist who led the nationwide experiment that resulted in this supposed breakthrough.

Can you imagine how such a report would effect tens of millions of people with heart problems? Well, it just "shows to go ya"... because if you bother to do some basic research about this study, you'll discover that it was paid for by AstraZeneca PLC, the maker of Crestor. Need I say more?

There are simpler ways of misleading the public: All you have to do is altogether neglect to inform them of an important aspect of what you're selling them.

As an example:

PATIENTS NOT TOLD OF DEVICE'S FLAW
College student dies when defibrillator fails, which makers knew could happen

Barry Meier, *The New York Times*—May 24, 2005

A medical device maker, Guidant Corp., did not tell doctors or patients for three years that a unit implanted in an estimated 24,000 people that is designed to shock a faltering heart contains a flaw that has caused a small number of those units to short-circuit and malfunction.

The matter came to light after the death in March of a 21-year-old-college student from Minnesota, Joshua Oukrop, with a genetic heart disease. Guidant acknowledges that his device, which is known as a defibrillator, short-circuited. The young man was in Moab, Utah, on a spring break bicycling trip with his girlfriend when he got off his bicycle complaining of fatigue. He then fell to the ground and died of cardiac arrest. ...

As if that weren't bad enough,

GUIDANT RECALLS HEART DEFIBRILLATORS
More than 38,000 implanted devices could malfunction

The Associated Press—June 18, 2005

A company under fire for not telling heart patients about a problem with its implanted defibrillators said yesterday that 50,000 of the devices could be flawed and offered to replace more than half of them.

At least two patients with defibrillators made by Guidant Corp. have died, and the company said its devices had failed at least 45 times. Guidant said it was advising physicians about the safety of several models. ...

Here's the latest on that story:

FDA HAD REPORT OF SHORT CIRCUIT IN HEART DEVICES

Barry Meier, *The New York Times*—September 12, 2005

Months before the Food and Drug Administration issued a safety alert in June about problems with Guidant Corporation heart devices, the agency received a report from the company showing that some of those units were short-circuiting, agency records obtained by The New York Times *show.*

But the agency did not make that data public at the time because it treats the information it receives in such reports as confidential. ...

... Guidant, which knew about the model's flaw for three years but did not tell physicians about it until May, has recently found

itself in the spotlight. But the disclosure that the FDA also had data that might have alerted doctors is likely to increase scrutiny of the agency's policy of not releasing the information it requires heart device makers to submit, as well as how quickly it reviews such reports.

Dr. Daniel G. Schultz, the director of the FDA's Center for Devices and Radiological Health, said in an interview Friday that it would tie up too many resources to review hundreds of filings the FDA receives each year and determine which data could be routinely released and what should be treated as confidential. ...

Can you believe this?! How transparent must the situation be before the public sees through the childish nonsense that it is so willing to accept on face value? First we are told that such things are confidential. But no one asks why. Then we are told that it would tie up too many resources to review the filings. What absolute claptrap! It's nothing more than another flagrant example of how the FDA covers up for the conglomerate, nothing less than corporate gangsterism that is worse than anything the Mafia could ever try to get away with.

Here's another related story:

DRUG STUDIES UNDER THE INFLUENCE
Medical schools may give sponsors control over results
Alicia Chang, The Associated Press—May 26, 2005

Many U.S. medical schools are willing to give companies that sponsor studies of new drugs and treatments considerable control over the results, according to survey results that some doctors found troubling.

Half of the schools said they would let pharmaceutical companies and makers of medical devices draft articles that appear in medical journals, and a quarter would allow them to supply the actual results. But academics draw the line at gag orders that keep researchers from publishing negative findings. ...

As usual, the conglomerate tries to cover its scandalous behavior with contradictions like the aforementioned "Half of the schools said they would let pharmaceutical companies draft articles that appear in medical journals ... But academics draw the line at gag orders."

You gotta be kidding! Anyone who can't see through this camouflage must be deaf, dumb, and blind. Recent controversies involving companies such as drug manufacturers GlaxoSmithKline and Merck, who were accused of suppressing unfavorable results about the antidepressant Paxil and the painkiller Vioxx, bear this out.

✻ ✻ ✻

To add to the deceitful practices of the conglomerate, we have this report by a second-year medical student at the University of Washington School of Medicine:

MEDICAL SCHOOLS SHOULD BE IMMUNE TO INFLUENCE

Guest Columnist Jake Donaldson, *Seattle Post-Intelligencer*—February 20, 2006

> *Bribes by drug and medical device companies have become a serious threat to physician integrity. The threat has infiltrated all corners of the medical profession, including its clinics and medical schools. The University of Washington School of Medicine and its affiliated hospitals are no exception. It is long past time for the institution to adopt policies banning all industry gifts to physicians, including free meals, free drug samples and direct support for medical education. ...*

Bravo Jake! You're onto the truth. However, just exposing and complaining about the bribes will do little good because the masterminds who do the bribing really have their acts together. They know that greed is one of humankind's three greatest weaknesses, and they take full advantage of that universal reality. Furthermore, these wise guys wouldn't be able to peddle their wares at the University of Washington School of Medicine and its affiliated hospitals IF there weren't a big market for them. So pull up the carpet and do some sweeping! While you're at it, get the other goodnicks on campus together and start chasing the gift-givers off the lot. But be mighty careful of the UW administrators who might not appreciate what you're trying to do.

A closing thought on this sick cover-up: I've read thousands of articles and reports over my adult lifetime in which study results were revealed to the public. They must have all been written by the same Hollywood writers because they contain the same ambiguities and catch phrases—no matter what the study is about. It's all remarkably formulaic, the biggest and most obvious statement reading, "A recent discovery of blah, blah, blah may lead to new ways to treat blah, blah, blah."

You know what? It doesn't happen. That's because most of these so-called breakthroughs are nothing more than research conducted for the benefit of that researcher's bank account. Heart attacks, arthritis drugs, new lip balm that prevents skin cancer, dog poops on the moon—who's to believe these studies? Most of them are bogus.

Here's a recent report that barely scratches the surface of what's going on with these studies:

REPORT FINDS OLD HEALTH STUDIES WRONG
Experts warn to not put too much stock in a single study

Lindsey Tanner, The Associated Press—July 13, 2005

Here's some medical news you can trust: A new study confirms that what doctors once said was good for you often turns out to be bad— or at least not as great as initially thought.

The report is a review of major studies published in three influential medical journals between 1990 and 2003, including 45 highly publicized studies that initially claimed a drug or other treatment worked.

Subsequent research contradicted results of seven studies—16 percent—and reported weaker results for seven others, an additional 16 percent. That means nearly one-third of the original results did not hold up, according to the study in today's Journal of the American Medical Association. ...

Take most of your studies and shove them!

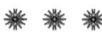

One last thought before moving on: Along with all the misleading studies that muddle the medical environment, we also have what I generally classify as "cockamamie studies." These are prize attempts to make a statement that is patently ridiculous, and would be ridiculed as such, were it not for the fact that the public doesn't bother to analyze what it's being told.

Here's a prime example:

OBESE MAY BE MORE SENSITIVE TO PAIN

Lee Bowman, Scripps Howard News Service—March 2, 2006

Obese people appear to be more sensitive to pain than people who aren't carrying extra pounds, according to a small study of older adults suffering from osteoarthritis of the knee. ...

I don't have to go any further than that before laughing out loud at this preposterous study! Dear reader—do you know why I'm reacting this way? It should be as plain as the nose on your face. In fact, I'm going to test your basic logic skills by asking you to put this book aside for a few minutes while you write down at least four reasons that would show that this study is an absurdity. Okay? Go to it—then come right back to this page.

All done? Now let's compare our analysis of the cockamamie study in question. Here are my reasons:

1. Someone suffering from osteoarthritis would certainly be more sensitive to pain, even if s/he wasn't obese.

2. Someone suffering from osteoarthritis, who also happens to be obese, would certainly be more sensitive to pain.

3. Someone suffering from osteoarthritis, who's obese AND older, would certainly be more sensitive to pain.

4. There are dozens of obvious reasons why older obese people suffering from any degenerative disease are more sensitive to pain. I could fill this page with them! We can start with the following:

   a. Obese people (with or without osteoarthritis) feel more pressure on their joints, which causes them to be more pain-sensitive.

   b. Older obese people with osteoarthritis are most likely not in good health, which will make them even more pain-sensitive.

   c. These same people are more than likely taking a number of drugs, which, combined with their already weakened physical condition, will make them more pain-sensitive.

   d. In all likelihood, these people are not exercising much, which makes them relatively brittle and more susceptible to pain.

Can you begin to imagine the pain threshold of the people who were studied? Obese, elderly, suffering from osteoarthritis of the knee, on medications, and so on. And you need a study to explain that they are more pain-sensitive?!

If you're wondering why I went off on one of my tangents, the people wasting their time and someone's money on such a cockamamie study are certainly part of the network of weak-minded individuals and organizations that help make up the American healthcare system. They mock basic intelligence and contribute to the conglomerate's scheme of things in more ways than you can imagine. And the more of them that we expose—the better off we are.

How did you come out on your test score? Were you with me on this? I hope so!

I couldn't let myself pass on this: A new study found a clear link between obesity and mood disorders. Readers, I haven't used the following old (standby) term in a long time, but I will now—NO SHIT! And did the aforementioned study indicate whether depression leads to obesity or obesity leads to depression?! You really have to laugh at such a study. It's an insult to intelligence.

※ ※ ※

One last comment on studies in general: Starting with the Air Force motto of "believe nothing that you hear and only half of what you see," you should graduate to this time-honored truth: ***Do not believe any report or study made by government agencies***—especially in this corrupt day and age. The Bush administration practically mandates that agency heads falsify data and information; that's one of the few existing ways of maintaining the fake spins that emanate from the White House on a daily basis. It's like dog poops on the moon! Hardly probable.

In support of this highly biased opinion about information released to the public by the government, you will take into account the fact that President Bush hardly ever gives press conferences (and the press seems to accept this policy unchallenged), while the Democratic members of Congress don't even bother to question it)!

In fact, I can't think of a president in recent history who has made fewer appearances before the nation's reporters. The reason should be as obvious: By not facing the press and the nation, he appears to hold himself exempt for any of his deceitful actions.

And while you're at it, you can be sure that governmental agency officials sidetrack the information process by creating scam studies that make our president's administration look a hundred percent better than it actually is.

As an example:

LIFE FOR OLDER AMERICANS IMPROVING, REPORT SAYS

Lee Bowman, Scripps Howard News Service—March 10, 2006

Life is getting better for American seniors, according to a new government snapshot that depicts a group getting healthier and

better educated, one growing in numbers and less likely to be poor.
*   The report, "65+ in the United States—2005," was compiled*
by the Census Bureau last year for the National Institute on Aging,
and released Thursday. ...

····   ····

This report, accurately labeled a "snapshot" (indeed it is—from an
old box camera that has seen better days!), goes on to list sets of
statistics primarily related to the numbers of Americans aged 65
and older living in various parts of the country, the states with the
largest and smallest elderly population, and details about ethnic
composition. It also *captures trends* (that's as ridiculous as the
snapshot label), and gives generalized opinions like, "Many people
have an image of aging that may be 20 years out of date."

    This is another classic example of how easily we are mislead
and how weak-minded the press is; any damn fool could read that
study and throw it in the garbage can where it belongs, but chances
are that it will slip by unnoticed, except by the president, who no
doubt will manage to quote from it and give the utterly false impression that things are actually getting better for older Americans.

    Nothing could be further from the truth. It's a spurious lie at
best.

If all the studies are spurious,
then how can you use some of them
to highlight a point you're making?

Great question! The answer lies in my ability to *discern* between those studies that
are obviously meant to support a viewpoint or product—regardless of the existing
evidence to the contrary—and those studies that are actually undertaken without
prior commitment to a hypothesis, or a patron to whom one is obligated.

    This is not necessarily a science, nor is it foolproof. However, if you first es-
tablish a criteria for your objective analysis of studies in general and then follow

its implications, quantum chances are that you will indeed separate the spurious from the authentic. As an example, here is the criteria that I use when I examine any particular study:

- What was the reason for the study? Is it meant to settle an outstanding issue, or was it made on behalf of a client, organization, or institution?

- Was the study undertaken independently, or was it funded by an outside source?

- Was the outside source in any manner, shape, or form directly or indirectly connected to or otherwise personally or professionally involved in the study?

- Were there financial incentives to prove or dispel the theory, product, or hypothesis in question?

- How will various market forces be influenced by the outcome of the study?

- Were there any other possible hidden motives for the study?

- What are the possible long-range effects of the study? Will it alter a present condition, create a new standard, or result in greater commerce?

- Whose interests will be served or defeated by the study?

- Over how long a period of time was the study conducted?

- How many people were involved in the study?

- How were the people chosen? Randomly or selectively?

- Were those people paid?

Unless you are incapable of analyzing data, facts, motives, and persuasions, these general criteria will give you a relatively clear picture of the purpose, intent, justification, objectivity, and validity of the study in question.

You can recognize certain obvious red flags if you know how to look for them. For instance, if a study is obviously meant to drastically alter the persuasion of millions of people and strongly influence market results, then the buyer should beware.

Here's a good example: A recent saw palmetto study concluded that the herbal treatment used by millions of men with enlarged prostates did not improve their conditions.

When I analyzed this study, certain things popped out of the page:

1. The study involved only 225 men. Hardly a significant number when you consider the ramifications of such a study.

2. The men received only 160 milligrams of saw palmetto or a placebo for one year. This is suspect because the recommended daily dosage is 500 milligrams.

3. I seriously question whether a one-year study is adequate in determining results because saw palmetto normally accrues greater effectiveness over a longer period of use.

4. There were twice as many serious adverse events in the placebo group as in the saw palmetto group, indicating that other serious health issues may have been present in the men involved—all the more so when you consider that only 225 men participated. That was all I needed to convince me that this study was spurious.

This study can easily be contradicted by other studies made over a longer period of time, including my own personal study. Seven years ago, my PSA[12] registered 6.9 (anything above 4 is considered problematic), and instead of opting for a biopsy (which physicians almost always push for), I decided to use the herbal extract in question. Long story short: on a year-by-year basis, my PSA has gradually lowered, and today stands at a safe 3.1. That's a significant change for the better.

I also know of dozens of other men who have benefited from the use of saw palmetto, which by the way *costs barely 20 cents a day.* That's a far cry from the costs of other forms of prostate treatment. It's also a damn good reason why the powers that be would try to undermine its reputation.

The conglomerate has always had a steady track record when it comes to challenging the efficacy of herbal products, because they represent the number-one enemy. It wants the public to use expensive drugs, not inexpensive herbal remedies. To insure their products' dominance, conglomerate operatives have infiltrated every government department that scrutinizes unregulated health remedies, with the intent of discrediting these remedies. And the public quickly buys into it.

What makes these government-conglomerate scams all the more shocking and insidious is that *the studies are often conducted by doctors and researchers who*

---

[12] PSA: Prostate-specific antigen is a protein produced by the cells of the prostate gland. The PSA test measures the amount of PSA in the blood.

are receiving consultation fees or grants from drug companies that will benefit from negative reports about unregulated health remedies. These people make the Mafia look like innocent amateurs!

✳ ✳ ✳

> *Was there a turning point in the impairment of the American healthcare system?*

The system had been heading downhill for a long time, but the final nail in the coffin was driven home when President and Mrs. Clinton's Health Security Act[13] was defeated in 1993. From that moment, America truly surrendered its health to the conglomerate, which has been in the driver's seat ever since.

Besides the complete capitulation (the Clintons never took up the fight again), what struck me as another "sign of the times" was that the press suddenly regarded Hillary Clinton as the second coming of Eleanor Roosevelt. **How anyone in his right mind could speak of Hillary Clinton in the same breath as Eleanor Roosevelt is beyond imagination.** It's an insult to human intelligence and goes to prove that the Fourth Estate is completely out of touch with reality as well as history.

To set the record straight, Hillary Clinton couldn't hold a candle to one of the greatest Americans of the 20th century on any level whatsoever. Whereas Hillary Clinton is basically nothing more than a clever lawyer-politician with little genuine dedication to a cause (as clearly proven by her quick withdrawal from the American healthcare scene), Eleanor Roosevelt championed causes against all odds at a time when a woman's voice was rarely considered (even if she was the First Lady), and she did whatever was necessary to win the battle—no matter how long it took or how strong the opposition. She was a fighter—not a quitter.

I believe we will never see the like of Eleanor Roosevelt again. We will witness only the growing lack of dedication and high values as personified by the Hillary Clintons and the hacks of both political parties in America.

As a concrete example, with Senator Hillary Clinton's well-known 2008 presidential ambitions at stake, you would think that she would now be championing universal healthcare (as she attempted to do in 1993). But that's not the case: She's spending her time supporting a law to ban desecration of the American flag.

---

[13] A sweeping piece of legislation to guarantee lifetime healthcare for every American and bring coherence to the Medicare and Medicaid system.

And she's doing it alongside a Republican senator from Utah. If that doesn't take the cake!

A note to Hillary Clinton (and all other "split-the-difference" politicians): I believe it was Franklin Delano Roosevelt who said, "You don't want to be compromised by your compromises."

> *Regarding vaccinations, do you suggest that people at high risk of contracting influenza should not have an annual flu shot?*

This is like asking about craters on Mars! Depending on your field of study and why you're asking the question, the answer is many different things for people of various persuasions.

First of all, let's examine the issue of vaccinations in general:

In spite of all the apparent good attributed to most vaccines (many childhood diseases are a thing of the past in America), a limited but meaningful body of evidence shows that these shots are doing more damage than good. *These inoculations may actually be injuring our immune system and leading to various diseases as we get older.*

In other words, as unlikely as it may seem to the uninformed, vaccines are not sure things. And you can bet your bottom dollar that the conglomerate would do everything in its power to conceal any evidence to that effect.

So we are basically on our own to do the research and discern accordingly. Along those lines, here's some food for thought from Dr. Joseph Mercola, author of *Total Health Program:*

> *All vaccines are immune depressing to some extent and that is the trade-off we are risking. The medical thought is that we trade a small immune depression for an immunity to one disease. Now let me repeat, we are trading a total immune system depression (our only defense against all known disease—including millions of pathogens—for a temporary immunity against one disease, usually an innocuous childhood disease. Therefore, the trade is not at all fair. Mullins puts it this way, "Are we trading mumps and measles for cancer and AIDS."*
>
> *The trade-off is not worth the risk. We are risking getting many more diseases than we are "preventing" from getting. (Later we will see that there is literally no prevention.) Another good example is*

the ritual of the yearly flu shot. There may be only two or three varieties of flu viruses in each shot, hence the names "Asian-Flu," "Japanese-Flu," "Indian-Flu," or "Swine-Flu." But there are literally thousands, maybe millions of flu-causing viruses.

Taking one or two does not make sense and many people report getting the flu after taking a flu shot. We do not know which variety of flu will affect us each year and in each locale. Therefore, the best method to avoid the flu is to strengthen our immune system by eating properly and getting all the essential vitamins and minerals that our body needs. Only nutrition can build and support a strong immune system, while vaccines help to tear our immunity down. Vaccines have been linked to AIDS and other immuno-deficient disorders as well. ...

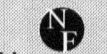

....

This makes sense to me, but the conglomerate easily overrides it by creating new spins on the issue year to year. And the public immediately buys into this tactic, especially if it's attached to a heightened sense of fear of some type of flu pandemic—such as the recent and ongoing bird-flu reports.

I must also point out—very vigorously—that exercise (as well as nutrition) also helps build and support a strong immune system.

What evidence is there to support doubts about the efficacy of flu shots? The following two reports shed light on the entire flu shot issue and also illustrate just how sinister and manipulative the conglomerate is:

REPORT: FLU SHOTS FOR ELDERLY NOT SAVING LIVES

Carla K. Johnson, The Associated Press—February 15, 2005

A new study based on more than three decades of U.S. data suggests that giving flu shots to the elderly has not saved any lives.

Led by National Institutes of Health researchers, the study challenges standard government dogma and is bound to confuse senior citizens. During last fall's flu vaccine shortage, thousands of older Americans, heeding the government's public health message, stood in long lines to get their shots.

"There is a sense that we're all going to die if we don't get the flu shot," said the study's lead author, Lone Simonsen, a senior epidemiologist at the National Institute of Allergy and Infectious Diseases in Bethesda, Md. "Maybe that's a little much."

The study should influence the nation's flu prevention strategy, Simonsen said, perhaps by expanding vaccination to schoolchildren, the biggest spreaders of the virus. However, the U.S. Centers for Disease Control and Prevention in Atlanta plans no change in its advice on who should get flu shots, saying the NIH research isn't enough to shift gears. ...

Another crock of nonsense from beginning to end! Massive confusion, manipulation, and stupidity from all sectors—and the elderly still don't know what to believe. That's the way the conglomerate operates. What will it take to make people see the obvious?

As for vaccinating schoolchildren, we would be better off developing a sophisticated educational program—for students, parents, and teachers—that would help avoid the spread of flu in school environments, in addition to teaching children about the overall dangers of prescription drug use, abuse, and addiction. (And once again, I don't mean "Just say no to drugs.")

But you can be sure of this: This conglomerate's members will not allow such a progressive approach—that is, unless they can cash in on it and control it for their own long-range purposes.

Here's the second report:

STUDY CASTS MORE DOUBT ON FLU SHOTS
Vaccinating children not very effective, scientists say

Lee Bowman, Scripps Howard News Service—February 25, 2005

On the heels of reports that cast doubt on whether annual flu shots for the elderly actually save lives, a new study calls into question whether the vaccinations are effective among children, particularly very young children.

The study, published today in the British journal, The Lancet, found that vaccines were effective in reducing long school absences but had little effect on other outcomes, such as hospital stays and pneumonia, compared with not getting shots. ...

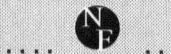

Vaccinations may or may not be effective among children because doctors fail to diagnose flu in the vast majority of young children, often diagnosing the symptoms as anything from asthma to pneumonia. Consequently, many of these children are not given medicines that might shorten their illness and keep them from spreading it to others.

As with many healthcare questions and issues, there are associated factors that play a large but unrecognized part in the overall scheme of things. In this case, I'm highlighting the loaded reality that doctors' misdiagnosis of symptoms, ailments, and disease is profoundly underestimated and extremely dangerous. This widespread failure to recognize the true nature of the medical problem is due in large part to medicine's present-day focus on specialization, which limits doctors' ability to respond to medical situations outside of their distinctive fields.

Needless to say, this study casting doubt on flu shots will soon be contradicted by the powers that be, leaving the American public in the same position that it has been in since the conglomerate's emergence—confused and thoroughly prepared to follow misleading, unsubstantiated medical advice.

Now let's bring the flu issue up-to-date. The 2004–2005 flu season produced a fiasco over flu vaccinations, with a shortage caused by a major source's contaminated vaccine, repeated statements by the government and the FDA that supplies would be very limited, and then a sudden reversal of the supposed shortage and a widespread availability of the shots.

It was a colossal example of national healthcare confusion and contradictions from all involved sectors. And the nation's press and media simply reported the issue at hand without any serious level of investigatory reporting.

With the 2005–2006 flu season, we faced an entirely new set of spins, beginning with this report:

NEW FLU-SHOT SUPPLIER APPROVED
AS VACCINE SEASON NEARS

John J. Lumpkin, The Associated Press—August 31, 2005

Mindful of last year's flu vaccine shortage, the Food and Drug Administration approved a new shot on Wednesday in an attempt to ensure adequate supplies during the upcoming flu season.

It remained uncertain, however, whether there would be enough shots for all who wanted them.

The FDA approved the vaccine Fluarix for people 18 years and older. The shots, made in Germany by a subsidiary of GlaxoSmith-Kline, have been available in other countries for years.

A spokesman said the company expects to supply 8 million doses to the U.S. market this flu season, at a price comparable to other flu shots. Flu vaccine typically costs less than $20 a dose. ...

. . . . 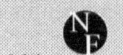 . . . .

To make a long story short, the government went through its usual machinations about how much flu vaccine the nation would have on hand. A year earlier, after the discovery of the contaminated vaccine, British regulators shut down a U.S. supplier, Chiron Corp., creating a surprise shortage.

But I sensed that the new flu season would be entirely different. That was putting it mildly!

As flu vaccine is dispensed at a nominal fee (usually $20), that doesn't leave much room for finagling and profiteering. Consequently, the conglomerate's operatives (including various agencies such as the FDA and the national Centers for Disease Control and Prevention) act as shills for the conglomerate by urging people (especially those over 65) to get their shots. However, this type of encouragement doesn't go far enough to rev up the profit scheme.

But that doesn't prevent the conglomerate from figuring out how to squeeze more money out of the flu market. Have a look:

FLU PREPARATIONS EXPECTED TO COST
AT LEAST $6.5 BILLION

The Associated Press—November 1, 2005

Vaccine improvement is expected to take center stage in the Bush administration's preparations for a worldwide flu outbreak, with a potential travel ban and restrictions on global commerce part of the contingency planning.

President Bush today will announce his strategy on how to prepare for the next flu pandemic—preparations expected to cost at least $6.5 billion. ...

A key element: States and cities will get their first specific instructions from federal health officials on such matters as who should get limited doses of vaccines and the antiviral medications Tamiflu or Relenza. ...

This is absolutely hilarious! Emperor Bush is now creating another "Iraq has weapons of mass destruction" scheme. You bet! This time the enemy about to launch the attack on the U.S. is a supposed flu pandemic. Somebody's going to clean up—big time!

The big spender in the White House will see to it that the conglomerate wets its whistle on the largesse, dispensing billions—on drugs that have not even been adequately tested! And the public will buy into the scheme without thinking twice because the media will have prepped the gullible masses for the grand rip-off.

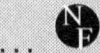

····   ····

With all the White House gibberish about bird flu, it should be noted that according to a World Bank draft report, although the United States pledged $334 million to fight bird flu worldwide, it has only disbursed about $71 million out of that pledge. This reminds me of how America refuses to pay its United Nations dues.

When the White House Overlord unveiled his "plan," it actually called for a $7.1 billion strategy to prepare for a possible worldwide outbreak, or "pandemic" as it is now being spun. And guess where most of that money will be spent—**research and a national stockpile of vaccines and antiviral drugs.** Another unfunded (individual states would fund the greater part of the plan) and unfounded mandate, just like the Iraq war—and a bonanza for the conglomerate.

Note: I am not pooh-poohing the whole concept of a flu pandemic as something to be ignored or merely a Bush contrivance. I have no crystal ball or verses from Nostradamus to dispel the apparent dangers of such a pandemic.

However, I do believe our media, government, and conglomerate will do everything it can to bungle this one up, should a pandemic occur (or even the distinct threat of one), and the public had better beware of being panicked into believing or doing something that only benefits the conglomerate.

One should recognize that, in spite of any national plan instituted by the government, IF a bird flu pandemic were to happen, our government will not be prepared to deal with its consequences. And if you think our lack of preparedness for Hurricane Katrina was a prime example of just how badly things can go when state and government agencies are neither prepared or capable of working together, a pandemic will prove to be a crushing catastrophe that might leave millions dead.

And just as various state and federal agencies were caught with their pants down when Hurricane Katrina hit, quickly jockeying for defensive positions when accusations were hurled, you can expect the same anemic response to any pandemic.

To be sure, major conflicts will arise among the government agencies responsible for the country's response, made worse by the fact that the Homeland Security Council will be in charge. The nation's health advocacy groups will turn to the Department of Health and Human Services (which includes the CDC, the FDA, and the National Institute of Health) for guidance and assistance, only to find that decision making will be in the hands of inept bureaucrats.

Instead of finding where the buck stops, advocacy groups will discover it being passed from one bewildered agency head to another.

And as usual with bureaucratic mismanagement, the process will take precedent over the outcome. In this case, the process will insure that liability protection to vaccine manufacturers that make the products needed to battle a pandemic is granted first and foremost.

As for the availability of bird flu vaccine, on November 20, 2005, Health and Human Services Secretary Mike Leavitt announced that the U.S. has only enough doses now for 4.3 million people, and that the nation lacks the manufacturing capacity to provide 300 million doses of a vaccine for three to five more years.

To add to the confusion (political spin), on June 7, 2006, Secretary Leavitt told the Associated Press, "Let's acknowledge the fact that for the first six months of any pandemic, we're not going to have a vaccine."

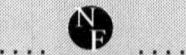

Besides the fact that this statement did not receive noteworthy press attention, if one takes this at face value, it means that we will not only be unprepared for a flu pandemic, but millions will die without any hope of securing a vaccination.

All of which goes to show you that the assortment of reports emanating from the various government agencies dealing with the flu amount to little more than words, words, words. In fact, after all was said and done, the 2006 flu season in America was extremely mild, with flu and pneumonia deaths below those of a typical flu season. Nary a whimper. Once again, believe nothing that you hear and only half of what you see.

Meanwhile, the death toll in Iraq continues to climb (often relegated to the inconsequential news pages), environment destruction worsens on a daily basis, and in spite of all the scientific evidence piling up about global warming, government officials pay little heed to this building cataclysm.

But everybody's alerted to the bird flu! And everyone is being told to get their flu shots. Great sales tactic. Not only does it keep the unsuspecting public focused on a pandemic that is highly unlikely (as there is no evidence of it being spread from human to human), it also helps to sell people on the idea of getting the added protection of a flu shot.

The 2006–2007 flu season will be a repeat performance of the same rigmarole that is typical of the way in which the conglomerate produces, markets, and distributes flu vaccine. In fact, as early as November 10, 2006, doctors and hospitals throughout the country were reporting that even though drug manufacturers have produced millions more doses than ever before—they have not received flu vaccines that were preordered more than six months ago.

Notwithstanding the difficulty of health providers finding enough vaccine to immunize even clinic and hospital staff, it appears that retail stores such as Safeway, Wal-Mart, Costco, and Rite-Aid that buy in bulk have access to the vaccine. Big business as usual—all under the guise of providing healthcare. What a mess!

* * *

We should also recognize that if a flu pandemic should occur, not only will we be unprepared for it, but the aftermath will be much worse than anything we can presently envision because THERE WILL BE NO FUNDS TO DEAL WITH THE DISASTER. Why? Because the money will already have been allocated and paid off to the pharmaceutical companies—for their next-to-worthless drugs. If you think I'm selling our country short, take a good look at what STILL hasn't happened in New Orleans since Hurricane Katrina.

On another level, one must wonder why the media focuses so much attention on the flu issue every year, yet fails to properly research and report on the overall state of American health, which is a far greater crisis than any singular issue. As I love to illustrate with personal stories, let me offer you this strange juxtaposition:

In the Seattle area, as a public service, Bartell drugstores offer flu, pneumonia, and tetanus shot vaccinations every October at nominal fees of $20, $35, and $40. I walked into one of their drugstores last year, and as I passed the table set up for the purpose of enrolling people for the shots, a visiting nurse service representative, who administers the vaccinations, beckoned me to listen to her advice about taking a flu shot.

As I do not get flu shots, I hardly needed to hear her pearls of wisdom. But I turned to listen because I was struck by her deplorable physical condition—she was at least 80 pounds overweight, her eyes were droopy, and her baggy face was marked by serious acne problems. Her cigarette-stained fingers and hands shook almost violently as she tried to explain why I should be protected against influenza. As I listened to her speak, I realized that she was probably around 40 years of age but looked more like a dilapidated 65.

I wanted to physically pick her up, shake her out of her stupor, and shout, "What are you talking about? Just look at you! You're dying before my eyes—and you're telling someone who's in great health that they're in danger of getting the flu if they don't take the cockamamie shot!"

Behind that poor woman's weak mentality and physical dilapidation are a legion of doctors who are themselves in terrible physical condition, suffering from lack of exercise, pot bellies, drug abuse, and rotting teeth. These medical schleps are giving us advice!

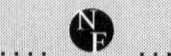

Along with doctors, the physical condition of healthcare workers
in general is deplorable—they are horrendously bad role models.
I find them depressing to look at. And to make matters worse, a
shockingly large number of them still smoke.

No wonder tens of millions of Americans are overweight, abuse drugs, suffer from depression, or are screwed-up enough to think that their annual flu shot is so damn important. The conglomerate leads their mindless followers and gets richer every day.

In closing out this issue of flu vaccinations, you must remember that we're dealing with vaccines of a very dubious nature, along with a healthcare situation that churns from serious to potentially catastrophic from day to day, both nationally and internationally. In fact, by the time you read this, the flu status may have traveled many different paths and mutated several times without discernable conclusions. We'll have to have an ongoing blog to adequately keep you up to date.

Regarding the central question of how to guard against the flu (whether you take a flu shot or not), here are my recommendations:

1. **Wash your hands with soap and water as often as you come into direct physical contact with people and objects.** Don't be afraid if someone thinks you're paranoid because you're better off coming across that way than getting the flu. I wash my hands immediately after I shake hands with someone, touch a door handle or object previously touched by someone, and any other time my instinct tells me that I should.

    The result of this behavior is that I don't ever get sick any more—no colds, flu, disorders, etc. It really works! (Note: Old-fashioned hand washing kills germs better than new-fangled antibacterial gels. That's a fact. But if you can't wash your hands, then do what politicians do on the stump—use Purell, the antiseptic goop of choice and self-proclaimed killer of 99.99 percent of most common germs that may cause illness.)

    And if you're wondering what to guard against before washing your hands, the worst germ carriers are cafeteria trays (10 times the germs found on toilet seats), headphones, and computer keyboards. The highest number of bacteria is found on the spigot of a drinking fountain—2.7 million bacterial cells per square inch.

2. **If you work in a profession where you come in contact with lots of people every day,** such as a schoolteacher or restaurant worker, then you must take special precautions to avoid direct contact with them.

3. **As a rule, don't hug, kiss, or stand close to them.** You can do this without making anyone feel badly—simply by using tact, common sense, and a good dose of humor. If the person you're talking to or serving is suffering from a cold or the flu, it's quite all right to stand away from them and say, "Man, I love you—but I don't love your cold!" If I'm working out at a health club where people have colds, I stay as far away from them as possible. I also do not drink water from the same fountain they use because people's mouths often come directly in contact with the spigot. And if I must use the same equipment as that person, I wipe it down thoroughly (all clubs provide antiseptic spray and towels) before I put my hands on it.

4. **If you ride the bus or subway,** you have the dual problem of close proximity with people with colds and repeatedly coming in direct contact with seats, rails, etc., that have been touched by hundreds of people that day. You've really got to be on your toes and stay clear of danger; always prepare to change your seat at the first sight of someone coughing nearby, while avoiding touching those seats and rails. If it's flu season and you're on a crowded bus or subway with numerous people coughing—get off, walk to work, or take a taxi, after calling your boss and saying that you're going to be late. Anything to avoid getting the flu—as it could lay you up for weeks.

5. **And if you can't really do any of these protective things—carry gloves with you everywhere.** They're one of the best medicines around. And a lot cheaper than meds! Also, carry disinfecting wipes (but note that sanitizers with an alcohol concentration of under 60 percent won't kill microbes).

6. **Whenever you push open a door, avoid using your hands.** Use your forearm or your wrist. You'll have much less chance of making contact with germs and viruses and transmitting them from your hands to your mouth, nose, or eyes.

7. **When you use an ATM machine or a PIN pad in a grocery store, don't key in your data with the tip of your index finger**—use the second joint in the finger, as there's much less chance of it coming in contact with your mouth, nose, or eyes.

Overall, just remember that good hygiene and individual responsibility are the most valuable tools available and can do more to control the spread of flu than any drug or vaccine.

Along these same lines, you should do everything in your power to reinforce your immune system throughout the year: Keep away from drugs, maintain a good diet, don't shy away from vitamin supplements, and, without fail, exercise regularly.

✳ ✳ ✳

As for treating the flu: Strange as it may sound, the old-fashioned remedies used when I was a child are still the best medicines. Drink lots of water, have tea with honey and lemon, eat chicken soup, and gargle with saltwater. You don't need antibiotics because they are no more effective than the tea, soup, etc., and they continually wear down your immune system, as their excessive use promotes resistant bacteria. (Actually, antibiotics won't work against flu because they don't have any effect on viruses, only bacteria.)

Something else to be aware of: The flu season receives significant attention in schools, giving the conglomerate billions of dollars in free and highly dangerous publicity. What tens of millions of parents don't realize is that while their children are repeatedly made aware of their "shots," they are also being indoctrinated into the drug lifestyle.

No one seems to understand that a flu shot is not the same thing as getting hooked on Prozac or ADHD drugs. But because of the drug companies' robust public relations machine and our nation's mentality of across-the-board acceptance of any pill that's prescribed—we treat all prescribed drugs as A-okay.

As I've said from the beginning, you're either in support of your immune system or working against it. It's that basic. The rest is all common sense—and being an informed, discerning person.

> *Should states have the right to dictate*
> *medical treatment for children?*

This is a loaded question because there are hundreds of potential scenarios; the healthcare agencies and courts responsible must first turn to state laws for such situations, interpret them accordingly, and finally discern—which takes as much wisdom as Solomon could allow for.

Most often these cases revolve around religious teachings such as the Jehovah's Witnesses, who refuse to accept whole blood transfusions (in current medical practice, whole blood transfusions are very rare, and blood derivatives are used instead), or Christian Scientists, who disavow medical interference in the course of a child's ailment, relying instead on God's healing power through prayer. (This teaching is the foundation of the Christian Science principle that disease and any other adversity can be cured through prayerful efforts, made possible only by God's grace.)

Some lawyers and courts are squabbling over the right of parents to stick to their religious guns, while state agencies are trying to protect the child and mandate medical treatment. Of course, in many cases this means blood transfusions, surgery, or drug treatment, any of which may put the child in as much danger as no treatment at all.

To insure the child's safety and the parents' personal and religious rights, this question can be answered only on a case-by-case basis.

Unfortunately, an added potential interference comes from the conglomerate itself, who would dictate medical treatment and drugs in every instance, as well as the courts that go along with that decision, with no concern for parents' rights.

As an example, on June 24, 2006, a nine-month-old Washington State baby, Riley Rogers, became the center of controversy when he was returned to Children's Hospital and Regional Medical Center, after being allegedly kidnapped by his mother, Tina Carlsen, to prevent the infant from undergoing surgery to treat a kidney ailment. Doctors insisted that the baby needed surgery to insert a tube so that he could undergo dialysis to treat the kidney ailment. The doctors were supported by the Child Protective Services (CPS), who urged a Pierce County judge to authorize the surgery.

The parents had mistrusted doctors because when the baby was born, they were told they should "take him home and love him" because he would live only for a few weeks.

The father's lawyer defended the right of the parents to look into other treatment options, but the judge ordered the surgery and limited the father to four hours of supervised visits with the baby each week. Meanwhile, the mother faced a second-degree kidnapping charge and could have been sentenced to up to a year in jail.

A local group, Citizens for Safe Birth, came to Carlsen's aid, asking for an emergency injunction to prevent the surgery from going ahead until a full hearing could be conducted. Despite this, and his mother's tearful courtroom objections, Riley Rogers had surgery the following day.

Afterward, the child's father, Todd Rogers, who petitioned for custody and said that he remains angry with state officials for forcing his partner into taking such desperate action, told reporters that "I am still not happy with the doctors at Children's, particularly the nephrologists. They don't tell you any of the things that might go wrong, just, 'This is what we're doing and if you don't like it, we'll call CPS.' If you don't cooperate, the state just takes control."

This case drew national attention and controversy over whether parents or doctors should decide what's best for an ailing child—even in cases that are not deemed emergencies—and highlights the ever-present danger of officials and courts following bureaucratic guidelines instead of truly looking after the needs of the child.

Whose interests have been served in this case?

> ### *Should children be used in clinical research?*

This is another loaded question. We must first determine when it is appropriate to put children at risk to test experimental drugs or devices. We must also ask whether doctors and pharmaceutical companies have an obligation to conduct research that could ultimately help sick children. In most cases, the federal government thinks so.

The big problem is that drug companies often test their products on children, regardless of how they conduct studies and report results. And more often than not, the children who are exposed to this testing come from poorer and less well-educated families, which allows for a greater opportunity for exploitation.

In an overall sense, federal laws and regulations permit doctors to use approved drugs and devices for unapproved procedures and patients, thus putting children at great risk. This is one of the gray areas that allows doctors to dispense antidepressants and sleeping pills to children that have been approved for use only in adults.

Without stronger regulations and an effective means of enforcing them, studies should be approved only if the risk is minimal. Otherwise, the conglomerate will abuse the privilege. That's a given.

Similarly, the FDA fails to adequately monitor the safety of medical devices after they are licensed for use in children. Although many children benefit from these devices (including shunts that drain fluid from the brain, breathing monitors, and instruments for correcting heart valve defects, etc.), there is hardly enough oversight on the part of the FDA or the American public.

> ### *What about all the medical questions of the day?*
> ### *When will they be answered?*

They won't be! **The last thing that the conglomerate wants is the resolution of outstanding medical questions and issues**—because that would seriously tamper with its commerce. It's like the old story of the guy who came up with a cure to the common cold, and when he refuses to turn it over to the conglomerate, he suddenly dies of a heart attack. And you better believe that it would happen that way!

Same goes for the guy who can show the automotive industry how to get 200 miles out of a gallon of gas (which *is* possible), or the person who can create energy out of air (also possible). If their work were to be recognized, they would either die quick deaths or be thrown in prison for supposed tax evasion.

By the way, the same holds true for cancer (and other killer diseases). **There's just too much money to be made from drugs and surgical procedures to allow it to be cured.** Don't you get it? Even if cures were to turn up, there's every likelihood that they might be withheld.

Another big reason looms as to why the conglomerate wants the serious medical questions to remain unanswered. The healthcare industry is similar to politics in that two major political parties are battling it out for votes and public support—and all the while they remain neck-and-neck down to the wire—which keeps everything polarized. And you know what? This polarization serves both parties because it generally splits issues (and political donations and bribes) down the middle, dividing American opinion with nothing getting solved in the process.

Think about it: You're either for abortion rights or against abortion rights, for gun control or against it, for capital punishment or against it, for legalized marijuana or against it, for the rights of a sex offender who's served his time to live in your neighborhood or against it, for the war in Iraq or against it.

It's pro or con, right or wrong, the devil or God, hell or heaven—everything is polarized. And this thinking is the perfect way to keep people from finding answers. In fact, it goes a lot further than simply polarizing people and issues—this mentality prevents people, institutions, and governments from seeking other alternatives. It practically mandates that we keep one foot or the other in the mud—and never break free from our collective restraints. No wonder our imagination is so limited. And no wonder we haven't solved any of our national issues.

It's no different with our nation's healthcare. We haven't cured cancer, AIDS, or any number of other diseases. And we are unable—so it would seem—to resolve medical issues that have been studied and researched for decades. These outstanding questions are never answered. And anytime that it seems we're about to at least come up with a consensus (much less seek other opinions and alternatives)—someone throws in the monkey wrench—*the new study or contradiction!*

Yeah, the conglomerate keeps you coming and going with one study and contradiction after another. That keeps everything on an even-steven basis, and the conglomerate continues to rake in the cash from all sides—a foolproof game plan.

Want some examples? Here goes:

1. STUDY: ESTROGEN PILLS RAISE RISK OF DEMENTIA
Hormone therapy was earlier believed to help older women avert forgetfulness

Lindsey Tanner, The Associated Press—June 22, 2004

Estrogen pills appear to slightly increase the risk of Alzheimer's disease and other forms of dementia in postmenopausal women, a study found, echoing recent findings involving estrogen-progestin supplements.

The findings contradict the long-held belief that estrogen pills can help keep older women's minds sharp.

The results came from a government study called the Women's Health Initiative and were published in today's Journal of the American Medical Association. ...

2. HOT FLASHES? NIGHT SWEATS?
HORMONE THERAPY STILL RATED BEST

Lauran Neergaard, The Associated Press—September 30, 2004

Hormone therapy comes with clear risks but remains the most effective treatment for hot flashes and night sweats, according to medical recommendations issued yesterday. ...

... The American College of Obstetricians and Gynecologists issued the new guide because of continuing confusion stemming from a major 2002 study that found hormones not only didn't keep postmenopausal women generally healthy—once a top reason for using them—but they could spur heart attacks, strokes and other illnesses. ...

3. ESTROGEN MAY HELP IN PREVENTING HEART DISEASE

Susan Phinney, *Seattle Post-Intelligencer*—February 14, 2006

Women who have avoided or dropped hormone replacement therapy may want to reconsider their options.

A new analysis of data from an earlier study, the Women's Health Initiative, hints that estrogen might help prevent heart disease when used early in menopause. ...

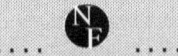

These three reports dealing with the estrogen issue highlight just how evasive and inconsistent these studies are; everything is generally neutralized and left in question, loaded down with words like "*appear* to slightly increase," "*could* spur heart attacks," "*hints* that estrogen might," all of which are meant to keep women from having a clear picture of the health issues involved.

And new studies keep coming up; on April 12, 2006, *The New York Times* released the latest one, which (again!) challenged conventional thoughts about women taking estrogen to relieve symptoms of menopause without increasing their risk of breast cancer. So whose findings do women follow?!

4. BIRTH CONTROL PILLS CUT RISK OF HEART DISEASE, CANCER
Contrary to previous studies, findings cite benefits for women
The Associated Press—October 20, 2004

The same huge federal study that led millions of women to abandon use of hormones after menopause now provides reassurance that another hormone concoction—the birth control pill—is safe.

In fact, women on The Pill had surprisingly lower risks of heart disease and stroke and no increased risk of breast cancer, contrary to what many previous studies have found. ...

Once again we read the familiar words, "contrary to what many previous studies have found." You would think that the media and the public would finally catch on to that endless game and put all these supposed studies and contradictions under the proper category of "Hollywood spins."

5. DENTAL AMALGAMS (MERCURY-METAL FILLINGS)
Inside Dentistry—Everything You Need to Know
Dr. Randall Nozawa, DDS—2000

In the mid-1800s, in the United States, a crude mercury-silver conglomerate called amalgam was introduced as an inexpensive dental filling material for people with modest incomes. Even in those times, dentists argued over the efficacious use of these mercury-metal fillings. Some said they were toxic, poisonous, a health detriment. Others vehemently denied such claims and promoted the use of amalgams as an affordable filling material for the masses. These advocates joined together to form an organization called the American Dental Association (ADA). Nearly 150 years later, the same arguments for and against the use of amalgams have not been resolved. ...

Those opposed to the use of amalgams cite a report by the American Academy of Neural Therapy (AANT) which states that mercury leaks out of its amalgam mixture while chewing, with removal and placement of the amalgam in teeth, and toxically affects the entire body, especially the brain, central nervous system, kidneys, lungs, and gastrointestinal tract. Also noted is the possibility of bacterial antibiotic resistance, which is due to the continual presence of mercury in the system. ...

... Those in support of the use of amalgams (the primary advocate being the ADA) insist that there isn't any evidence of mercury causing sickness. Their rationale for this stance is that amalgams have been used for over 100 years and the mixture is still the filling of choice for the masses.

True to form, insurance companies prefer to pay for amalgam fillings because the material is cheaper.

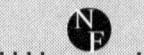

....

The amalgam issue periodically brings forth new studies that are as dubious as any I have ever read. The latest one was made by the University of Washington and involved orphans in Portugal (would you believe it!). The results found no evidence of IQ or other neurological impairment caused by dental fillings made with mercury. However, it also stated that those children in the group that used amalgam fillings did have higher levels of mercury in their urine. As I said earlier—take most of your studies and shove them!

6. LIMBERING UP? IT MAY BE A STRETCH TO FIND BENEFITS
Increasing flexibility doesn't prevent injuries, study says

Ira Dreyfuss, The Associated Press—August 14, 2004

Stretching does not live up to its reputation as an injury preventer, a study has found.

"We could not find a benefit," said Stephen Thacker, director of the epidemiology program office at the Centers for Disease Control and Prevention. ...

... Thacker and four CDC colleagues combed research databases for studies that had compared stretching with other ways to prevent training injuries. ...

... Their report is in the March issue of the American College of Sports Medicine journal, Medicine and Science in Sports and Exercise. ...

Of all the medical reports I have read over the years, this one easily takes the cake for stupidity and ignorance beyond imagination. It proves that many of the people who create these reports don't have the slightest idea of what they are talking about.

Nonetheless, this cockamamie report, which contradicts everything known to science and man about the benefits of stretching, flying in the face of common sense, will be read by countless people who will accept its findings and pass along its ill-advised attitude to thousands of others—many of whom will suffer the consequences. Most importantly, it adds to the public's confusion, which plays right into the hands of the conglomerate.

To set the record straight: Stretching improves flexibility and gives you a better range of motion of your joints; improves circulation and helps shorten recovery time after a muscle injury; reduces risk of injury in sports and helps protect your muscles and joints; allows you to improve and maintain proper posture, which minimizes aches and pains; relaxes tight muscles, helps reduce stress; improves reflexes; and enhances overall physical coordination, especially as you get older.

Stretching benefits also multiply significantly when done in conjunction with an effective warmup before exercising.

The CDC would be better off if it examined Nickolas Vassili's stretching routine on page 354 (which keeps him perfectly limber and helps prevent him from suffering any strains, cramps, and injuries) and threw its databases in the garbage can!

Stretching feels a lot better than arthritis! And it doesn't cost anything!

7. MILLIONS GET NEEDLESS PAP TESTS, SAYS RESEARCHERS

The Associated Press—October 8, 2004

Nearly 10 million U.S. women who have had hysterectomies are needlessly getting routine Pap tests, researchers say. ...

... In 1996, the U.S. Preventive Services Task Force said routine Pap tests are unnecessary for women who have had both their cervix and uterus removed for reasons other than cervical cancer.

That recommendation was recently echoed by the American Cancer Society and the American College of Obstetricians and Gynecologists.

But Veterans Affairs researchers found that nearly 46 percent of such women were still getting Pap tests in 2002.

"I actually was quite surprised because, in this case, women are being screened for cancer in an organ they don't have," said Dr. Brenda Sirovich of the VA Medical Center in White River Junction, Vt., and Dartmouth College. ...

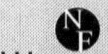

Can you begin to estimate what the overall costs for those 10 million Pap tests were? And who got paid for these unnecessary tests? And why they took place? If you think that it's all just an unintentional mistake, then you might as well get a lobotomy because you're not using your mind. The answer to all of these questions is the same: the conglomerate!

8. ASPIRIN ISN'T ALWAYS WHAT DOCTOR ORDERED

Andrew Pollack, *The New York Times*—July 20, 2004

More than 20 million Americans take aspirin regularly to help prevent heart attacks and strokes. But new evidence suggests that for many of them, the pills do little if any good.

Recent studies have found that anywhere from 5 percent to more than 40 percent of aspirin users are "non-responsive" or "resistant" to the medicine. That means that aspirin does not inhibit their blood from clotting, as it is supposed to.

"They are taking it for stroke and heart attack prevention, and it's not going to work," said Dr. Daniel Simon, the associate director of interventional cardiology at Brigham and Women's Hospital in Boston and an associate professor at Harvard University. ...

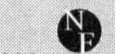

This study indicates that millions of people (within that 5 to 40 percent group) are going down the wrong medical path to preventing stroke and heart attack, and chances are that their doctors will not inform them of such.

9. NEW THINKING ON GULF WAR ILLNESSES
Latest study blames troops' exposure to neurotoxins

Scott Shane, *The New York Times*—September 24, 2004

A federal panel of medical experts studying illnesses among veterans of the war in the Persian Gulf has broken with earlier studies and concluded that many suffer from neurological damage caused by exposure to toxic chemicals, rejecting past findings that the ailments resulted mostly from wartime stress. ...

It's been 13 years since the Gulf War ended, and these Warren Commission-type studies still haven't revealed the truth about the myriad of illnesses suffered by these veterans. These studies have different answers to fit different agendas, and it's unlikely we'll ever be told what really happened.

Nearly 200,000 ailing veterans of the Gulf War are receiving disability benefits—twice the rate as vets from World War II, Korea, and Vietnam. In fact, according to Julie Mock, an Army veteran with multiple sclerosis and president of the National Gulf War Veterans Resource Center, 25 percent of the nearly 700,000 veterans who served in the 1991 Persian Gulf War are ill.

If that doesn't tell you something. ...

10. OBESITY SURGERY CAN CURE OTHER PROBLEMS, TOO, RE-SEARCH FINDS

Lindsey Tanner, The Associated Press—November 5, 2004

Obesity surgery helps patients do more than shed weight—it often cures their diabetes, high blood pressure and high cholesterol, researchers say. ...

11. LIPOSUCTION MAY NOT MAKE YOU HEALTHIER

Jeff Donn, The Associated Press—June 17, 2004

Liposuctioning your waistline can make you look just fabulous, but it won't necessarily make you healthier.

In a study, obese women who dropped up to 23 pounds of belly fat by way of liposuction did not appear to lower their risk of diabetes or heart disease, both of which are fat-related. ...

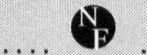

These last two examples directly contradict each other. Both studies were conducted within months of each other and prove that most studies represent nothing more than whatever someone is trying to prove—in order to make gobs of money. Study sponsers will manipulate, falsify, misquote, mislead, pad, or hide statistics and data, doing whatever is necessary to verify their contentions.

And don't believe for a moment that it's far-fetched for the conglomerate to pay people to devise studies that will support their financial objectives. For instance, there's big money in liposuction—so it's to be expected that "studies" will show all sorts of positive things about this vacuum-cleaner procedure and downplay any negative effects.

12. ONCE-TOUTED VITAMIN E FAILS AS A MAGIC BULLET

Stephen Smith, *The Boston Globe*—November 26, 2004

In a world hungry for medical magic bullets, vitamin E seemed to have it all. It's cheap. It's available. And, for years, doctors and patients alike believed it really worked, showing particular promise as ammunition against heart disease. There were even studies that appeared to prove it. ...

... Now, luminaries in cardiology are issuing a very different advisory to patients: Vitamin E won't help your heart condition, they said in August. And if you take too much, they added this month, it could hurt you. ...

It's a crying shame that the so-called medical experts can't even come to consensus about a single vitamin! No wonder the more complex issues remain unresolved.

13. MOM'S ANTI-DEPRESSANT USE MAY CAUSE BABIES TO HAVE WITHDRAWAL

Benedict Carey, *The New York Times*—February 4, 2005

After a yearlong debate over the risks of anti-depressants to minors, an analysis of World Health Organization medical records has found that infants whose mothers took the drugs while pregnant may suffer withdrawal symptoms.

The study challenges the assurances that many doctors have long given pregnant women with depression that taking drugs will not affect their babies. ...

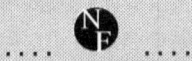

If this weren't so heartbreaking, I'd want to laugh hysterically—both at the filthy scoundrel doctors and the rest of their conglomerate cohorts who have the nerve to tell pregnant women and their husbands that these drugs will not affect their babies. **It's an absolute lie.**

It's the same distortion of truth and reality that is perpetrated prior to childbirth, when the doctor tells the laboring woman that drugs must be used to induce labor and will have no effect on the child. You have to be crazy to blindly accept this falsehood. Nan and I were among the millions who didn't recognize how foolish and dangerous a decision it was.

The sole purpose of this gargantuan treachery is to keep the doctor on schedule to pocket his fees without having to extend himself. It also provides the pharmaceutical beasts with steady cash flow.

If you think there's any hope that pregnant women will one day be alerted to the dangers of drug use, here's another example of the constant treachery of the doctors and drugmakers:

14. CHILDBIRTH STUDY SAYS NO NEED TO DELAY EPIDURALS

Denise Grady, *The New York Times*—February 17, 2005

Women in labor may suffer needlessly because doctors mistakenly advise them to delay a common pain treatment for fear that it will impede contractions and lead to a Caesarean section, researchers are reporting.

A new study of the treatment—a type of anesthesia that injects painkiller into the spinal fluid and the epidural area around the spinal cord to numb the pelvic region—finds that giving it early or late in labor makes no difference in Caesarian rates among women having first babies.

There is no reason for women to deny themselves the medicine or for the doctors to withhold it, the study says.

Other researchers urged caution, noting that not all hospitals offered such combined anesthesia and that the findings might not apply to all epidural treatments.

About 60 percent of American women have epidural anesthesia during childbirth. Dr. Cynthia Wong, the lead author of the new study and an obstetric anesthesiologist at Northwestern Memorial

Hospital in Chicago, said women were often pressured to delay the treatment and made to feel guilty or weak if they asked for one too soon.

Wong said: "Woman say: 'I must be a wimp. I had to ask for pain medication so early.' If they're wimps, we're all wimps."

The study appears today in The New England Journal of Medicine. ...

What a truckload of nonsense. First of all, we're easily tricked into accepting the word "medicine" in place of the word "drugs." Yeah, "take your medicine" isn't quite the same thing as being drugged. **And being pregnant doesn't mean you're sick—does it?**

So why must 60 percent of pregnant women opt for an injection of painkiller? The reason is basic in the minds of the conglomerate. Their number-one game plan is to get you into the drug lifestyle right from birth—which is exactly what happens with the greater percentage of pregnant woman who are enticed by the clever manipulations and scare tactics of the doctor with the big wristwatch.

And YES—you are a wimp if you acquiesce without good reason.

Much worse, you have now enrolled as a permanent wimp at the disposal of the conglomerate for the rest of your life, along with your newborn child.

Wake up! You don't need painkillers to have a baby. Women have been having babies for thousands of years without them. DON'T GET YOURSELF AND YOUR CHILD STARTED ON DRUGS! Once you get into them—you're hooked!

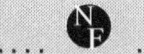

....

Over the course of the last 33 years (ever since the birth of our first child), I have been very direct in telling pregnant women (at least 30 of them) of the dangers involved in the use of painkillers during birth. These were all open-ended and very extensive discussions, and in every single instance the women expressed a strong need to experience the birth process without drugs.

What happened? *Every one* of these women ended up taking a painkiller—sometimes within less than three hours after going into labor. The reasons varied from simple weakness of mind to fighting the good fight for many hours and finally giving in to extreme agony.

In other words, all of these women were not wimps. However, upon further discussion with these women, it became apparent that in most cases their decisions were swayed by the attendant physician.

15. MORE RESEARCH CASTS DOUBTS ON BENEFITS OF EPISIOTOMIES

Carla K. Johnson, The Associated Press—May 4, 2005

For years, some doctors believed than an episiotomy, an incision to enlarge the vaginal opening during childbirth, would prevent spontaneous tearing that would be hard to repair.

They also believed the procedure would help women avoid incontinence and improve their sex lives.

It turns out those beliefs were myths.

A new review of 26 research studies shows that episiotomies are linked with a higher risk of injury, more trouble healing and more pain. ...

"This review puts together in one place all the evidence that we're not getting the results we want," said Dr. Katherine Hartman, the study's lead author and a researcher at the University of North Carolina.

The review was published in today's Journal of the American Medical Association. ...

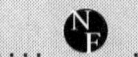

How many more studies do you need to prove a contention? Aren't 26 enough?! Since 1983, the American College of Obstetricians and Gynecologists has said episiotomies should not be done routinely. However, an Associated Press analysis of hospital data found that 616,702 episiotomies were performed in 2002.

It is estimated that one million women each year have unnecessary episiotomies.

16. OVARY LOSS MAY HURT WOMEN, STUDY SAYS
Removal during hysterectomy called unnecessary

The Associated Press—August 1, 2005

Most women getting a hysterectomy should keep their ovaries because the common extra step of removing them seems to do no good and might decrease their long-term survival, researchers report.

The study, being published today in the journal Obstetrics & Gynecology, *does not settle the issue. It does not track actual patients but uses other data to create a model of the surgery's effects.*

Still, the work promises to raise questions from women and their doctors about a procedure long accepted despite little evidence to back it. ...

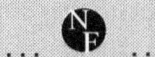

....

Three thoughts on the study: (1) Why doesn't the study track actual patients? (2) Why has the procedure been accepted despite little evidence to back it? (3) The conglomerate benefits because the procedures and subsequent treatment generate more money for the doctors and the drug industry.

Note that the study says, "the work promises to raise questions," which only goes to prove that this study is a lot of hogwash, just an excuse to obtain money under fraudulent pretenses.

17. BREAST IMPLANT BAN MAY BE LIFTED
In a surprise, FDA advisers accept safety
of firm's newer silicone devices

Lauran Neergaard, The Associated Press—April 14, 2005

In a surprising turnaround, federal health advisers yesterday recommended allowing silicone-gel breast implants to return to the U.S. market after a 13-year ban on most uses of the devices—but only under strict conditions that will limit how easily women can get them. ...

... The 7 to 2 vote came just one day after a rival manufacturer,

Inamed Corp., failed to satisfy lingering concerns about how often the implants break apart and leak inside women's bodies. ...

... Prospective patients must sign consent forms acknowledging implant risks, including that they ultimately may break and require removal or replacement. ...

Little wonder that this "surprise turnaround" happened, nor does the requirement of patients to sign a consent form seem unusual when you consider the way that the FDA often handles these issues. It follows the dictates of the conglomerate operatives, who of course are driven by market potential. To cover their misguided decisions and protect doctors from lawsuits, they ask patients to sign consent forms. Business as usual. And the public continues to blindly accept distortions of truth and their accompanying ambiguities.

18. TEENS TAKING DEPO-PROVERA
CAN RECOVER LOST BONE DENSITY
Rebound occurs after they stop using the contraceptive

Julie Davidow, *Seattle Post-Intelligencer*—February 8, 2005

Teenagers recover bone loss from taking Depo-Provera once they stop using the injectable contraceptive, according to a new study from Seattle researchers.

Three months ago, the Food and Drug Administration added a black-box warning to the packaging, advising consumers that bone loss associated with Depo-Provera may be irreversible. ...

Again and again, we bear witness to the strange and utterly confusing machinations of FDA studies and contradictions. The only relative characteristic about FDA data and its conclusions is that rarely enough research has been conducted to determine a drug's or procedure's true impacts.

The FDA constantly backtracks (often years too late to protect the public), either adding warnings or ordering a product be pulled from the shelves. In either case, the public ends up being the unwitting guinea pig, and drug users are left in the lurch, wondering about the true safety of a product.

19. HIGH-FIBER DIET AND CANCER:
PREVENTION CLAIMS DISPUTED
But findings are at odds with those of other studies

Michelle Fay Cortez, Bloomberg News—December 14, 2005

Eating plenty of fruits, vegetables and cereal fiber, proved to ward off

*heart disease and diabetes, doesn't help prevent colorectal cancer,
new research shows. ...*

Of course the findings are at odds with other studies! That's the way the game is
played.

20. BIG STUDY FINDS NO CLEAR BENEFIT OF CALCIUM PILLS

Gina Kolata, *The New York Times*—February 16, 2006

*A large, seven-year study of healthy women over age 50 found no
broad benefit from calcium and vitamin D supplements in preventing
broken bones, despite widespread endorsement by doctors for the
supplements. ...*

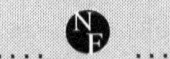

Needless to say, this report supports my general attitude about the
way in which most studies contradict one another and leave outstanding medical issues in the twilight zone. In fact, this $18 million
study, which was part of the Women's Health Initiative (a federal
project) that recently reported findings that low-fat diets do not protect against breast or colorectal cancer or heart disease, presented
even stronger evidence against health messages in general: The
results from the new study on calcium and Vitamin D, like the
others, confound popular beliefs and raise questions about public
health messages that had been addressed to the entire population.

No kidding! Just what I've been saying all along! It's one big (gigantic!) conglomerate deception that the public almost always falls for.

21. WOMEN WITH LUPUS CAN USE
BIRTH CONTROL PILL, STUDIES SAY

Linda A. Johnson, The Associated Press—December 15, 2005

*Upending the conventional medical wisdom, two studies found that
birth control pills do not worsen lupus and appear to be safe for the
tens of thousands of women with the crippling immune disorder.*

"For 30 years, we were all wrong," said Dr. Michelle Petri, lead researcher on one of the studies and director of the Lupus Center at Johns Hopkins University School of Medicine. ...

Dr. Petri says, "For 30 years, we were all wrong." My response is: How come? What were the mistakes? Who made them? And how do we know that the new studies are any better than all the others?

22. STUDY TYING LONGER LIFE
TO EXTRA POUNDS DRAWS FIRE

Gina Kolata, *The New York Times*—May 27, 2005

The new federal study suggesting that people tend to live longer if they are slightly overweight was challenged yesterday by scientists from the Harvard School of Public Health and the American Cancer Society, as well as a heart disease researcher.

But authors of the federal research said in interviews that they stood by their conclusions and that the criticisms were based on misrepresentations of what they had done.

The study under attack was published last month by researchers at the Centers for Disease Control and Prevention and the National Cancer Institute. It concluded that people who are overweight but not obese have a lower death risk than people of normal weight. The scientists also reported that being very thin increased the risk of death, even if the thinness was long-standing and not due to illness.

In a seminar and news conference yesterday at the public health school, in Boston, the critics said other studies, including their own, had found that the death risk from excess pounds increased continuously from normal weight to overweight to obesity. ...

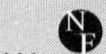

Yada, yada, yada... it goes on forever with these studies. Here you have the American Cancer Society challenging the study by the National Cancer Institute. You would think that both organizations would be responsible enough to do a combined study to provide the public with some reliable and acceptable data on the subject.

But that's not in the cards because these people aren't of a mind to cooperate and be progressive. Each has to defend its own turf—at the expense of millions of people who are left in the dark.

And when the press, the public, or concerned officials jump on a bandwagon against a given report, its findings are quickly disowned.

Take a look:

23. HEALTH AND FAT DON'T MIX, CDC CHIEF SAYS
Agency backtracks on report that the slightly overweight live longer

Marilynn Marchione, The Associated Press—June 3, 2005

Weighing a little too much might not kill you, but there's nothing healthy about it, the head of the nation's health agency said yesterday, distancing herself from a controversial report suggesting that being overweight isn't so bad. ...

... At a news conference, Dr. Julie Gerberding, CDC chief, acknowledged potential flaws in the study and pledged to get scientists and the public back on track.

"It is not OK to be overweight. People need to be fit, they need to have a healthy diet, they need to exercise," she said. "I'm very sorry for the confusion that these scientific discussions have had.". ...

Bravo Julie! Nice to see you come clean. However, the serious question remains on how much damage occurred as a result of the original report, and the CDC's support thereof. The case also reminds us once again that few true experts exist. It also highlights—as always—"Believe nothing of what you hear and half of what you see."

To close this section about medical questions of the day, here are two reports that further exemplify my point of view:

24. VITAMIN C WON'T STOP A COLD—UNLESS YOU RUN MILES

Lee Bowman, Scripps Howard News Service—June 28, 2005

A new review of 65 years of research on colds and vitamin C concludes there's little evidence that 200 milligrams or more a day wards off or shortens the duration of the common cold—with the possible exception of people exposed to extreme cold or physical stress. ...

... A best-selling book, Vitamin C and the Common Cold, *by Nobel Laureate chemist Linus Pauling, published in 1970, and several subsequent books popularized the notion that large doses of the vitamin (1000 mg or more) could reduce the incidence of colds by almost half. The government's recommended daily allowance for vitamin C is 60 mg.*

The review, published yesterday in the journal Public Library of Science Medicine, *considered studies that compared people taking vitamin C with those who took a placebo. ...*

No wonder the public doesn't know what to believe or which way to turn! Even a Nobel Laureate chemist's work is suddenly dismissed. Once again, the experts can't come together about a single vitamin!

25. DOCTORS, U.S. PANEL AT ODDS OVER WORTH OF YEARLY EXAMS

Lindsey Tanner, The Associated Press—June 28, 2005

Many adults think a yearly checkup is just part of staying healthy, and a new survey shows doctors do, too.

But that practice isn't endorsed by a panel of experts that says there's no evidence annual physicals for healthy people are useful. ...

... It [the survey] renews a debate over annual physicals that dates back at least nine years. That's when the U.S. Preventive Services Task Force declared there is insufficient evidence of any benefit from many of the tests often given with yearly checkups.

The task force is a respected non-government panel of researchers commissioned by Congress to develop evidence-based recommendations for medical care. It doesn't recommend for or against annual physicals, and neither does the American Medical Association. ...

Needless to say, both the panel of respected nongovernment researchers and the AMA prefer to sit on the fence, rather than go on record for or against yearly physicals. That insures that the public won't know what is best for them. It also keeps the merry-go-round going round and round and never getting anywhere.

* * *

Always one to add another kicker, here are some more recent contradictory studies:

- **Fish oil doesn't cut cancer risk.**

- **Maybe tofu isn't so great after all.**

- **Low-fat diets didn't lower cancer risks.**

- **The surprising relationship between beta-carotene and heightened lung cancer risk.**

- **Do meat and dairy harm aging bones?**

- **Inhaling nitric oxide helps patients with respiratory failure.**

- **Drinking a glass of wine each day prolongs life.**

Will toothpaste and flossing, bathing, fastening seatbelts, and using toilet paper be the next things to come under attack? Is nothing sacred?

I have mentioned these examples of polarization and contradiction, which cover a variety of medical topics and issues, to clearly illustrate that the conglomerate's standard methodology of dividing and conquering is alive and well and in permanent residency in America. But this does not scratch the surface of the overwhelming number of outstanding medical problems that are buried in the conglomerate's deceitful practices (I would need a separate book to cover those).

And if you multiply all these studies and contradictions by the number of people directly affected by them—you would see a broader picture of our nation's catastrophic healthcare system.

To add to the complexity of the overall national healthcare crisis, the press barely skims the top of the myriad problems, issues, and conflicts, choosing to restrict its focus to bare-bones reporting and analysis. The result is hardly enough to persuade Americans to pay more attention to what's going on.

Even worse, the press can easily, often unintentionally, slant a study one way or the other, casting more ambiguity onto an already unclear picture. This often happens because the newspaper reporter hasn't done the prerequisite homework needed to understand the background of the issue, consequently doing a sloppy job of writing about the study.

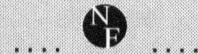

In my many years of researching healthcare facts, documents, studies, etc., I have found that, generally speaking, the factual information presented in news reports has been taken from other "original" sources and passed along to the public without any in-depth research, study, or follow-up. This results in little more than basic news reporting—which I then have to backtrack on to come up with a clear sense of what the report truly represents. This is one of the reasons that I review and critique these studies and reports.

> ### *Are our hospitals safe?*

That's like asking if our roads are safe. Statistically speaking, 43,000 people are killed on American roads each year, with a high percentage of those deaths caused by speeding and drunk-driving. And although the statistical research is very limited, the use of cell phones is obviously adding to the carnage.

Now, you would think that accidental deaths in hospitals because of medical errors rank well below that figure, wouldn't you? HealthGrades, an organization that publishes rankings of hospitals and doctors, said in 2004 that mistakes in hospitals may kill twice as many people as previously thought. It estimated **195,000 deaths a year!!!**

I ask you to stop and consider what this reality represents. *Think carefully.* We're talking about more than 65 times the number of people killed on 9/11. That's on a yearly basis. Can you visualize this carnage? Do you understand what it represents? It's not just a statistic, an inconsequential number.

By that reckoning, medical error ranks just behind heart disease and cancer as the leading causes of death.

The HealthGrades report goes on to say:

> ... *"There is little evidence that patient safety has improved in the last five years," according to Dr. Samantha Collier, vice president*

of medical affairs at HealthGrades, which publishes rankings of hospitals and doctors. "The equivalent of 390 jumbo jets full of people are dying each year due to likely preventable, in-hospital medical errors, making this one of the leading killers in the U.S.". ...

... "This should give you pause when you go to a hospital," said Dr. Kenneth Kizer of the National Quality Forum, a Washington-based group that develops quality measurements for health care. He said the HealthGrades' death estimate did not shock him, adding that the tally would be even larger if researchers factored in errors at nursing homes, private doctors' offices and other outpatient settings.

HealthGrades officials say their study is particularly gloomy because it suggests there has been no improvement in the death rate following several high-profile mistakes. ...

On that note, surgeons are infamous for removing the wrong foot, breast, or organ, drilling into the wrong side of a skull, giving the wrong patient a heart catheterization, or committing a range of wrong site, procedure, or patient surgeries.

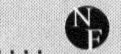

The aforementioned HealthGrades report is indicative of the general state of our harmful healthcare system, underscoring the incredible reality that **although America pays more than half of the total amount of money spent worldwide on healthcare, it ranks 37th among industrialized nations.**

Think about this: As of October 17, 2006, not only are we as a nation of 300 million—which is only about five percent of the world's population—spending more money on healthcare than the rest of the world's population of 6,525,170,264, but we are also far behind so many other nations when it comes to the quality of our healthcare.

Here's another noteworthy report on the subject:

MEDICAL WORKERS ARE OFTEN MUM ON MISTAKES
Nurses, doctors rarely speak up
when they see patient care problems, study finds

Lee Bowman, Scripps Howard News Service—January 27, 2005

Doctors, nurses and other health care workers seldom challenge a colleague when they see mistakes being made in patient care, according to a new study.

Researchers spent more than 10,000 hours observing and interviewing more than 2,000 health workers at 19 hospitals around the country.

Among the stories they heard were of a nurse who gave up reminding a colleague to put up safety rails on a child's bed; a pharmacist who gave a patient an inadequate amount of pain medicine because the doctor who prescribed it is a "jerk" and gives the pharmacy a hard time if challenged; and a nurse who watched a colon-surgery patient die after failing to convince a doctor who intimidated her that the man was in trouble. ...

... The study, released yesterday, was co-sponsored by the American Association of Critical-Care nurses and VitalSmarts, a California firm that consults on leadership and organizational performance. ...

... Among the findings in the report, titled: "Silence Kills: The Seven Crucial Conversations for Healthcare":

- *Eighty-four percent of doctors and 62 percent of nurses and other care providers have seen co-workers repeatedly taking shortcuts that could endanger patients.*

- *Eighty-eight percent of doctors and 48 percent of nurses and other providers work with people who show poor clinical judgment, although the problems seem concentrated among a small percentage of colleagues—about 10 percent.*

- *Fewer than 10 percent of doctors, nurses and other caregivers said they directly confront colleagues about their concerns. And a fifth of the doctors said they've seen harm come to patients as a result of the behavior of these colleagues.*

Overall, researchers found that health workers were reluctant to talk with colleagues about matters concerning competence, broken rules, mistakes, teamwork, lack of support, disrespect and micromanagement from doctors and supervisors. ...

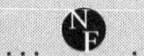

. . . .

I should point out that, by and large, because of the way that the medical profession investigates itself (it is similar to most police departments in that internal investigations are shams) and the laws that protect it, **no one outside the hospital—not the public, the state, or even the organization that accredits hospitals—is entitled to know what really happens when something goes awry.** This helps explain why 195,000 people needlessly die in hospitals every year. Wholesale murder! And wholesale cover-up.

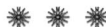

I hardly need to remind myself again about my personal experience at St. Vincent's Hospital in New York City, when our highly paid obstetrician came very close to killing my son and wife. In that light, the above study comes as no surprise. However, considering the defensive posture of doctors and the massive number of yearly deaths in hospitals as a result of medical mistakes, you can bet that this study reveals only the tip of the iceberg.

As part of this deadly equation, here's a report that would make most people cringe in horror:

CLEAN UP HYGIENE IN U.S. HOSPITALS

Betsy McCaughey, guest columnist,
***Seattle Post-Intelligencer*—June 7, 2005**

Infections that have been nearly eradicated in some other countries are raging through hospitals here in the United States. The major reason? Poor hygiene. In fact, hygiene is so inadequate in most U.S. hospitals that one of every 20 patients contracts an infection during a hospital stay. Hospital infections kill an estimated 103,000 people in the United States a year, as many as AIDS, breast cancer and auto accidents combined.

And the danger is worsening as many hospital infections can no longer be cured with common antibiotics. One of the deadliest germs is a staph bacteria called MRSA, short for methicillin-resistant Staphylococcus aureus, *which lives harmlessly on the skin but causes havoc when it enters the body ... Today, experts estimate that more than 60 percent of staph infections are MRSA.*

Hospitals in Denmark, Finland and the Netherlands once faced similar rates, but brought them down to below 1 percent. How? Through the rigorous enforcement of rules on hand washing, the meticulous cleaning of equipment and hospital rooms, the use of gowns and disposable aprons to prevent doctors and nurses from spreading germs on clothing and the testing of incoming patients to identify and isolate those carrying germs. ...

... Hospital infections can be stopped, but most hospital administrators have not made prevention a top priority. The Centers for Disease Control and Prevention are also to blame. While the CDC has made some efforts to curb hospital infections, it has failed to follow the rigorous precautions that are working in other countries and in those U.S. hospitals where they have been tried.

In 2003, a task force for the Society of Healthcare Epidemiologists of America chastised the CDC for the failure, but the CDC has still not acted. Every year of delay is costing thousands of lives. ...

.... 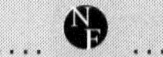 ....

In February, the CDC declared that it will not support the growing demand to make hospital infection rates public. That's criminal because if you need to be hospitalized, you should be able to find out which hospitals in your area have the worst infection problems. This secrecy may allow some hospitals to save face, but it won't save lives or money. But then, like the FDA and its criminal posturing over confidentiality, the CDC goes the same route with its secrecy. And, once again, the public be damned!

Here's another report that makes one wonder:

SURGICAL TOOLS WASHED IN HYDRAULIC FLUID
An estimated 3,800 patients put in jeopardy
The Associated Press—June 13, 2005

About 3,800 patients at two hospitals run by Duke University Health System were operated on last year with instruments that were washed in hydraulic fluid instead of detergent, hospital regulators said.

Duke Health Raleigh and Durham Regional hospitals put patients in "immediate jeopardy" in November and December by not detecting the problem, despite complaints from medical staff about slick tools, according to a report by the Centers for Medicare & Medicaid Services. ...

... Duke Health officials assured patients in January that the likelihood of infection from the tools was "no more than the risk normally associated" with the procedures that the patients underwent.

However, dozens of patients who were exposed to the surgical instruments have reported lingering health concerns ranging from fatigue and joint pain to problems requiring hospitalization, the The (Raleigh) News & Observer *reported Sunday. ...*

Making such a mistake was bad enough, but the hospital officials also ignored warnings from medical staff for many weeks, and then had the colossal nerve to say there was no more risk to patients than under normal conditions.

More of the same kind of news:

HOSPITAL'S BOTTOM LINE TIED TO SURGICAL MISTAKES
Lee Bowman, Scripps Howard News Service—June 8, 2005

Did the hospital where you're having that operation next week turn a profit last year? If not, the odds are higher that the medical staff will make a significant mistake during or after your surgery, according to a study published yesterday.

Researchers from the U.S. Agency for Healthcare Research and Quality reviewed medical errors in the files of about 1 million patients who underwent major surgery in 176 Florida hospitals between 1996 and 2000.

They found that over time, a decrease in a hospital's financial profit margin leads to a higher risk for mistakes in the treatment of adult surgical patients. ...

... Patients who had surgery in the bottom-tiered hospitals were:

- *Nearly 6 percent more likely to have a medical error occur during the procedure, such as having an instrument left in the body, a reaction to a blood transfusion or complications from anesthesia.*

- *Almost 15 percent more likely to have a post-surgical medical error, such as the development of bedsores.*

- *About 12 percent more likely to experience any of 24 preventable patient safety events arising from surgery, nursing care or problems such as nerve compression injuries or the reopening of a surgical site. ...*

This correlation between hospital profit margins and patient safety once again points out that the bottom line for the conglomerate is money.

Yet another report on the dismal state of our patient care:

U.S. LEADS WAY IN MEDICAL ERRORS
Susan Heavey, Reuters—November 3, 2005

Patients in the United States reported higher rates of medical errors and more disorganized doctor visits and out-of-pocket costs than people in Canada, Britain and three other developed countries, according to a survey released on Thursday.

Thirty-four percent of U.S. patients received wrong medication, improper treatment or incorrect or delayed test results during the last two years, the Commonwealth Fund found. ...

With the preponderance of documented facts like these, hospitals are very dangerous places, even if you're relatively healthy. It is commonplace for someone to die unexpectedly in one of them because of neglect or "failure to rescue" a patient.

While I'm still on the topic, here's a related issue:

HOSPITALS TAKE ADVANTAGE OF THE UNINSURED
Steve W. Berman, guest columnist,
Seattle Post-Intelligencer—June 2, 2005

Walking into an emergency room with a sick child is a terrifying experience for any parent. But for many Washingtonians, that visit can be made worse by hospital business practices that condemn the uninsured to huge debt.

The practice—charging uninsured the highest rate—is ethically and morally wrong, and state officials need to take action to put an end to it.

Here's how it works. Large payers use their economic clout to negotiate deep discounts with hospitals. Since insurers and HMOs can exert such economic muscle in these negotiations, hospitals have little choice but to agree to markdowns.

While HMOs pay pennies for the proverbial $10 aspirin, often that same hospital will charge uninsured patients absurdly high prices for the same pill.

Recently, an uninsured patient was charged $174,107 to fix a broken leg. Included in the charges was a $1,600 X-ray, which should have cost around $130. Another hospital in the same chain charged an uninsured patient $48,374 for a two-hour visit to treat an infection.

This is big business: One national hospital chain collected about $400 million from uninsured patients in a five-year period, much of that coming from excessive charges. ...

... The impact on the working poor is staggering. A recent Harvard University study found that 50 percent of the personal bankruptcies in the United States are due to health care debt. In Washington state, Physicians for a National Health Program reports that in 2004, more than 19,000 bankruptcies were caused by medical issues. ...

As this article indicates, one obvious aspect of this deplorable American institution is that an unmistakable caste system is embedded in its very nature. Not only do poor people go into debt to pay their hospital bills, they end up at the back of the waiting line (where they will be penalized further with higher prices and inferior service). They also must accept the painful reality that those who are fortunate enough to be privately insured will be given better overall care, as well as quick follow-up care.

This is no surprise, as most clinics first inquire about patients' insurance status before they ask about their conditions, which pretty much shatters the myth that "when you're sick, you'll get the needed care." Hardly. In fact, according to a 2005 study published in *The Journal of the American Medical Association,* only

28 percent of clinics even attempt to find out how sick callers were, whereas 98 percent ask about their insurance.

Once again, power and deceit reign supreme for the conglomerate, who preys on the poor and makes hospitals unsafe for anyone who is uninsured.

A closing note related to the subject of hospital safety: Our nation's emergency care is at a breaking point. Poor people without insurance are forced to come to emergency rooms, which must treat them regardless of their ability to pay. According to a study by the Institute of Medicine, there were nearly 114 million emergency room visits in 2003, compared to 90 million a decade earlier. During that same 10-year period, the total number of U.S. hospitals decreased by 703, the number of ERs by 425, and the number of hospital beds dropped nationwide by 198,000.

Needless to say, things can only get worse.

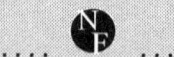

. . . .

In conclusion, any intelligent person examining the number of annual road deaths (approximately 43,000) and the yearly preventable hospital deaths (195,000) might wonder why our society fails to take greater notice of these avoidable deaths *(2.4 million over a 10-year period!)* and institute massive prevention campaigns.

The answer is quite simple: Whereas the deaths of 3,000 people on September 11, 2001, resulted in a national call-to-arms that will cost U.S. taxpayers potentially trillions of dollars in government spending and national deficit, the deaths of millions on the road and in hospitals warrants little attention in comparison.

Here's another way of looking at this inhuman fact of American life: **Only politically correct dead bodies count.** Whereas the relatives of those who died on 9/11 are entitled to hefty government payments, those who die in hospitals or on the roads are not so deserving.

You might ask yourself, why is that? Is one body less dead than another? Is one human being less deserving than another? Is one person's suffering greater than another's suffering?

Examine these questions honestly… and you can see the game plan of the conglomerate and our present administration in Washington as well as the level of ignorance (and acceptance) on the part of the American public.

To beat a dead horse, politicians in both political parties and conglomerate members can gain little in the way of power or money from the prevention of the greater number of needless deaths. In other words, *they really don't give a damn about human life unless they can milk it for their own personal or political benefit.* (This same mentality showed its ugly face in the aftermath of Hurricane Katrina.)

> *How can a patient be sure if surgery is necessary?*

To begin with, you must assume that the surgeon wants to cut and that s/he will do everything in his power to convince you that this is the way to go. S/he will forcefully encourage, manipulate, and pressure you to have a Caesarean[14] (the surgeon's bread-and-butter operation), to remove your prostate gland, or to undergo drastic cosmetic surgery. And should you get a call from the doctor's office telling you that you must have an organ excised or risk death, I guarantee that your first instinct will be to surrender yourself posthaste—without bothering to get a second opinion.

As for getting another opinion, by all means obtain at least three opinions before allowing yourself to go under the knife for anything more serious than a biopsy. (Even then, think twice because a large percentage of biopsies are carried out solely to protect the doctor from a malpractice suit.) I know that it's costly, but your health is far more important than a vacation or a new car.

You must also seek out opinions from *different types of doctors* with *different medical approaches.* There's no point in asking three doctors who do little else than liposuction if this is the right procedure for you.

If you really care about upholding your existence, you will take the time to research your medical and health problems *before* going ahead with any procedure. I previously indicated that tens of thousands of men diagnosed with prostate cancer almost immediately opt for surgery, chemotherapy, or radiation treatment, and yet many alternatives exist that have proven just as effective with far less devastating effects on the body's own immune system: dendreon amino therapy, cryotherapy, various herbal and homeopathic treatments, and robotic surgery.

---

[14] On November 16, 2005, the government reported that the rate of Caesarean sections in the U.S. climbed to an all-time high, despite efforts by public health officials to bring down the number of such deliveries.

Unfortunately, these men rarely take the time to explore these alternative forms of treatment. What's even more suspect about their rush to do surgery, chemo, or radiation is the fact that prostate cancer's slow development usually affords more than enough time to examine all these options.

So why do so few men acquaint themselves with the alternatives to the standard trio of surgery-chemo-radiation? Because they are encouraged from all sides to "do something about it right away." Besides, how could someone as honest and sincere as Joe Torre (the manager of the New York Yankees) be wrong?

While I'm addressing this specific issue of prostate cancer, I'm going to get very personal with a statement by my friend Neil Selden.

> Ten years ago I was told by my family doctor that my prostate PSA was 93 (anything above four is considered dangerous), and that it was a case of aggressive cancer. This was confirmed by the head of urology at a well-known hospital, who gave me a life expectancy of two to three years if I began taking a chemical estrogen; he claimed that my X-rays and other tests supported that.
>
> My wife and I pursued possible alternative treatments, including dietary supports by Dr. Jack Taylor in Chicago, and the use of PC SPES, an herbal estrogen supplement recommended by Frank Wiewel, director of People Against Cancer, a grassroots organization in Otho, Iowa.
>
> At the same time, by a miracle, we connected with the most loving, huggy, brilliant, and well-respected oncologist probably in the world, who reinterpreted my data in a positive light and who was totally supportive of our herbal and dietary approach.
>
> Within three months of using PC SPES, we received a phone call from our oncologist, who told us in amazement and delight that my PSA had fallen to below 1.
>
> We used PC SPES for some years until it was taken off the market, then tried "pulsing" the chemical estrogen Lupron, which worked acceptably, and now we have returned to a new herbal approach recommended by People Against Cancer. My PSA continues to be below 1.
>
> My dietary approach at this time, recommended by People Against Cancer, is 70 percent vegetables, 10 percent fruit, 10 percent protein, and 10 percent grains, plus supplementary minerals and vitamins, plus yoga, exercise, meditation, and much, much giving and receiving of love.

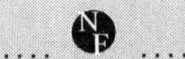

On several occasions I have met individuals who have been diagnosed with prostate cancer, and I offered to arrange for them to contact Neil before deciding on any medical procedure. However, these gentlemen would not as much as chance a telephone call to Neil. Instead, within short order, they opted for invasive surgery and chemo.

Make no mistake about this—surgeons earn their keep by cutting and not by advising caution or suggesting you research the problem before undergoing surgery. Furthermore, our friend Edmond Spencer went under the knife for prostate cancer at the age of 81, which was medically unsound, and died shortly thereafter. If you think that's an isolated case—you're absolutely nuts!

Don't you get it? A poultry farmer wants you to eat poultry, not fish; Ford Motor Company is going to sell you a Ford, not a Chevy; Safeway doesn't suggest you visit Trader Joe's; and no commercial entity is going out of its way to support someone else's product or service. They want you to buy from them. So when you consider any medical procedure, *remember that it's not about health—it's all about money.*

Note: For those readers (surgeon-inspired) who might take my views about surgery as highly unfair and lacking objectivity, understand that I'm aware of the great advances in surgical procedures over the past 50 years. (In the 1950s the word "cancer" couldn't be mentioned on the radio; today 4 out of every 10 cancer patients are likely to survive for at least 5 years). But my purpose is not to praise or downgrade but to enlighten and inform about the problems that are not being dealt with at the expense of millions of lives.

When I was about seven years old, my mother took me to Thom McCann's shoe store and bought me a pair of shoes that must have been two sizes too small for my feet. The salesman nearly broke the shoehorn forcing my feet into those ill-chosen shoes, and I still remember how painful it was to walk in them. Consequently, I developed large bunions on the first joints of both big toes. These disfigurements still make it quite difficult to find shoes that fit comfortably—even with a 4E, I need shoes stretched an additional two sizes.

I still curse the day that my mother bought those shoes, setting in motion a lifetime problem. However, notwithstanding the way that my feet look (people regard them as slightly grotesque, while I relate to them as aristocratic!), and the problem of finding shoes that fit, I've never had a problem with my feet. I walk 12 to 15 miles a week at a fast pace, jog four times a week, skip rope, box, and zap about like a dancer with springs beneath his soles.

The reason I relate this story is that three different podiatrists have strongly urged that I have cosmetic surgery on these bunions. Guess what I told them? And you can guess what I've told eight different people (mostly friends) who were pushed to have this type of surgery. Unfortunately, all eight of them, assured by surgeons that they would be back to their normal stride within three months, went under the knife, only to suffer severe consequences.

On average, 14 months passed before they were able to walk normally, and even then for limited distances. Although their feet gained a measure of cosmetic improvement, they will never be completely healthy again because it is impossible to cut through so many essential, delicate veins and nerves in the foot and restore them completely.

And why did this happen? The bastard surgeons! Cut, cut, cut—and keep cutting! That's what they're paid to do—and that's what they do whether it's advisable or not. And if you think that I'm harping on this because I hold grudges against Thom McCann's or the surgeons, my concern is with all the people who make the mistake of having surgery on their bunions, only to end up leading sedentary lives as a result. They'll never be able to walk, run, and exercise properly, and that's a permanent handicap.

Apropos of the aforementioned history of my bunions, I went to a podiatrist regularly when I worked at Arthur Murray's so many years ago, and it was a light, pleasant experience that I always looked forward to. The service included a foot bath, cutting away corns, trimming toenails, powdering, some light cushioning over the areas that had been cut, and the best of service.

I mention this because I recently went to a podiatrist to have a corn on the bottom of my foot removed. It had started to impede my boxing skills, and as it is nothing more than cutting away some dead skin (a very simple procedure), I made the appointment.

After arriving at the doctor's office, which includes a sales showroom of footwear, etc., and filling out some paperwork for Medicare, I was taken into a tiny room—actually a small broom closet that had been converted into an office. *This was the doctor's operating room!* It had an old barber's chair and not much more. And it was freezing!

The doctor provided nothing along the lines of what I had experienced years ago. In fact, this was like a Keystone Kops comedy. No place to sit and take your shoes off (I had to do it in the cramped barber's chair), no foot bath, or other extended service.

This doctor spent all of 90 seconds cutting away a bit of the corn, slicing enough of it to cause some bleeding; then she searched through a cardboard box for a Band-Aid—and that was it.

Quite a contrast from my earlier experiences with a podiatrist, but par for the course in this day and age—**a microcosm of the entire healthcare demise in America.**

✳ ✳ ✳

There is also the question of high costs of surgery. Some patients are traveling overseas to get it done, not only for lower costs but better care and more communicative doctors.

FOREIGN SURGEONS ATTRACT U.S. PATIENTS
**Americans say they find top-quality orthopedic surgery and
other health care in foreign lands, such as India,
with far lower costs, little delay and more personal attention**

Ramola Talwar Badam—The Associated Press, September 25, 2005

*Bradley Thayer, a retired apple farmer from Okanogan, Wash.,
traveled 7,500 miles to get his torn knee ligament fixed, and says he
paid a third of what it would cost him in a U.S. hospital.*

And that included airfare to Bombay.

*Thayer, 60, had no health insurance when he fell and injured
himself while vacationing in British Columbia. He says his U.S.
doctors told him he would have to wait six months for surgery and
pay bills totaling $35,000. So he joined a rising tide of American
and European patients heading to India, Thailand and Singapore
for top-class orthopedic surgery, plastic surgery, infertility treatment
and cardiology that come much cheaper than in the West. ...*

This helps debunk any American assumption that you won't find quality healthcare outside of the U.S. Quite to the contrary.

✳ ✳ ✳

Of special note regarding surgery: On my way to work out recently, I passed a huge billboard with before and after photographs of a woman who originally weighed over 300 pounds and became a slim charmer with a big smile. The caption below the photographs read, "I lost 150 pounds with the safest weight-loss surgery."

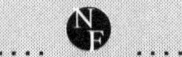

Well, bravo for her. I'm glad she's looking good and hopefully feeling good, BUT... many dangers are involved in gastric-bypass and other stomach-shrinking cosmetic surgeries, including risk of death. In other words, you play with fire when you opt for any form of surgical abdominal reduction, and you play right into the hands of the brigades of surgeons who gladly risk *your* life to benefit their wallets.

What is arguably strange about this level of surgical procedures is that the media have accepted obesity surgery as a normal procedure, while at the same time they would surely deride my method of "tupping" (see pages 317–346), which is basically nothing more than a water cure. They would label me a threat to society while they support the rearrangement of your intestinal tract by these scalpel-wielding physicians. It only goes to show you how ignorant and crazy we are.

I have mentioned the culpability of the media, which work as paid lackeys for the conglomerate—just as they promote violence on TV and in films—because it sells. In this regard, I find that TV programming centered on cosmetic surgery is degenerate and as dangerous as it gets, feeding into the needs and half-baked views of the bloodthirsty public.

Among these conglomerate shticks are *The Swan* and *Extreme Plastic Surgery*, both of which lure the general public into a state of mindless acceptance of these surgical procedures, providing nothing in the way of objectivity or safeguarding the public. American-style healthcare madness, as only we can do it! (In case you're wondering, the only TV program that scored even lower on my ratings chart for sick, sick, sick is *Nip/Tuck*).

The Swan combines elements of *Iron Chef* and *This Is Your Life*, setting up a competition between two women who will undergo drastic surgery to achieve the self-esteem that has eluded them because of physical impairment or disability early in life. This contest is played out to the hilt, with both gals undergoing all the necessary procedures, including liposuction, facial uplifts, nose jobs, new teeth ... the works.

At the end of the show, each contestant looks in a mirror and sees how she's been transformed into a new person for the first time. Then the host (a very hot young woman herself) does the Oscar bit and opens an envelope that contains the name of the winner who will go on to the finals and perhaps become The Swan.

Dramatic, well-scripted, and filmed, with nary a doubt as to how the (now beautiful) women will fare in the future—so what's wrong with it? Why am I agitating against this production?

First of all, I'm happy for anyone whose life is changed for the better. I love happy endings! But this carnival performance, with all its supportive and smiling medical personnel (cast), does not uphold existence because it completely ignores the fact that these women are given $60- to $70,000 in cosmetic surgery to act as shills for the conglomerate.

Sure, the contestants may profit enormously on a personal level (if they get the rest of their act together), but nonetheless they are helping to promote drastic surgical procedures that are often unnecessary, dangerous, and extremely costly.

The Swan conveniently links the hideous aims of the conglomerate and the weak mentality of our unhealthy society. It's a big showcase for a select group of women (who may or may not get the follow-up treatment and support they will need) at the expense of tens of millions of men and women who will never be able to come to terms with their bodies and lack of self-esteem, and who will continue to think that they haven't got what it takes to be beautiful people. How shameful.

By offering yourself up to these scumbags (that's what they are!) you show utter disrespect for yourself and your body. You allow yourself to be treated like a piece of meat on a slab, nothing more than another bank deposit for these mentally disfigured frauds, whose smiles and positive feedback are as false as the procedures they sell you. Their real intent is to persuade you to return and pay them more money to cut out your entrails.

Yeah, line up folks and be part of the conglomerate's world—where good health and intelligence have been replaced by the shylocks of schlock, where supposed metamorphosis destroys all vestiges of common sense and decency.

To add to the freakish nature of this type of programming, they've now added a kicker: The "Miss Plastic Surgery" contest. I just can't wait!

The TV presentation called *Extreme Plastic Surgery* recently showed an actual operation on a woman having cosmetic surgery on her stomach. The show's crack team of stomach reconstructors performed like a group of plumbers working on a stuffed toilet. They used all sorts of tools, gadgets, and scalpels; they stuck probes and tubes into the woman's belly; then they cut her open from stem to stern, before slicing out God knows how many pounds of fat cells—**just like a butcher gutting and filleting a piece of meat or fish.** I'm not exaggerating.

I watched this medical procedure, wondering if I was watching a science-fiction movie instead, but it was quite for real. And when I juxtaposed it with my own form of weight reducing, I had to wonder what planet I was living on.

How could anyone in his right mind accept this slicing and dicing of one's stomach over my simple water cure? It's easy. Television programs like *Extreme Plastic Surgery* and *The Swan* are bonanzas for the conglomerate, while the simple act of tupping has no commercial value. No pills, bills, or therapy—it would only cut into the huge profits of the people who drive the engines for the bosses at the conglomerate.

Here's a significant report that backs up my attitudes:

OBESITY PROCEDURES RISKIER THAN THOUGHT
Death rates in study provide 'a reality check'
Lindsey Tanner, The Associated Press—October 24, 2005

The chances of dying within a year after obesity surgery are much higher than previously thought, even among people in their 30s and 40s, a study of more than 16,000 Medicare patients found.

Some previous studies of people in their 30s to their 50s—the most common ages for obesity surgery—found death rates well under 1 percent. But among 35- to 44-year-olds in the Medicare study, more than 5 percent of men and nearly 3 percent of women were dead within a year, and slightly higher rates were seen in patients 45 to 54.

Among patients 65 to 74, nearly 13 percent of men and about 6 percent of women died. In patients 75 and older, half of the men and 40 percent of the women died.

"The risk of death is much higher than has been reported," said University of Washington surgeon Dr. David Flum, the Medicare study's lead author. "It's a reality check for those patients who are considering these operations." ...

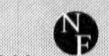

. . . .

It's much more than a reality check—it's a dire warning to BE SHARP, GET IN GEAR, AND STOP IN YOUR TRACKS BEFORE THEY MURDER YOU! Listen up guys and gals, I'm not spouting at the mouth these hundreds of pages just to make some noise and gain some attention for my method of dealing with obesity. I'm trying to save lives. Perhaps yours.

To further add to this cosmetic madness, the demand for plastic surgery for pets is increasing, despite objections from animal-rights activists and some dog breeders. You can bet that it's only a matter of time before you read about the new television series called *Face-Lift for Fido* and *Kitty Tummy-Tuck.*

> *Are you against all types of cosmetic surgery?*

Society's unreasonably rabid attitude of striving for the perfect, unattainable images that it sees in magazines and pop culture (which are mostly the result of digital manipulation anyhow) produces untold personal misery, emptiness, and lack of self-esteem, both in men and women. I recently watched a *Larry King Live* show on which he had a female guest who had spent $80,000 on 30 cosmetic procedures—and she may have more. A cosmetic surgery addict! It should be noted that this individual—having undertaken so many procedures to improve her appearance—looked awful, almost grotesque, from battle scars.

But if it upholds your existence to have a nose job, reduce the size of your jowls, correct a disfigurement, or you've had an accident and need reconstructive surgery, by all means, go for it! **But don't confuse safe and necessary surgical improvement with unnecessary and dangerous surgical procedures** that only benefit the conglomerate and further contribute to the madness of our quick-fix, image-driven society.

Use your brains before giving in to the commercials and testimonials. Think before you act irrationally. And do your homework before you make a decision that could permanently and adversely affect your life. Be safe!

When I say "Do your homework," I mean GET WITH IT! Act as if you were responsible for an important research study. All too often, people spend a few minutes online, reading one or two reports on the subject of interest, then call it a day. That won't cut the mustard, especially with decisions that could significantly alter—or end—your life.

As an example, if you were to go online and research Botox, you would probably come away with a favorable opinion of this cosmetic fad. In fact, you would have to dig a bit to learn that Botox comes from the single most deadly toxin known to man. With that reality in mind, you might think twice before becoming a user.

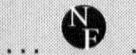

Some people who call themselves plastic surgeons may not have the training that supposedly goes with the title. In fact, some states don't regulate who can call themselves a plastic or cosmetic surgeon. Doesn't that grab you!

A final thought on cosmetic surgery: It should only be a last resort. Before opting for it, try some old-fashioned methods of improving your self-esteem: Plan and execute some project that you have always dreamed of doing; buy some new clothes that make you look good; improve your personality and disposition by engaging in some form of meditation; work out—and get into great shape and condition; practice loving yourself in as many ways as possible; recognize and improve upon your best qualities; and change your lifestyle for the better.

> *I'm always reading about the*
> *medical liability crisis. What's it really about?*

It's about GREED. Only here we're talking about the two greediest pigs of all, the doctors and the lawyers, vultures who are pitted against each other. While these two villains are at each other's throats, the ever-sinister insurance companies are enjoying a field day.

Neither side really gives a damn about the person in the middle—the patient and client. The results are predictable: Doctors pay more and more for liability insurance, lawyers collect more and more in damages, and medical costs keep rising.

A government report found that the Medicare program alone pays $60 to $120 billion each year because of the medical liability crisis. The majority of these costs are related to "defensive medicine" practices: doctors who are afraid of lawsuits order every test possible, including biopsies. No one has ever been sued for ordering too many tests.

Here's a relevant report:

FEARING SUITS, DOCTORS PRACTICE
ALARMING RATE OF 'DEFENSIVE MEDICINE'
Lindsey Tanner, The Associated Press—June 1, 2005

Fear of getting sued leads an alarming number of doctors to practice "defensive medicine," such as ordering unnecessary tests and avoiding risky procedures, a survey found.

The practice has been around for decades and is no secret to many patients. But the survey of 824 Pennsylvania doctors suggests it is surprisingly common, researchers said. ...

... The studies were published in today's Journal of the American Medical Association.

Ninety-three percent of the Pennsylvania doctors surveyed in 2003 said they sometimes or often practiced defensive medicine because of malpractice concerns.

That means they engaged in unsound practices that exposed patients to potential harm, said Dr. Peter Budetti, a physician-lawyer and public health professor at University of Oklahoma Health Sciences Center.

"Perhaps the greatest irony is that defensive medicine may be counterproductive and actually might increase malpractice risk," said Budetti, who wrote an accompanying editorial.

Examples include performing breast biopsies in women with lumps unlikely to be cancer, hospitalizing low-risk patients with chest pain and eliminating high-risk procedures or abandoning the practice of medicine altogether. ...

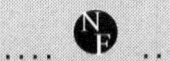

· · · ·   · · · ·

As much as I am tempted to feel a bit sorry for doctors who practice defensive medicine to protect themselves from malpractice claims, when you get right down to the bare bones of basic human values, if we are our brothers' and sisters' keepers in the truest sense of the word, then we have no right to take risks with other people's lives. All the more so if we have taken an oath to "First, do no harm."

As modern medicine is controlled by the insurance industry (which makes most of its profits from investment, not premiums), where procedures are assigned a certain fee, one must also be aware of unnecessary tests performed merely because they are covered by insurance. Here's an actual account provided by my friend, Dr. Randall Nozawa, DDS.

> *My wife went into the emergency room with a bout of serious food poisoning. The attending ER doctor decided a pregnancy test was warranted, even though she assured the doctor she was on schedule with her cycle, and at the age of 39 years, after three pregnancies, she knew her body well enough to guarantee she was indeed **not** pregnant. He **insisted**, so she took the test.*
>
> *Of course it came back negative, but his claim at that point was, "Well, you must be having a miscarriage, so then the next thing he did was order a catheter inserted, an ultrasound, and a CAT scan.*
>
> *After poking two poorly inserted IVs in each of her arms, they prepared to sent her home with a shot of pain medicine. Then the ER doctor asked her, "How do you feel knowing you're pregnant at **your** age?" Her response was, "How do you feel knowing you are WRONG, and you've caused me a lot of unnecessary pain, suffering, and expenses?*
>
> *Two days later, she ended up back in another hospital with a staph infection from the poorly inserted IVs. She demanded that her records from the first hospital be faxed to the new hospital. Nowhere on their records did they indicate that she was pregnant.*

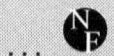

• • • •   • • • •

Needless to say, if doctors paid proper attention to their medical responsibilities and less to their watches or bank accounts, there would be far fewer malpractice lawsuits. Simply put, doctors are not heeding their sworn oath to "First, do no harm." They are doing great harm, resulting in a multitude of malpractice cases, as well as contributing to those 195,000 unnecessary and preventable deaths yearly in hospitals.

An example:

$17.1 MILLION AWARDED IN MALPRACTICE SUIT
Brain damage to baby results in huge verdict
The Associated Press—April 19, 2005

A woman who sued a hospital and two doctors over brain damage to her son, who nearly bled to death in the womb, has been awarded $17.1 million by a Snohomish County Superior Court jury. ...

... [The] case centered on an ultrasound examination that was performed before she gave birth to her son, Benjamin.

Because of a rare medical condition called fetal maternal hemorrhage, the child lost 75 percent of his blood before birth, had to be resuscitated after an emergency delivery by Caesarean section and was left with serious brain damage, impaired vision and cerebral palsy. ...

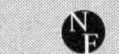

And in Florida, a judge recently awarded parents of a disabled child $60.9 million because doctors waited too long to perform a Cesarean section to deliver a child, The boy, now two, cannot see or swallow, or move his arms or legs. Doctors say he will not live past 21.

So don't climb on the sympathy bandwagon for doctors complaining about the high cost of insurance.

Furthermore, for all of you doctor lovers—and so many millions of you are out there—the next time you immediately come to their defense, ask yourself how many homeless, uninsured, poverty-stricken physicians you know.

Then think about the *one million* innocent individuals who died needlessly in hospitals in the last five years. Think about them. Visualize them: **Almost twice the number of people who live in the city of Seattle**—all lifeless because doctors didn't give a damn about the sworn oath they took. Where is your compassion for these people? They had as much right to life as the doctors and all others responsible for this slaughter.

* * *

I also have a closing thought on the question of malpractice awards and tort reform. According to a 2004 study by the Congressional Budget Office, malpractice costs account for less than 2 percent of total healthcare spending. The same study estimates that even a reduction of 25 to 30 percent in malpractice costs would lower healthcare costs by less than half of 1 percent.

This proves that the issue is really a gigantic bone used to cover up essential problems.

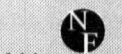

. . . .

The answers to lowering the fiscal effects of medical malpractice lie not with arbitrarily limiting compensation to injured patients, but with bolstering identification and discipline of corrupt doctors and better regulation of the medical malpractice insurance industry.

Pardon me (again) but I have an added thought on this subject of malpractice liability: In November 2005, Washingtonian doctors and lawyers went at it hot and heavy over voter initiatives (I-330 and I-336) that offered Washingtonians new guidelines favorable to their particular malpractice liability needs. It was a typical catfight between the two greedy rascals, filled with accusations, overbearing judgments supported by allied factions, and an all-out attempt to look good at the opposition's expense.

And did the doctors ever spend money on these underdone initiatives that hardly addressed the essential problems related to liability claims! They invested huge amounts in the hope of winning over votes.

In case you don't know, both initiatives were soundly defeated. And wouldn't you know it, three months later a compromise was reached in Olympia (the capital of the state of Washington). House Bill 2292 will not cap pain and suffering damages or automatically revoke the licenses of bad doctors, but it might help to settle some cases before they go to trial. This was hailed as a breakthrough.

Big deal! Just some cleverly constructed political nonsense that accomplishes next to nothing in the overall malpractice scheme of things.

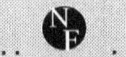

> I guarantee that the amount of time, energy, and money spent by doctors on their 2005 initiative campaign in the state of Washington alone far exceeds all the efforts that have ever been made by the entire medical profession in the last 100 years to protect the American public from the deadly pathology of smoking. That's a fact. An ugly one to look at, but a fact nonetheless. It reveals the true nature of their worldly goals.

Don't for a moment think that the aforementioned indictment is meant to absolve the lawyers of their unending devotion to making big bucks instead of being primarily concerned with such basic things as truth and justice. After all, the legal profession shares the overall responsibility for the deaths of millions of smokers from cancer and emphysema because it was the one who protected the tobacco industry from prosecution. And it did it for the holy dollar—just like the doctors who ignored their noble oath because they were too busy raking in the money.

Just to give you a clear perspective on the true nature of malpractice insurance, for every one report I've seen on the vastly more important issue of the lack of adequate health insurance for Americans (85 million uninsured or underinsured—and the number continues to grow!), there have been 40 to 50 reports on malpractice insurance. Do you get the picture?

I must add another jarring note to the healthcare insurance issue: Did you know that the banking industry is now positioning to cut a slice of the healthcare business for itself? In fact, it wants to become big players in the business of healthcare. And left to its own devious devices, it will corner a new market—health savings accounts. That's what's on the horizon. **Move over conglomerate, and make room for another bunch of profit-fixated devils to add to the sick picture of American healthcare.**

> *Judging from the tone of your accusations, you reduce the entire medical profession and the conglomerate to little more than a scandalous breed of charlatans, killers, and drug dealers. Is this the case?*

You got it! My tone and attitudes reflect the truth about the medical profession and the conglomerate as a whole. And the quotes contained in this section of the book reflect the opinions of many doctors and medical organizations that are equally appalled by these existing conditions and realities.

As I've already accused the conglomerate of mass murder and labeled them the most dangerous drug dealers in the world, let us look at their lesser crimes, which fall under the category of medical scandals.

You might read up on one case at the University of Washington (UW) in 2004, where more than a decade after whistleblowers began trying to expose and end a fraudulent medical billing system, and just days after news reports focused on the failure of its top medical school officials to end illegal practices, the medical school announced plans for an "independent" internal review of its Medicare rip-offs.

This reminded me of many independent investigations of dozens of prison facilities throughout America, most notably the infamous Women's House of Detention in Greenwich Village during the 1960s (when I was heavily involved in prison reform). My comparison lies in the corrupt scheme to whitewash the truth by means of a supposed internal investigation or review. The results of these findings always end up the same way, showing that conditions are not nearly as bad as reported and that great progress has been made to remedy the problems. That's what's known as "the Blarney spin."

Here's the way the University of Washington scandal unfolded:

SELF-DIAGNOSIS
UW launches a lessons-learned probe
of a medical scandal that just won't go away
Rick Anderson, *Seattle Weekly*—June 16–22, 2004

... University Vice President for Medical Affairs Paul Ramsey says he wants a committee to determine what lessons can be learned from the scandal—although one of those lessons is already painfully obvious: On the same day Ramsey announced his review, last Thursday, June 10, the university paid $35 million to the government to settle a civil lawsuit resulting from record-setting Medicare fraud. ...

... Nonetheless, the university, which also spent at least $25 million in legal fees the past five years and watched two of its doctors admit to felonies in connection with the billings, maintains that the "vast majority" of questioned billings "were unintentional mistakes," and admits no wrongdoing.

Can you imagine this colossal scam described as "unintentional mistakes?" This proved to be a well-organized machine designed to overbill Medicare for procedures that were not performed, **often by doctors who weren't even there!**

Here's another connection to this scandal:

DOCTOR CONVICTED IN UW BILLING FRAUD
LOSES BID TO END PROBATION

Seattle Post-Intelligencer staff and news services—May 10, 2005

Judge Robert Lasnik refused yesterday to end the probation of a former University of Washington physician convicted as part of a major investigation into billing fraud at the university.

Lasnik ruled that Dr. H. Richard Winn would have to serve the 2½ years remaining on his probation.

However, Lasnik offered to write a letter to New York State's medical board encouraging it to allow the neurosurgeon to practice there. Winn is working as a researcher at the Mount Sinai School of Medicine.

In his 2003 guilty plea, Winn admitted to obstructing justice by asking UW employees to keep information from investigators looking into overbilling of Medicare and Medicaid at the UW.

How does that grab you? This character doesn't even serve any hard time for a felony crime, but he's got a judge offering to help him avoid the full measure of his probation. Yeah, babe, we've got two systems of justice in America—one for the conglomerate, the other for Mr. and Mrs. John Q. Public. Better believe it!

The conglomerate, like all the despots in history, believes that "might is right" and will yield nothing to the common man, woman, and child seeking truth, justice, and peace.

The aforementioned scandal not only illustrates the extent to which the conglomerate's charter members will go to defraud the public, but it also highlights the fact that a major university, even when convicted of fraud involving tens of millions of dollars, will not admit to any wrongdoing. Beyond that wholesale denial of indisputable facts, thousands of UW students were exposed to this decade-long scandal—and you can wonder about the negative lessons they learned.

Here's another true story about the henchmen of the conglomerate:

BIG DRUG MAKER TO PLEAD GUILTY IN MEDICAID CASE

Gardiner Harris, *The New York Times*—July 16, 2004

The drug giant Schering-Plough has agreed to pay $350 million in fines and plead guilty to criminal charges that it cheated the federal Medicaid program, according to people close to the negotiations.

The settlement, expected to be announced next week with federal prosecutors in Philadelphia, stems from a six-year investigation prompted by three whistle-blowers who accused Schering-Plough of selling its products to private health care providers for far less than it sold them to Medicaid. Federal law requires drug makers to offer their lowest prices to Medicaid, the federal and state health program for the poor.

Although the settlement is not yet final, Schering-Plough is expected to admit that it gave grants to the private providers to conduct patient education and marketing programs as part of a kickback scheme to induce them to buy Schering-Plough's drugs at relatively high prices.

Schering-Plough then billed Medicaid authorities at those higher prices—without giving the offsetting grants. ...

Although this is a criminal case that involves $350 million in fines, there's no mention of anyone going to prison, is there? Why not? Some poor slob who tries to hoodwink people out of a couple of thousand bucks will serve hard time, but conglomerate members merely pay fines, go home to their mansions, and try to figure out their next multimillion-dollar scheme. Another example of the American caste system at work.

And as for the $350 million in fines, who benefits from it? The same conglomerate. What goes around comes around.

A further note on the Schering-Plough case:

FEDS PROBE "PAYOFFS" BY DRUG COMPANY

Gardiner Harris, *The New York Times*—June 27, 2004

... Details of the Schering-Plough tactics, gleaned from interviews with 20 doctors, as well as industry executives and people close to the investigation, shed light on the shadowy system of financial lures that pharmaceutical companies have used to persuade physicians to favor their drugs.

Schering-Plough's tactics, these people said, included paying doctors large sums to prescribe its drug for hepatitis C and to take part in company-sponsored clinical trials that were little more than thinly disguised marketing efforts that required little effort on the doctors' part. Doctors who showed disloyalty by testing other company's drugs, or even talking favorably about them, risked being barred from the Schering-Plough money stream. ...

... At the heart of the investigations into drug-industry marketing is the question of whether drug companies are persuading doctors—often through payoffs—to prescribe drugs that patients do not need, or should not use, or for which there may be cheaper alternatives. Investigators also are seeking to determine whether companies manipulate prices to cheat the federal Medicaid and Medicare health programs. ...

... In many ways, the investigations are a response to the evolution of the pharmaceutical business, which has grown into a $400 billion behemoth that is among the most profitable industries on earth.

... Offering treatments for almost any affliction and facing competition in which each percentage point of market share can represent tens of millions of dollars, most drug makers now spend twice as much on marketing medicines as they do researching them. ...

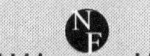

If you really want perspective on just how rich and powerful these drug companies are, try this on for size: Although the lawsuits and criminal charges regarding the weight-reducing drug Fen-Phen have yet to hit the courts, we can expect those fines and awards to total billions of dollars. In fact, Fen-Phen's manufacturer, Wyeth, has put aside more than $16 billion to compensate victims. The lawyers are salivating!

Can you imagine how much money this company rakes in—to have $16 billion in reserve to pay claims? It must be its petty cash fund!

Just in case you haven't figured out why these companies have such large cash reserves for these claims, **it's because they knew—all along—that their product was dangerous.**

To continue with this story ...

> *... Pfizer agreed last month to pay $430 million and pleaded guilty to criminal charges involving the marketing of the pain drug Nuerontin by the company's Warner-Lambert unit. AstraZeneca paid $355 million last year, and TAP Pharmaceuticals paid $875 million in 2001; each pleaded guilty to criminal charges of fraud for inducing physicians to bill the government for some drugs that the company gave the doctors free. ...*

Unless you can't read or are afflicted with a serious mind disorder (and I attack the general mentality of the public because of the extent to which it continues to ignore the conglomerate's monumental deceit and criminality), the above stories spell out three things:

1. Drug companies manipulate prices to cheat federal Medicaid and Medicare health programs.
2. Doctors are bribed to prescribe drugs that patients do not need, or should not use, or can be purchased at a cheaper cost. Talk about undermining health-care!
3. Drug makers are more interested in marketing than research.

The conglomerate fully expects the American public to go along with its scandalous affairs. And you know what? The public will. The reasons for this are quite elemental: By and large, the public refuses to confront those who participate in the conglomerate's criminal actions because it is afraid to get on the "wrong side"; doctors are treated as "special people"; and the general view is that physicians can do no wrong—even when they're caught stealing millions of dollars or amputating the wrong limb of a patient.

We let doctors get away with murder and defend them with vehemence—while at the same time we would condemn almost anyone else for a slight infraction of the law. Another grotesque aspect of the American caste system in action. The conglomerate knows this and takes full advantage, to the tune of hundreds of billions of dollars and the loss of millions of innocent lives.

✳ ✳ ✳

While we're on the subject of medical scandal, let us examine another highly revealing reality about our hospitals.

CHARITY HEADS' SALARIES SOAR ABOVE INFLATION RATE, STUDY SAYS

Siobhan McDonough, The Associated Press—September 20, 2004

... Salaries of leaders of 309 of the largest non-profit organizations were reviewed in 2003. ...

... The four top earners surveyed worked at hospitals: Harold Varmus, president of the Memorial Sloan-Kettering Cancer Center in New York, and Floyd Loop, chief executive of Cleveland Clinic Foundation, both of whom earned $1.7 million in 2003; Herbert Pardes, chief executive of New York-Presbyterian Hospital, $1.3 million; and Peter Traber, president of the Baylor College of Medicine, $1.2 million. ...

Besides the fact that these salaries don't include perks, this is the message that comes across:

1. These are not true nonprofit organizations in any sense of the term, yet profit-making in an all-but-legal definition.

2. These "heads" need not worry that their donors will stop giving to their charities because of such high salaries. Not knowing any better, the ignorant public will shell out its bucks any day of the week and twice on Sundays to support these charlatan institutions, or simply to gain a tax deduction.

3. The conglomerate will observe all the little ruckuses made by these revelations, only to continue to look down at the public and treat them as swine to be had.

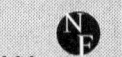

Here's an interesting comparison: While these nonprofit hospitals

pay their chief executives millions of dollars a year, Jim Sinegal, the chief executive of Costco Wholesale Club, the fifth-largest retailer in the U.S., receives a yearly salary of only $350,000.
Way to go, Jim!

While I'm on this subject, I should point out some startling facts:

- The current salary gap between CEOs and workers stands at 431 to 1, which compares to a gap of 107 to 1 in 1990.

- If salaries of workers kept up with the paychecks of CEOs, the average worker would be paid over $110,000.

- If the minimum wage had risen at the same rate, workers would now earn $23 an hour.

- Since 1997 the federal minimum wage has remained at $5.15 per hour. While this continues, on June 13, 2006, House lawmakers approved a $3,300 pay raise that increases their salaries to $168,500. This 2-percent cost-of-living raise is the seventh straight for members of both houses of Congress (in spite of their record low approval ratings)!

- On June 21, 2006, by a 52–46 vote, the Republican-controlled Senate defeated a proposed increase in the minimum wage from $5.15 to $5.85. The vote was 8 short of the 60 needed for approval.

All of this speaks volumes about the overall living standards of people of different classes, not to mention the disparity in healthcare. Beyond that, it clearly illustrates that our present political system, with its range of slogans about patriotism, fighting terrorism, and concern for the American public, tolerates a living standard that condemns tens of millions of Americans (including veterans) to living in near-poverty conditions—with no hope to achieve the American Dream.

So please—someone—tell me who our GIs are fighting for?

Here's another recent report that caught my attention:

EXPERIMENT VOLUNTEERS KEPT IN DARK BY SCIENTISTS
Patients not told of NIH researcher's financial interests

John Solomon, The Associated Press—January 4, 2005

Government scientists have collected millions of dollars in royalties for experimental treatments without having to tell patients testing the treatments that the researchers had a financial connection, according to documents and interviews.

The personal royalties are legal, though the researchers developed the treatments at government expense. But the Health and Human Services Department promised in May 2000 that scientists' financial stakes would be disclosed to patients, a pledge that followed an uproar over conflicts of interest and mistakes in federal experiments.

The National Institutes of Health says it didn't implement a policy to order the disclosure until last week, shortly after the Associated Press filed a Freedom of Information Act request. ...

... The nearly five-year delay means hundreds, perhaps thousands, of patients in NIH experiments made decisions to participate in experiments that often carry risks without full knowledge about the researchers' financial interests.

"It's hard for patients to make an informed decision when they don't have all the information," said Bill Allison of the Center for Public Integrity, which monitors the ethics of government employees. ...

... In all, 916 current and former NIH researchers are receiving royalty payments for drugs and other inventions they developed while working for the government, according to information obtained by AP. ... In 2004, these researchers collected a total of $8.9 million. ...

... The government owns the patents and the scientists are listed as inventors so they can share in licensing deals struck with private manufacturers. ...

... The arrangements can create concerns about conflicts. ...

Another illustration of just how much deceit and corruption exists within the overall structure of the American healthcare system. And as always—the ignorant public be damned!

And yet another scandalous story:

EXCESSIVE MEDICAL EXPENSES:
STUDY FINDS THAT HALF OF
HEALTH CARE DOLLARS ARE WASTED

Victoria Colliver, *San Francisco Chronicle*—February 9, 2005

About 50 percent of health care spending is eaten up by waste, excessive prices and fraud, according to a report set for release today by Boston University researchers. ...

... "If half of health care spending is wasted now, that's $950 billion this year. If we could save even a third of waste, we'd save over $300 billion this year," said Alan Sager, co-director of the health reform program at Boston University's School of Public Health and co-author of the report. ...

... "We know there is enough money to take care of everyone, but not if we keep practicing blank-check mentality and using cost controls that have failed for decades," he said. ...

There certainly is more than enough money to take care of everyone. The problem, however, is that America must first manifest a desire and will to be *its brothers' and sisters' keepers*. Then we must parcel out its services in a fair and responsible way. But that's impossible under present conditions—no matter how much money is available. There's just too much corruption.

A closing medical scandal:

SCAM COSTS INSURERS MILLIONS
Thousands have unneeded surgery, tests in health fraud

Robert Pear, *The New York Times*—March 12, 2005

Twelve Blue Cross and Blue Shield plans, working with the FBI, said yesterday they had broken up an elaborate insurance scam in which thousands of patients from 47 states were sent to California to undergo unnecessary surgical and diagnostic procedures, for which doctors filed more than $1 billion of fraudulent insurance claims.

Insurance executives and law enforcement officials said that surgery clinics in Southern California typically paid recruiters $2,000 to $4,000 for each patient who received a medical procedure. The patients, they said, received rewards in the form of cash or discounts on cosmetic surgery. ...

... The Blue Cross and Blue Shield plans filed a civil lawsuit Thursday against nine surgery clinics, 21 doctors and 13 people

described as owners, employees or administrators of the clinics. The Justice Department and the district attorney in Orange County, Calif., have filed criminal charges against some of the defendants. ...

You just gotta love those doctors!

I know I said "closing medical scandal," but I couldn't possibly leave this one out because it's another incredible example of just how far the conglomerate goes next to rake money in from every possible source—no matter how outrageous and corrupt the practice is.

DRUG RESEARCHERS LEAK SECRETS TO WALL ST.

Luke Timmerman and David Heath, *Seattle Times*—August 7, 2005

Despite confidentiality contracts, doctors are divulging details of their ongoing drug research—for a fee—to elite investors eager to get an edge in the market. Experts say the practice breaks insider-trading laws, violates medical ethics and jeopardizes vital research. And the government regulators seem to know nothing about it.

Doctors testing new drugs are sworn to keep their research secret until drug companies announce the final results. But elite Wall Street firms—looking to make quick profits—have found a way to harvest these secrets:

They pay doctors to divulge the details early.

A Seattle Times *investigation found at least 26 cases in which doctors have leaked confidential and critical details of their ongoing drug research to Wall Street firms.*

The practice involves doctors at top research universities from UCLA to the University of Pennsylvania, and powerful financial firms including Citigroup Smith Barney, UBS and Wachovia Securities.

In 24 of the 26 cases, the firms issued reports to select clients with detailed information obtained from doctors involved in confidential studies. The reports advised clients whether to buy or sell a drug stock.

Trading stock based on secret information bought from medical researchers is illegal, say legal experts who were told of The Times' *findings.*

"That's a good way to go to jail," said lawyer Thomas Newkirk, former associate director of enforcement at the Securities and Exchange Commission (SEC). ...

... Until now, the selling of drug secrets has been hidden from securities regulators and the public, but biotech and Wall Street insiders said the practice is widespread.

The investigation also revealed this statement by Arthur Caplan, Director, Center for Bioethics, University of Pennsylvania:

"The practice is a moral cesspool."

Hah, hah, hah! The doctors are at it again. Off and running. And considering their behavior from the starting gate to the finish line, it's time we changed their sworn oath from "First, do no harm" to "First, grab the dough and run!"

As for the drug research leak practice being a moral cesspool, you bet it is. And not unlike typical conglomerate "outreach," the doctors—bless their corrupt hearts—are right up to their necks in the slime.

The big question: Will these people do hard time in prison? That's if you call Martha Stewart's form of captivity hard time. Sounds more like a slap on the wrist instead, and another way of telling America that two forms of justice rule: one for the rich, another for the poor.

As for this insider practice being widespread, you would have to be a complete fool to believe otherwise.

> *From your earliest mention of your family physician Dr. Warpick to your present attitude about doctors, I wonder if you have ever met a doctor you liked and respected?*

You bet I have—he was one of the finest human beings I have ever had the pleasure to know. Dr. Abraham Shiffman operated a small private clinic on Spring Street in New York (just a few blocks from where I worked at the headquarters of Encounter) back in the 1960s. He ministered to everyone who walked in the door, no matter who you were or how much money you had.

His waiting room was always crowded with people of all ages and social and economic standing and backgrounds, from laborers to pregnant women to children with dozens of different ailments. From morning to night, Dr. Shiffman welcomed them with open arms. In between treating patients he came into the waiting room and gave everyone a fond hello, a warm hug, or a joke to lighten their burden.

I remember him approaching a middle-aged man with the flu and asking him a series of questions. "Are you feverish? Coughing a lot? Headachy? Feeling miserable?" The man answered "yes" to all these questions. Dr. Shiffman put his arm around the man and said, "Then what are you doing here? You should go and find a good doctor!"

This self-effacing, gregarious physician was one of the most discerning and generous individuals you'd ever meet. He regarded each person with understanding and compassion, never making anyone concerned about the cost for treatment. He would size you up and when it came time to pay your bill, he would make it a fun experience by saying something like, "You look like you're flush today—so I want 100 pennies—and not a penny less!" or "When was the last time you brought me a pastrami on rye?"

When it came time to give a prescription, more often than not he would reach into his private pharmacy and give you pills at no cost.

This mensch not only lived by the Hippocratic oath, but he also gave of himself tirelessly and loved his work and his patients.

Dr. Shiffman was a joy to know and it's a joy remembering him. I say to all of you doctors out there—*you should be just like him!*

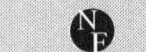

Don't think that I don't know that lots of good doctors are out there who are just as dedicated to their patients as Dr. Shiffman was—I salute each and every one of them.

But you must remember—this book wasn't written for the purpose of praising anyone, but for dealing with serious problems, specifically obesity. And after examining the obesity topic and other related issues for so many years, I've expanded it to include the overall healthcare issue in America.

I also want to emphasize that there are 5,000 praise-givers for every one whistleblower and confronter. I am the confronter. That's my calling.

Furthermore, for those doctors who take offense at my confrontational attitude, I wouldn't have to be writing these words or feeling so much anger toward your profession if you were doing your jobs and upholding your sworn oath. **So blame yourselves!**

> ### *Where did these doctors go wrong?*

Most of their professional and personal problems can be traced to parents who drove them to be successful doctors—in much the same way that stage mothers drive their children to be famous stars. Starting early on, these kids study like crazy to attain the good grades that will get them into the best medical schools. In the process, they miss out on the normal social activities that would give them the balance they badly need.

By the time they start the long process of becoming physicians, they are already in harm's way, faced with endless, brutal study and continued social deprivation, and are caught up in their incessant need to succeed.

But this is only the beginning of their troubles. Once they graduate, they have to fulfill their internship requirements. In case you don't know, we're talking about work schedules that are gruesome. Whoever invented these torturous training programs should be thrown in a cage with some angry pit bulls!

. . . .

I recently talked with an acquaintance whose wife is serving her internship in a Washington state hospital. He told me that his wife, who's a surgeon, was working 120 hours a week! That's roughly 18 hours a day, if you're counting it as a seven-day week. Needless to say, no one should be working 18 hours a day, especially someone who is operating on patients. It's dangerous! And there are laws against it.

However, the administrators running these hospitals circumvent the laws and do as they damn well please, in spite of the severe risks involved for the patients as well as the overworked doctors. No wonder 195,000 people are killed in hospitals yearly. I said *killed*, not *died*—because that's what it is.

By the time these interns receive their credentials and begin to practice medicine, they are, for the most part, miserable human beings who will, with few exceptions, do great harm and damage to themselves and society. If you doubt this, then ask yourself why so many of them abuse drugs, lead unhappy lives in spite of their success, and commit suicide.

The same goes for the dentists and lawyers who are put through the same sequence of schooling and are just as full of themselves as the doctors. *They're all badly damaged goods.*

Thank God that some of them manage to right their misguided course and recover their souls.

A closing thought on doctors: I think that there was a major shift in patient treatment when doctors became "specialists." Until then, the general practitioner, also regarded (affectionately, at that) as the "family doctor," had to stay up- to-date on his knowledge and connected to the latest medical advancements—or else lose patients.

In the process, if a doctor was treating you for a particular ailment, he also had to be prepared for whatever else he might come across. If you came to him complaining of chest pain, and the doctor discovered that you had an ulcer, he could (and would) do something about it. That's no longer the case.

In fact, today's specialists will ignore obvious signs of "other problems" and focus only on their special field. This is bad medicine.

To make matters much worse, these doctors who specialize in one area of medicine often do not keep abreast of other fields of medicine. Thus they are no longer equipped to recognize other medical problems, which could result in the neglect of a potentially life-threatening illness. It's one reason why we have so many emergency situations that could have been avoided had the individual received timely treatment.

Coupled with the confusing maze of interconnected regulations and insurance obstacles, this modern-day form of medical practice adds considerably to the decline of healthcare in America.

We need to get back to basics.

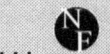

Specialized medicine, as practiced by most doctors (including dentists) is a financial bonanza for everyone but the patient. All the doctors get their slice of the medical action, and the patient needs to visit any number of specialists to deal with his varied ailments. That's very costly. Even more so if you're among the many millions who are uninsured or underinsured. In a word, it's a racket.

> *Since you lump all doctors together,*
> *do you have any choice words about dentists?*

My first memorable encounter with one of them came at the age of 11, just after my family moved to Brooklyn. My father walked me over to a dentist's office just a few blocks from his restaurant. This dentist was young, friendly, and had a big smile on his face. He gave me a thorough dental exam and asked my father to step into his private office, while I remained in the dental chair.

I realized that my father, with his poor English, might not understand everything the dentist would say, so I got out of the chair and listened to the conversation. I could hardly forget a word of it!

"Mr. Karpodines, your son has perfect teeth. They are a remarkable specimen. Not one child in a million has teeth like that. The reason I'm telling you this is that I'm attending a dental convention in Chicago this summer, and as part of the convention the American Dental Association is putting together an exhibit of perfect teeth from every age group. And if you agree to it... I can arrange to pay you a good sum of money for your son's teeth. And you have nothing to worry about because we'll provide him with a set of dentures. What do you think?"

I didn't wait to hear my father's response, as I knew he would refuse the offer. I just walked out of the office and roamed around Brooklyn, all the while wishing that dentist would drop dead. Imagine, he wanted to pull all of my teeth and exhibit them at a convention. That fucking ghoul.

The experience had a terrible psychological effect on me. I stopped caring for my teeth and when I started having serious dental problems, I wouldn't think of going to a dentist. I just toughed it out. Even on the day of my first wedding, when I had a badly abscessed wisdom tooth, I still wouldn't consider getting professional help.

The long-range effect of all this dental trauma was that my teeth gradually went to pot.

Before you get around to asking if I ever met a dentist I liked and respected, the answer is yes. The first one, believe it or not, was a distant second cousin whom I met in Athens, Greece, in 1968. She turned out to be a marvelous dental surgeon who served me a lovely continental breakfast every morning for 10 days and proceeded to cap my entire disheveled mouth—for less than $300! For all the years that we lived in Greece, she treated my family's dental needs as her own. A Greek mensch!

The second dental gem came to me by instinct alone. It happened 30 years after my Greek cousin capped my mouth. By this time, the crowns had completely deteriorated, and as Seattle dentists wanted between $27,000 and $33,000 to restore my mouth, I was at a loss.

One morning, I got one of those buzzes in my brain, which I've learned over the years to follow. It told me to look in the Yellow Pages under Dentists. Without knowing what to expect, I thumbed through the pages and when I came to "The Smile Guy," Dr. Randall Nozawa, I knew I had hit pay dirt. I called and explained my situation, including the important part about my lack of dental insurance. After some squabbling with the receptionist, I managed to schedule an appointment.

I was greeted by a powerful-looking man in dungarees, a bodybuilder and trainer, as well as a dentist, who, after an initial exam, asked me about myself. Learning that I had writing and publishing skills as well as a background in the movie industry, he offered to do my teeth in exchange for help in writing a book on dentistry *(Inside Dentistry—Everything You Need to Know)* and teaching him to write a movie. A barter arrangement with a dentist! Can you believe it? Thus I ended up with a perfect smile for the rest of my life, a book credit that I'm proud of, and a dear friend.

Randall is one of the few dentists who has treated the poor, AIDS victims, and those with HIV. He is a super dentist and an equally super human being, unlike 99 percent of his dental cohorts, who are as unfeeling and greedy as they come. Without hesitation I label them as thoughtless and uncaring about so many people in desperate need of dental care.

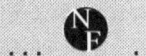

Dentists are, by and large, a shameless breed, even more so than medical practitioners; this is because most doctors, when put in a position of having to treat someone without insurance or cash, will at least try to do something. Not so for dentists. They'll just say "adios"—that is, if you're even lucky enough to get past their receptionists. **There are no emergency rooms for dental patients.** Another terrible weakness in our healthcare system.

You may think that I can't find worse things to say about dentists, but that's not the case. Here's something that really describes their lack of concern, decency, and humanity. Native Alaskan children suffer the pain of tooth decay and other serious mouth problems on a much greater scale than others with better access to dental treatment. But the American Dental Association (ADA) is steadfast in its opposition to dental therapists who would work with the Alaskan Native Tribal Health Consortium to train Alaskan natives to become dental therapists.

Although performance evaluations of dental therapists are uniformly favorable (in many cases the therapists are better trained to provide care to children than the dentists are), the ADA would rather see these children go without badly needed dental care.

To further illustrate the unyielding mentality of the ADA, no therapist program has ever seen the light of day in an American university. In fact, the Washington State Dental Association intimidated University of Washington officials who were supportive of such a dental therapist program by threatening to block donations by their members.

The rich and powerful conglomerate cohorts who control American dentistry are responsible for untold suffering among the indigenous peoples (as well as millions of others) and are therefore guilty of *crimes against humanity.*

The thought of having to find a dentist makes most Americans feel sick!

> ### *Where do nurses fit into*
> ### *your healthcare equation?*

Generally speaking, nurses are overworked, underpaid, and do not receive the respect they deserve. They are used by doctors, forced to work under duress and subjugation, do much of the dirty work (quite literally), and receive disproportionate blame for poor patient care.

Adding to their problems, laws exist that create dangerous working conditions for nurses, who bear the brunt of patient care, while the doctors make their leisurely rounds. Here's a major case in point: California's 1999 law,[15] which took effect in 2004, is the first in the nation to mandate fixed nurse-to-patient ratios after takeovers of community hospitals by for-profit chains led to cutbacks. But after the November 2004 election, California Governor Arnold Schwarzenegger's

---

[15] A regulation that was signed into law by former California Governor Gray Davis, which established a ratio of one nurse to every five patients in California hospitals.

officials loosened requirements for nurse staffing and emergency rooms, and delayed (until 2008) putting into effect a ruling requiring a one-to-five nurse-to-patient ratio for medical-surgical units.

In many ways, nursing can be a thankless profession, but thank God for it. Nurses are one saving grace in the midst of all the medical profession's chaos and greed. My only argument with nurses is that they have failed to join ranks sufficiently on a national level so that they might inform and better enlighten the public of the faltering conditions within hospitals. Their united voice could be a beacon of light within the darkness of the conglomerate's shameful world.

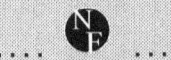

On November 11, 2005, acting on behalf of Governor Schwarzenegger, Attorney General Bill Lockyer dropped the legal battle over the state rule requiring one nurse for every five patients. That's a win for the good guys!

How do nursing homes fare in your estimation?

They range from excellent to infamous. Depending on location, staffing, and economic factors, they can provide adequate to exceptional healthcare services to our elderly and disabled—or they can be death camps. I've seen and heard of both these types.

This much I can state with assuredness: *Under most conditions, when a nursing home patient's money or insurance runs out—look out!*

Furthermore, we need to do a much better job of overseeing what goes on in nursing homes. Too much abuse and neglect go unreported. As a result, thousands of people who are unable to care for themselves fall through the cracks and never recover. What better example do you need than what happened as a result of Hurricane Katrina, when many nursing home patients were left behind to die. There were even numerous television reports and accusations of "putting patients to sleep." On July 18, 2006, a doctor and two nurses were arrested after the state attorney general accused them of using lethal injections to deliberately kill four elderly New Orleans hospital patients during the aftermath of Hurricane Katrina.

Once again, the American caste system is hard at work.

What about mental hospitals?

Here's a generality that unfortunately holds more water than Lake Superior: Most of these places should be shut down, and the staffs arrested for a wide assortment of criminal actions against their patients. Look, it's so damn easy to take complete advantage of people locked away in these terrible hell-holes—especially when these helpless patients are drugged and incapable of defending themselves.

To take it one grizzly step further, there's very little in the way of oversight because (1) it's a low priority, so funds are not available; (2) patients are usually left in the hands of underpaid and inexperienced attendants who are apt to take criminal advantage of these people; (3) medical staffs are limited, so they rely primarily on the use of drugs rather than trying to counsel patients; and (4) the public really doesn't give a damn! In fact, the only time any attention is given to this inhuman matter is when some reporter investigates and does a high-profile, award-winning story. Two weeks later, it's quickly forgotten.

Let's face it, millions of mentally and emotionally ill people have been abandoned. And those that are not locked away in the limited number of remaining institutions are wandering the streets. It's another national disgrace—and no one's going to do anything about it. Neither Republicans or Democrats are willing to take up the issue in earnest because they're all too busy feeding corporate thirst and war and terrorist efforts, as well as raising money for reelection.

Nursing homes and mental hospitals have numerous built-in problems that require renewed diligence and oversight. But we also have enormous problems related to outpatient services: One of the biggest is that registered counselors are guilty of professional misconduct on a grand scale. We're talking about widespread rape (politely referred to as "sexual misconduct") and any number of other crimes that are relatively easy for the counselors to get away with.

As hard as it may be to believe, in the state of Washington, you need only take a four-hour AIDS awareness class, pay a $40 registration fee—and you're a registered counselor! There's no other requirements, no intensive screening of applicants, no credentials necessary. Another healthcare fiasco.

> *Do you ever envision getting sick?*
> *And if so, who will treat you?*
>
> *Aren't you afraid that "they"*
> *will find out who you are and retaliate?*

All things being equal, there's every likelihood that I will eventually come down with something. But I expect it will be mild and that I'll get over it in a much shorter time than the average person because my strong immune system will go right to work on the problem. Unfettered from any drug weakness, it will do its job without any hassle.

As for any serious illness requiring actual medical assistance, my attitude is quite conceptual: I will do what upholds existence. If that means going to a doctor or hospital, I will take those measures as need be, as I did with the hernia operation.

I won't worry that some doctor will try to sabotage my recovery. I don't think they would want to set a live bomb like me loose. Can you imagine the headlines?!

> *If you did get sick,*
> *would you take prescription drugs?*

Again, I'll do what upholds existence. Needless to say, I want nothing to do with drugs, but if I have no other choice, I'll go with what I must do, which changes nothing concerning what I've said about medication.

As an example of my overall approach to this general question, in early November of 2005, I awoke one morning and found that the left side of my face was badly swollen. Apparently I had irritated an area of my gums with some overly aggressive flossing, and it had become infected and spread to the cheek area. Luckily, there was no pain, and I presumed that my teeth and gums were not infected.

I called my dentist friend Dr. Randall Nozawa for advice. After listening to my description of the problem, he outlined a simple treatment program involving swabbing the irritated gums with hydrogen peroxide and washing out my mouth with a mixture of lemon juice and salt.

There was no thought of medication. We would first try a number of other treatments. Drugs would only be a last resort.

The hydrogen peroxide and lemon and salt worked. Within 18 hours the swelling decreased considerably. And by the third day there was no sign of swelling and no other irritation.

Now here's my point: I'll bet you dollars to donuts that under the same conditions 99 percent of the American public would have immediately turned to their doctors and ended up at the prescription counter. That's how well-trained you have become.

Remember, if you take drugs indiscriminately, you're as much a junkie as any common street addict.

Do you ever think of death?

Yes, especially when I reached the age of 69. I suspect that it's a precursor to the age of 70, a number that, for whatever reason, conjures up one's mortality. In any case, when you're faced with serious illness, disease, or death, it often comes to us as a complete stranger and we refuse to let it into our lives. But if it's there, we must face it. As the famous Hollywood line goes, "everyone dies."

Having said that, "Out of X" something happened to me in mid-December, 2005, which made me all the more aware of my own mortality. I discovered blood in my stool, which is often an indicator of colorectal cancer, especially for someone who was 69 years old.

Luckily, I had already done research on the subject of colon cancer, which is the third most common cancer in both men and women. I decided on having a colonoscopy, which is the most reliable way of detecting polyps, tumors, and cancer in the colon.

The procedure is almost painless: A colonoscope is inserted through the rectum into the colon, allowing the doctor to see the lining of your entire colon. The colonoscope is also connected to a video camera and a display monitor so the doctor can closely examine the inside of your colon. All the while, you are fully awake and able to watch the display monitor and see everything that's going on.

Over the course of about 25 minutes, six polyps were discovered and painlessly removed from my colon. During the procedure, I asked the doctor several questions, including the all-important one: "Are they cancerous or benign?" Although it was not possible to make an absolute determination right then, he was of the opinion that "they are probably benign."

. . . .

I behaved well during my medical procedure. You see, I'm not against
medicine and doctors; I'm against bad medicine and bad doctors.

I anxiously waited out the next six days, hoping that the lab results would show
that the polyps were all benign, and when my doctor's nurse called me and gave
me the good news, I was more than just relieved—I was over the top.

Needless to say, my exceptional physical condition gave me good reason to
believe that I was not suffering from any cancer. However, for the record, here's
some feedback to all of you—men AND women—about colorectal cancer:

1. Colorectal cancer is the second most common cause of cancer death among
   men and women.

2. About 150,000 Americans will be diagnosed with colorectal cancer this year,
   and more than 55,000 will die from the disease.

3. It usually starts with a small growth called a polyp. If found early, the polyp
   can be removed, thus preventing cancer before it starts.

4. African-American men and women are diagnosed with and die from colon
   cancer at a higher rate than any other U.S. racial or ethnic group.

5. More than 90 percent of colon cancer cases occur in people 50 and older, so
   you should get tested for the disease starting at age 50. However, those with a
   family history of the disease should begin testing at a younger age.

6. Colon cancer is often highly treatable, and if discovered early and treated, the
   five-year survival rate is 90 percent.

7. Most importantly—get over any hangup you have about dealing with a rectal
   problem; I know it may seem embarrassing, but unless you can put that behind you (isn't that a great pun!) **you may well be signing your own death
   certificate.** This is a killer, and often a silent one—with little detectable signs
   of a serious problem. So get screened and save a life!

By the way, a recent pooled analysis of 13 studies involving 725,000 people found little evidence of a protective benefit for dietary fiber against colon cancer—which is a reversal of prior studies. (Wouldn't you know it!)

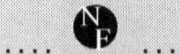

Something else I want to tag on to the general reality about the colon: Most medical people will tell you that death starts in the colon. I take exception to that; from everything that I have experienced, studied, and discovered, death begins in the mouth.

The mouth can be a safe haven for unwanted diseases and a focal point for disease transmission. Not only that, but it's the starting point for eating an unhealthy diet. It is where so many illnesses and lifelong problems begin, a distinct infection site for a germ invasion to enter to plunder the body. But we rarely pay attention to our mouths. We don't realize that it's where the action is! That opening allows the passage and circulation of things that can become systemic and do great harm to every part of the body. And, believe it or not, kissing can be more dangerous than sexual intercourse under certain conditions.

If you can visualize just how important your mouth is to your well-being, perhaps you can start treating it more appropriately and conscientiously. Give your mouth its due—and it will pay off for you like a jackpot!

If our healthcare system is so bad,
then how do you account for the fact
that our longevity continues to increase?

Any question of longevity is relative to what longevity represents—the number of years you live or the number of years of quality existence. My grandparents in Greece lived quality lives into their 90s. They lived without the benefit of drugs, doctors, clinics, or hospitals. Up until the end, they were robust and active, although they had lived through two dictatorships, two world wars, one civil war, and endured many deprivations over the years.

Their children, most of whom lived in Athens, lived quality lives into their 80s. Only my father, who immigrated to America, missed out on a quality life, dying of cancer at the age of 47. What does that tell you? Had he remained in Greece, he would have escaped his financial pressures, taken better care of himself, have been more in touch with his emotions (which were blunted by his American life-style), and not worked himself to death.

Because of drugs and other various medical procedures, we've managed to stretch out our lives well into our 70s, 80s, and even 90s, but at what cost to our *quality* of existence? How many of those years, especially after the age of 60, are quality years—free from illness, disease, drugs, medical procedures, and hospitalization?

And what do we look forward to in the closing years of our lives? I've had a good look at our senior citizens, and I'm not talking about the poor or downtrodden (we know how neglected they are). I'm talking about middle-class people who are fully insured and have the necessary means to exist under the best conditions. Better than 95 percent of them end up suffering from a variety of serious medical problems like obesity, diabetes, cancer, heart disease, stroke, arthritis, respiratory ailments, neurological disorders, Parkinson's disease, etc. They are placed on drug maintenance, remain under the constant care of their physicians, slipping in and out of hospitals, and **exhaust the remaining years of their lives for the conglomerate's benefit.**

And strange as it may seem (especially to younger people), these senior citizens accept this diminished quality of life as if it were normal. *No, no, no—it's not supposed to be that way!*

Because they have been programmed and trained from Day One to respect authority figures, especially their doctors, they will not complain or lift a finger in an attempt to change course and regain their lives. They will go to their graves believing that they've had a fair shake and that the powers that be provided them with the best medical treatment and care.

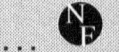

When our family lived in Greece, there was a slaughterhouse not far from our home. Whenever farmers brought their pigs to be dispatched, the poor animals knew what was going to happen even before they were taken into the abattoir, and they put up the fight of their lives. Not so for humans. We are willingly butchered by the conglomerate and never even complain, much less fight for our lives. That's because we have, over our lifetime, willingly given our bodies over to these killers and have been reduced to a shell of what we were meant to be—regardless of what the longevity charts tell us.

What madness! **We all deserve to live quality lives well into our 90s and beyond, free of the plethora of sicknesses that befall us.**

So you can stick your so-called longevity where it belongs—up the rectums of the bastards who infest our society with their drugs and medical procedures! I'll take 90 to 100 years of the good life, free of all junk and medical emergencies and insurance worries any day of the week and twice on Sunday—when I'll still be cooking roast chicken for my family and friends, and telling stories they've heard a hundred times.

A closing thought about longevity: Although the overall life expectancy for Americans has increased, we still trail many other countries, according to statistics from the World Health Organization, including Japan, Monaco, San Marino, Switzerland, Australia, Andorra, Iceland, Austria, Canada, Finland, France, Germany, Greece, Israel, Italy, Luxembourg, Malta, the Netherlands, New Zealand, Norway, Singapore, Spain, and the United Kingdom. What does that tell you?

Furthermore, if you factor in all the vital variables such as disabilities, living conditions, race and income, general lifestyle, future expectations, etc., and come up with an overall adjusted quality life expectancy, **you will find that ours is the worst of all the industrialized nations.**

As for the poor of America, life expectancy has little to do with a number; it's about having no life to live.

> ### *What's the secret of longevity?*

To begin with, we would do well to emulate those people who manage to live long, healthy, productive lives without drugs (including steroids and growth hormones), doctors, and hospitals. Who are these fortunate people? Well, if you research worldwide longevity charts, data, and other studies, you'll discover that most of them live in small, rural locations in either the Mediterranean region (like my grandparents) or in parts of rural Japan (like Okinawa) and Russia.

These long-lifers are usually married, eat good food (with a diet that includes lots of olive oil and red wine), are very active (lots of farmers and fishermen), and enjoy stress-free lives.

Needless to say, most Americans, especially those who live in big cities, can hardly subscribe to uncomplicated lifestyles; our desire for more money, goods, and materialistic security far outweighs thoughts of a simpler life. Consequently we suffer all the associated ills of a consumer society that requires more worldly things with which to encapsulate itself.

As we grow older, we pay a dear price for our indulgences, resulting in a diminishing quality of life that erodes any of the benefits we have accumulated over the course of our lives.

Does that mean we are necessarily doomed to such a pointless and hollow degeneration? My answer is no. Although we cannot regain that which we have missed out on during the decades of striving for the so-called American dream, we still have a good shot at settling for a much healthier form of survival in our later years. How? By following six basic rules:

- Do not use drugs unless there is absolutely no other option. In doing so, you will avoid the pitfalls that lead to serious illness and disease and open yourself to the possibility of quality longevity.

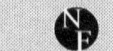

The cumulative effect of all the junk you've allowed (often "welcomed") into your body over the decades has, as I stated early in this book, reduced your immune system to a second-rate backup plan. Age further weakens it, leaving you susceptible to all manner of diseases.

This is partly why so many people in their late 40s to early 50s suddenly develop cancer and never again regain good health. Your only hope of countering that is to completely detoxify your body. That means NO DRUGS and a good cleansing program.

- Formulate a healthy, balanced diet that certainly should include lots of fruits and vegetables, olive oil, and red wine.

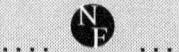

You don't have to be a health junkie to know what's good to eat and what's not. Hundreds of good books are available on the subject. All you need is common sense and the willpower to spend more time in the vegetable and fruit section of your grocer than in the snack department.

- Cleanse your system regularly.

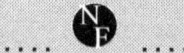

The toxins you've accumulated over a lifetime won't just go away. They'll kill you (in one way or another), even if you eat right, exercise, and abstain from drug use. They've got to be flushed out.

- Exercise! And I don't mean "moderately."

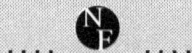

People who live the longest "quality" lives generally do not work out in health clubs, BUT they exercise strenuously on a daily basis. How? Their work provides them with a natural form of weightlifting and bodybuilding. That's what farming, fishing, construction work, and household chores are all about—heavy-duty labor.

Pushing, pulling, lifting, carrying, struggling with objects, and battling the elements—normal everyday activity that nourishes the soul and keeps the body at optimum strength and fitness. That's the stuff of good workouts! But if you're city-bound, join a club.

- Use supplements.

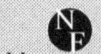

There are supplements, and there are supplements. Some (many!) are poor imitations of the real McCoys or even worthless fakes that are possibly dangerous to your health. How do you know which ones to use and which to keep away from? To be quite frank, you have to get off your butt and do some really serious research. That means spending many hours on the Internet reading up on the subject, talking with knowledgeable people, learning to decipher the labels on supplement containers and health food products, evaluating your personal needs, and then keeping track of the actual results. Lots of work. But infinitely worth all the hard effort, both to your health and pocketbook.

- **DON'T SMOKE!**

You don't need any more facts about smoking—it's deadly. Period. And there's little point talking about secrets to longevity if you're a smoker.

Aside from the fact that you should follow these basic rules because they uphold your existence, you should also realize that by practicing good health you are showing concern for those people to whom you have a lifetime commitment.

Understand this: Should you fail to do everything in your power to live a healthy existence—the people you love will pay for it. They are the ones who will bear the burden of your illnesses; they will have to care for you, devoting years of their lives to helping you survive, wheeling you around, taking you to hospitals, feeding you your drugs, staying with you while you go through the death routine, or just suffering the pain of committing you to a nursing home.

If you love your spouse, children, family, and dear friends, you have a greater responsibility to yourself and all of them as well. Don't deprive yourself and them of those years that should be golden ones filled with all the richness of life that every human being deserves.

Take it upon yourself—TODAY!—to turn things around. Those rules for a healthy survival are the right pill for you.

> ### *How do you feel about euthanasia?*

This is a hotly debatable topic because it touches on everything from religion to science. Unlike most topical issues, which remain polarized, the question of assisted suicide (or "mercy killing") goes way beyond a simple yes or no. Everyone has a different opinion or viewpoint, based on a maze of attitudes, emotions, and philosophies. Is suffering meaningless and degrading or does it somehow uphold existence? Consequently, no consensus exists on the subject, and laws vary from state to state, and country to country.

This is not surprising, as it relates to the broad question of "Who owns the body—the individual or the state?" Or put in political terms, the role of government versus the right of individual citizens. In a sense, the issue embodies the same personal and societal elements as the question of abortion rights.

The American public was taken on a huge social-political ride with the Terry Schiavo case, which not only pitted one political party against another but also established a battlefield between Terry Schiavo's husband and her parents. As such, it remained front-page news for many weeks, highlighting the extreme gulf and contrariety on all sides.

This ever-emerging issue has been fueled by many prominent cases, including those of Karen Anne Quinlan, who was the first modern icon of the right-to-die debate, and Dr. Jack Kevorkian, a retired pathologist who was sentenced in Michigan to two terms of imprisonment for helping a man suffering from ALS (Lou Gehrig's disease) to die.

In two 1997 decisions, the Supreme Court ruled that there is no constitutional right to physician-assisted suicide.

That may be constitutionally correct, but *I believe that the right to die is as fundamental as the right to live.* Note: The Oregon Death with Dignity Act has been on the books for eight years and has proven to give peaceful dying to 246 patients, with no evidence of abuse of the law.

I don't believe that we will solve the essential debate or arrive at some middle-ground approach to this controversial issue in the near future. Like the abortion issue, no one is willing to give any ground and agree to disagree. It will be used and abused by all sides, another hindrance to progress and human understanding.

Something happened recently "Out of X" that touched me personally about the euthanasia issue: Back in 1970, when I was directing our community project, Journey, a young Swedish gentleman named Stig Hjelmgaard joined our ranks. He was strong-willed and charming in a boyish way, and he met a 16-year-old girl name Lynne, whom he fell in love with and married. They moved to Sweden and led their lives to the fullest.

On July 2, 2006, I received this email from my friend Neil Selden:

> *You may recall Stig Hjelmgaard and Lynne. Don't know if you know, he died a few weeks ago, in Copenhagen. A contrarian to the end, he refused to die in bed. He secretly managed to get out of bed and into a chair to do his dying. Hooray for Stig!*

Yes, hooray for Stig! He had the right to choose how he wanted to die. We all do. Just as we have the right to decide how to live—and no institution or religion should interfere with that privilege.

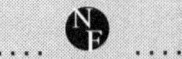

The one question related to this broad issue that all of us might ask ourselves is … does the conglomerate have a vested interest in needlessly keeping patients alive with drugs, feeding tubes, and artificial ventilators? From my point of view, the answer is yes. That is, until the individual's money or insurance runs out. Then it's time to simply turn its back on that person, or accidentally neglect to give him his painkiller.…

Are there any true experts in your book?

Very few indeed. But you wouldn't know it from the large number of people who claim to be. And that covers all walks of life. Give someone a title or position of authority and they go into Neverland, acting as if they really do have all the answers.

Because they have been spouting their great truths for so long, they actually believe what they're saying. What feeds this megalomaniac enterprise and believability gap is that the general public is dumb enough to actually accept and trust most of these "experts"—without actually studying their track records or doing any background research.

Here's a typical example of this expert mentality. Because someone manages a Major League baseball team, Mr. and Mrs. John Q. Public accept the idea that this person really knows baseball. Although his overall record in the major leagues is 155 wins and 473 losses—he's still treated like an expert and will be hired again and again!

The same goes for Hollywood executives and producers, most of whom have had more flops than you can count. The studios keep recycling those guys as if they were dormant geniuses who just need the right material to break new ground.

And the same mentality holds true for business. One idiot after another has had the chutzpah to push himself up the pecking order and gain control of a company long enough to run it into the ground. Each will soon be named to run another outfit, with the same results.

Speaking of business, since I was a child, I've read and heard all sorts of accounts and commentaries about economic theories that guide our country's destiny. Since these theories were created by a select number of prominent people (experts!) who seemed to know more about economy and finance than all others, you would presume that these authorities had a real grip on their subject of expertise, right?

Pardon me if I laugh out loud at the whole load of cockamamie nonsense from beginning to end. These great minds, larger-than-life figures who established these absolute theories for the world to follow, never knew what they were talking about—and as a nation, we've been dumb enough to hang with those theories in spite of the overwhelming truth that they are pure bunk. **They simply don't work.** No more than communism works.

If I were to bring together the greatest chefs in the world to create a menu of unsurpassed culinary delights, and they turned out little more than tasteless porridge and burnt toast, you would know that something was mighty wrong! But the brains behind our economic theories—all-knowing and accredited bankers, brokers, mathematicians, scholars, and theorists, who have devised their economic theories and principles from institutionalist and neoclassical economics to liberal and free market capitalism, from the mercantilist system to Keynesian economics, from quantitative science to supply-side economics, and all the other models you care to name in your economics encyclopedia—have all missed the boat.

Just take a good look at the overall economic conditions of the world—including our own—and any child could see it for what it's worth. It operates for only a select group of people and does not take the rest of the world (or America) into consideration. **IT'S A FAILURE.**

America is bankrupt, in debt to the tune of trillions of dollars;[16] can't afford to care for millions of poor, homeless, hurting citizens; is the only industrialized nation that does not provide healthcare to all members of society; and mismanages its affairs in much the same way an alcoholic, gambler, or drug addict handles his life.

These economic specialists not only don't know what they're talking about, they're also totally unwilling to look at any other economic theory that might produce better results. Here's one example: While all our financial experts, both in government and the private sector, maintain the importance of holding down wages (a minimum wage of $6.75 an hour is too high for these experts), Costco—whose CEO manages to survive pretty well on only $350,000 a year (a pittance compared to other CEOs of major companies)—pays its employees $17 and up an hour, plus benefits. Not only has this arrangement not broken the bank, but it works across the board for everyone, from the satisfied employees to the customers who receive great service from the efficient and caring workers. Not bad—huh?

And there's no reason—economic or otherwise—why Costco's hourly wage couldn't be paid to all workers. In fact, it's more feasible than any current plan or theory. Better than cutting taxes (mostly for the rich), a dramatic raise in pay for America's workforce would have far-reaching beneficial results for the entire nation; that extra cash would be spent on more goods, new cars, and homes; increase manufacturing; create new jobs; lower crime; reduce poverty and associated social problems; and all but eliminate the lower class in America.

But it can't happen because both political parties don't want it to happen. Why? Two fundamental reasons: First, raising the standard of living for all Americans would create a new balance of control and power within the framework of American politics—and neither the political forces or the conglomerates are willing to relinquish their upper hand. Second, by eliminating poverty and the lower-class, the banks could no longer feed off average workers' small salaries, the car manufacturers and their distributors would not be able to charge exorbitant interest rates, the insurance companies and the repo artists would have slimmer pickings, the healthcare industry would be forced to provide better services at more reasonable rates, conglomerates in general would be unable to maintain their present-day profiteering ways, and the politicians would find themselves out of "business as usual." There would actually be some "we" in "We the People."

---

[16] Foreigners own half of America's publicly traded debt. In fact, about $2.19 trillion in Treasury securities are held by central banks, including China. No wonder why we accept China's poor human rights record, while at the same time we maintain an embargo against Cuba. We behave like frightened bullies!

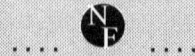

You must remember that the poor, lower classes pay the highest interest rates, are penalized the most by the courts, and are taken advantage of in every possible way. That's the biggest reason for keeping them in poverty or near-poverty. Trust this: If every wage earner made $20 an hour, business would thrive and so would the economy. But then things would be on an even plane, and that's what the upper classes and big shots are most afraid of.

You can guess what the Wall Street experts have to say about the way Costco handles its financial affairs, much less what they would express should anyone push for the same wages for all workers. They're up in arms against such salaries and other provisions and benefits that enrich the lives of employees. Of course, these meatheads have all the great economic theories to fall back on—every one but the success and well-being of the ordinary Joe and Jane. And they will stick to their guns no matter how many millions of people suffer as a result, not budging an inch—even if their expert theories were to lead the country into another depression.

Needless to say, these know-it-all experts, who make big bucks and receive all sorts of perks and stock options, and keep legions of people with real talent and ability from getting ahead, also go out of their fool way to heap praise on themselves.

These economic dodos do not stand alone in their mindless observance and dedication to their expert knowledge. The public believes them!

And, of course, the medical profession, with its vise on the public domain, contains more of these experts than all the other professions combined, except for the evangelists. They use their positions to ply their trade unfairly and often illegitimately, getting away with murder because they not only claim to be experts, but they also have the requisite, socially approved credentials. And the American public treats them as if they were infallible.

Some years ago, a friend spent eight years getting through graduate school, finally obtaining his Ph.D as a psychologist and setting up his first practice in New York City. He called me from his office and said, "Nickolas, I put my shingle on the door today, hung my credentials on the wall, and welcomed my first patient... who's sitting in my office waiting for me. And I'm afraid to sit with him because I don't think I can help him. I don't think I know what I'm doing—after all those fucking years!"

At least my friend was honest enough to realize that he didn't know too much at the time and called me for help. Most of the people who go through long years of schooling and end up with a title quickly get very full of themselves and start believing all sorts of things said about them that simply aren't true. Whereas that can be okay in some professions, it's not acceptable when dealing with someone's illness. (All those fool experts should be driving buses or selling shoes!)

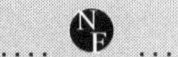

We would all be better off if we had fewer experts and more earnest people with a value system, with a concept of life that allows for true humility as well as continued growth and development. That's the only way we can nurture real experts and eventually see a higher class of humanity. Until then, we're stuck in a national rut with idiots and scoundrels who claim to know enough to advise us on health matters, education, religion, and politics. **In reality, they are guiding us to the brink of disaster and possible extinction.**

Medically speaking, don't necessarily trust any expert—especially doctors—who tell you that his diagnosis or prognosis is the absolute last word on the subject. I know some people who are alive today because they refused to accept a physician's expert opinion, and I knew lots of people who are dead because they trusted their doctor's absolute judgment.

Furthermore, anyone who tells you that you have only one option that can possibly alter your medical condition should automatically be regarded with suspicion because most doctors (especially those over 50) do not keep up with all the latest medical advances (which are not necessarily high-tech, bioenergetic stuff).

There is ALWAYS something new or experimental going on that might just be what you need. ALWAYS do your research and homework as if your life depended on it.

And taking a page from my old friend Lou Como, who frequently communicated (and communed!) with aliens, think as if you *were* an alien. What would *they* do if they came upon an earthling problem? With their far superior luminosity and omniscience, they would quickly cast aside our antiquated and finite thinking and methodology and propose any number of solutions to those everyday problems that plague our existence. Yes, they would have the answers ... because they are not encumbered by our cramped field of vision, nor bound by monetary concerns. And I believe that you would find far fewer experts among the truly enlightened of other worlds.

As a closing thought on experts, I'm sure you've noticed that I have treated supposed studies made by so-called experts (usually attached to research groups, government agencies, well-known nonprofits, and the conglomerate) with scorn.

Here's a perfect example of how my attitude is justified:

STUDY SHOWS OBESITY RISKS MAY HAVE BEEN OVERSTATED

Seattle Post-Intelligencer News Services—April 20, 2005

Obesity is less deadly now than in years past, and carrying a few extra pounds doesn't appear to increase mortality at all, a study in today's edition of the Journal of the American Medical Association *showed.*

The Centers for Disease Control and Prevention analysis also showed its own earlier estimates were overstated. Excess weight killed about 25,000 people in 2000, a dramatic drop from 365,000 deaths the CDC reported in January when the agency said excess weight and sedentary lifestyles may catch smoking as the leading cause of preventable death in the United States. ...

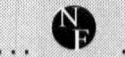

. . . .

These experts conveniently changed their figures from 365,000 to only 25,000 in less than four months, and the public is expected to trust them!

Unless you can't read between the lines, it's obvious that SOMEONE had good reason to spin this new finding out of whole cloth. Who? The conglomerate, for one. It would love nothing more than to have the public continue to dive headlong into the fat abyss, which this new report encouraged.

Joining ranks with the conglomerate, you have The Center for Consumer Freedom, an advocacy group financed by Coca-Cola, Wendy's, and Tyson Foods, among others. They proclaim, "Americans have been force-fed a steady diet of obesity myths by the 'food police,' trial lawyers, and even our own government."

On the Center's website, this group also declares that the Founding Fathers greatly enjoyed their food and drink, and that this important area of personal choice fought for by early American patriots is under attack. In other words, confronting obesity in America is unpatriotic!

None of the aforementioned comes as a surprise. It's all part of **the grand deception we call the American healthcare system.** Once again, it proves that "Believe nothing that you hear and half of what you see" is the correct way to approach these matters.

A parting note regarding weight-loss experts: Programs like Jenny Craig, eDiets, OPTIFAST, Weight Watchers, Health Management Resources, Medifast, and others in the business of providing supposedly expert medical supervision or low-calorie diets to millions of overweight and obese people have little to show for all their efforts, despite unsubstantiated claims to the contrary. Anyone who believes that these experts really know what they're talking about should take the time to read the daily headlines about the growing number of overweight and obese people in America.

Better yet, just take a broad look at any large group of people—in a stadium, theater, restaurant—and you'll see the true picture of obesity in America. Millions of these same overweight and obese people, who spend more than $46 billion a year on weight-reduction programs, have little to show for it. That doesn't mean that the weight-loss programs are responsible for their condition, but it does mean that these programs are not succeeding at curbing the problem. In other words, their effectiveness is not that great.

If it were, do you think that people would be willing to give up a year of their life rather than be fat? Or trim a decade off their lives for a thinner waistline? Or lose a limb than put on extra pounds? Those are some of the sacrifices overweight respondents recorded in a 2006 Yale University online survey. These people, like millions of others, have tried every kind of diet, gone to weight-loss clinics, pushed themselves in extreme ways—without lasting results.

The painful reality is that even under the best of circumstances, the vast majority of these people will regain the weight they've lost and repeatedly end up back at point one. So much for the weight-loss experts.

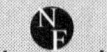

One of the most objectionable aspects of weight-loss clinics is their scandalous method of luring customers with supposedly low-price programs, only to hit up their trusting clients by forcefully selling them their food supplements and other products, many of which are unproven. Needless to say, if these clinics truly had faith in their ability to help their clients, they wouldn't need to devise a side racket. It's just another shameful part of the healthcare industry.

But what about experts who simply provide information to the public?

For instance, government agencies like the U.S. Department of Health and Human Services or the Department of Agriculture?

What about them? Are you suggesting that those experts actually know more than the average dumb dodo simply because they do not—like the conglomerate—personally profit from the pain and suffering of the general public? You're wrong on that count, because most of these agencies are run by political appointees who must toe the line, staying within the bounds of the current administration's dictates, or else, like the FDA, they are lapdogs for the conglomerate.

In addition, government agencies and the panels of doctors and scientists who collaborate with them on matters pertaining to exercise and nutrition are ordinary folk who know as much about those respective subjects as anyone else. In other words, most of their expertise is anecdotal, based on general assessments taken from a variety of other anecdotal sources, supported only by questionable statistics and a potpourri of out-of-date studies.

However, to be quite fair, they do manage to update things like federal dietary guidelines from time to time. But what good does that do? Now we are told to "Balance calories between the amount we eat and the amount of energy we burn" instead of "Aim for a healthy weight, based on body mass index." Or "Keep trans fat as low as possible. Get no more than 10 percent of your calories from saturated fat and no more than 300 milligrams of cholesterol daily," as opposed to the old guideline of "Keep your diet low in saturated fat and cholesterol and moderate in total fat."

Lot of good that does! All these guidelines plus $2.75 will get you a cup of coffee. In fact, the average obese person pays little attention to such expertise because it is far outweighed by the efforts of the conglomerate and all the other industries that profit tremendously by keeping him or her overweight.

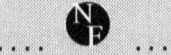

I can assure you that drugstores alone have a greater vested interest in the sales of over-the-counter weight-aid remedies and prescriptions than in promoting federal guidelines that might help people keep their weight off.

Where does "alternative medicine" fit into your equation for good health?

It fits in very well. I'm a believer in homeopathic medicine, thanks to Thakur,[17] who was a great advocate and specialist in homeopathy; hypnosis (long regarded as quackery but now approved by the American Medical Association [AMA]); and many forms of naturopathy.

For those of you without basic knowledge of homeopathy, here's a quick introduction from *Homeopathic Medicine At Home*, by Maesimund B. Panos and Jane Heimlich.

> *The term homeopathy (sometimes spelled homoeopathy) comes from the Greek* homoios *("similar") and* pathos *("suffering" or sickness"). The fundamental law upon which homeopathy is based is the* law of similars, *or "Like is cured by like"—in Latin,* similia similibus curentur. *The law of similars states that a remedy can cure a disease if it produces in a healthy person symptoms similar to those of the disease. ...*
>
> *... Homeopathy was "discovered" in the early 1800s by a German physician, Samuel Christian Friedrich Hahnemann. Shortly after setting up practice, he became disillusioned with medicine, and with good reason. Eighteenth- and nineteenth-century physicians believed that sickness was caused by humors, or fluids, that had*

---

[17] Sree Sree Thakur Anukul Chandra, Indian mystic and spiritual advisor (1888–1969).

to be expelled from the body by every possible means. To achieve this end, patients were cauterized, blistered, purged, and bled. Hahnemann protested against these brutal and senseless methods, and his colleagues quickly denounced him for heresy.

He was also opposed to the way doctors prescribed medicines. In those days, it was customary to mix a great number of drugs in one prescription. In his book, Who Is Your Doctor and Why?, *Dr. Alonzo J. Shadman mentions having seen, in the* Pharmacopoeia *of 1875, a prescription that contained fifty ingredients. Earlier, Hahnemann's outspoken criticism of this "degrading commerce in prescription" naturally enraged the chemists, who were as powerful as our drug companies today, and they were to hound him all of his life. ...*

The conglomerate goes back a lot further than we realize!

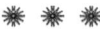

Although the AMA and the conglomerate goons still refuse to put their seal of approval on alternative treatments because they're threatened by anything they can't totally control for their own aggrandizement and power, the public is finally recognizing that there is more to medicine than human-made drugs and scalpels.

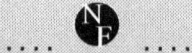

The only reason that the conglomerate has yet to attack the medicinal properties of the widely used aloe vera plant is that there's an unimpeachable 3,000-year history of its effectiveness. It's a remarkable healthcare product! Let's hope the medical racketeers never get their claws on it.

However, alternative medicine has failed to seek its own fully legitimate platform. Instead, it has fallen into a number of traps formerly reserved for conglomerate operatives. In the process, it is fast losing control of what should otherwise be inherent values—and is beginning to look, sound, and behave like its conventional counterparts. To be more precise:

1.   The higher echelons in alternative medicine have too many of their petty

jealousies and egos at stake. As such, they are playing it safe, as if they were more interested in gaining acceptance from the conglomerate than truly advancing the cause of alternative medicine and treatment.

2.   In an overall sense, alternative medicine is similar to the environmental industry in that it is fragmented, too full of itself to join hands in a common bond, and ill-equipped to inform the public of distinctions between conventional and alternative medicine and treatment. What a shame. And what a gigantic loss for an America in desperate need of healthcare alternatives.

3.   Not enough general information about alternative medicine is disseminated to the public. As such, the average person is kept in the dark about consulting alternative approaches when s/he becomes sick, which is why men diagnosed with prostate cancer immediately choose the better-known medical procedures and why tens of millions of people run to the drug counters instead of visiting a natural health store.

4.   The cost of natural remedies has skyrocketed in recent years, which means that alternative medicine has fallen into the same money trap as conventional medicine. If you doubt this, just walk into a natural health store and examine the prices for herbal remedies. In many cases, it rivals or exceeds the costs of over-the-counter drugs and prescriptions.

5.   Striving to increase its market potential, alternative medicine plays into the hands of the conglomerate, who not only chooses profit above good health but also knows how to control market forces and defeat the weak-minded opposition. And because of the conglomerate's powerful lobbies and political donations, the government is always on the side of the racketeering you-know-who. That's why natural remedies take such a lambasting from government agencies and their subordinates.

Before leaving the topic of alternative medicine, I must take off the kid gloves and say this—if you don't think that alternative medicine is going the way of all flesh—just like all the other money-grabbers—then tell me why you do not see or hear these people openly confronting the pharmaceutical industry and the entire conglomerate?

Whereas they should be at the forefront of the battle against the vultures that are thriving off the human bodies being destroyed by the tens of thousands every day, they have no united front, and thus no solidarity against the conglomerate. Shame on all of them. As healers, they have a responsibility to the public. That responsibility goes a lot further than just selling their wares.

❋ ❋ ❋

> ## What about traditional healing?

That's a broad topic that would take another book to cover, because it involves everything from native medicines of the world to witchcraft and voodoo. Needless to say, enormous time, energy, and money would be needed to evaluate the diverse approaches, medicines, instruments, and philosophies connected to this worldwide, nonconventional treatment.

Nonetheless, as millions of people are uninsured or underinsured, and millions more are unhappy with Western medical treatment and are seeking alternatives, it is safe to say that roughly two-thirds of Americans have sought something other than doctors and conventional Western medicine to treat their physical ills.

For instance, a growing number of Hawaii residents are using traditional healing methods long practiced in the Pacific Islands as an alternative to visiting a regular doctor. Looking further, the Chinese have brought their medicines to many countries, and their herbal shops can be found in the Chinatowns of the world.

An encouraging fact is that traditional healing methods, ranging from homeopathy, Chinese herbal medicine, and acupuncture to the yoga and Ayurvedic approaches commonly used in India, are being combined with conventional medical therapies in state-supported healthcare programs. For instance, the Global Academy (Institute for Integrative Medicine) has completed model integrative medical projects with the Albert Einstein School of Medicine in New York.

Generally speaking, Western society has much to learn from many forms of traditional healing. Unfortunately, as this vast knowledge becomes more accessible, it is vulnerable to falling into the hands of the conglomerate—who will of course use it only as a means to increase profits.

> ## What about "antiaging" drugs and antioxidants?

First of all, unless you're talking about human growth hormone (which I won't get into because I would first need to review hundreds of medical texts on the subject—but if you need insider stuff, get in touch with Jose Canseco!), typical antiaging products are not drugs but actual nutrients that have been fashioned into supplements, renewals, and cleansing programs. I'm personally familiar with the Isagenix Cleansing and Fat-burning System.

Countless more nutrient products and cleansing programs crowd the market, almost none of which are evaluated by the FDA but are nonetheless under the ever-watchful eyes of agencies (such as the FCC) that regulate the sales of products claiming to prevent or cure disease.

Unfortunately, although some have been known to cure disease, many only lay claim to such health improvements as elevating energy, improving eating habits, and increasing mental clarity and overall health awareness. Check out these claims before wasting your time talking to a doctor who knows next to nothing about nutrition. You'll be the better for it.

Before moving on, I want to mention that the entire process of aging is a very complex one that has not been researched properly and leaves many vital questions unanswered (except for anecdotal evidence). The only thing we can be sure of is that the process is not irreversible. There's no reason why molecular damage cannot be repaired, the biological clock cannot be reset, and we cannot recover strength and vitality.

People have been known to live 165 years, and the East has a long and venerable history that is devoted to the science of longevity. What you must realize is that the conglomerate will do all in its power to suppress anything that might prolong a quality life without drugs, doctors, hospitals, and insurance companies.

> *Do people somehow want to be ill?*

There's more truth to that than meets the eye. We suffer from both psychosomatic illness and a need to wear illness on our sleeves to gain sympathy and attention. In fact, being sick becomes a normal way of life for many people, another encapsulation like drugs, gambling, sex, and work.

Taking it a step further, many people would rather visit a doctor or be hospitalized than go on a vacation or learn a creative skill. And just as many prefer to use a walker, cane, or scooter to get around than to rehabilitate themselves.

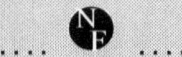

At least 60 percent of those people using ambulatory devices could be recharged and restored to normal activity—were it not for the doctors stultifying treatment, drugs, and the lack of physical therapy.

Being sick becomes a standard mentality, like practicing poor hygiene or a lack of personal dental care. I've seen it thousands of times among people of all ages and backgrounds.

Ever the great confronter, I want to grab these people and shout, "It's fun to be healthy!" But it would do little good because, instead of leading lives, the American public has become full-time patients. *Going to the doctor has become an American pastime,[18] a participatory and spectator sport.* And needless to say, it prevents people from honestly evaluating themselves and dealing with what really ails them.

Does stress kill?

This is another huge medical myth perpetrated by an ignorant establishment that has limited its studies to a narrow band of information that is more anecdotal than scientific. For one thing, there is good and bad stress. Specifically, short-term stress revs up the immune system, while chronic or long-term stress releases hormones that break down the system's ability to respond.

When we are bombarded by problems, conflicts, and a host of seemingly unending setbacks, this level of stress can seriously disrupt the immune system, make us sick, slow to heal, and run our emotions into the ground. However, people should break the habit of immediately relegating stress to an abnormality that causes death and for which drug treatment is necessary.

Millions of cases exist of people living under the most stressful conditions imaginable, such as prisons and concentration camps, who have not only survived but managed to grow and become healthier human beings in the process—and

---

[18] Americans went to the doctor more than a billion times in 2004. That's 3.8 visits for every man, woman and child, according to the CDC's National Health Statistics.

without drug treatment.

So the notion that stress is *the* killer, especially in men, is totally inaccurate and unsubstantiated, although everyone buys into it.

What often kills men is a combination of stress and unexpressed emotions. That's what's deadly, especially in this society, where we (especially men) are socially trained and programmed to bury our normal feelings. My father's death was attributed to Hodgkin's disease, but the underlying cause was directly related to his inability to express emotions. Many medical findings have reflected the same correlation between Hodgkin's disease and repressed emotions.

Let me put it another way: When you get right down to it, emotional pain, left to fester in our gut and mind and heart, does a lot more damage to our health than stress. They are not necessarily one and the same.

> *What's your take on anger management?*

Anger does not need any management. Like pain and fear, anger is a normal emotion that is vital to our survival and well-being. The experts (especially the psychologists and psychiatrists) who sell the public on the idea of anger as a problem have failed to distinguish between normal anger and hostility.

Hostility is a form of acting out that has little to do with normal anger and lots to do with a cowboy mentality of aggressiveness and a need to prove ourselves as strong men and women (an American tradition).

Simply put, there is a huge difference between telling someone that you're angry at them and taking a tire-iron and breaking it over his skull. One is a feeling, the other an action or threatened action ("Shut up—or I'll kick your teeth in!")

As I am an advocate for the expression of normal feelings—which conflicts with the uptight American attitude—I must point out that our frame of reference is so distorted that it's criminal and barbaric. Because we are so repelled by normal anger (as much as raise your voice and people are ready to call the police!), we force people to repress these normal urges. In turn these urges fester within us and eventually lead to hostile actions. That's why we have so many cases of sudden unexplainable acts of violence, such as road rage, which is a growing menace to tens of millions of people.

On March 26, 2006, at a Capitol Hill location in Seattle, six young people, including two girls aged 15 and 14, were slaughtered in cold blood in what was the second-largest mass murder in the city's history. Using a pistol-grip shotgun and semiautomatic handgun, the 28-year-old killer taunted his victims as he fired, "There's plenty for everyone." Shortly thereafter, as the first police officer arrived, the gunman shot himself in the head.

There was this reaction from the family of the killer: "He was very nonviolent and he loved his friends as much as he loved his family." And from friends, he was described as "polite" and "respectful," while neighbors commented, "This is a total shock." There were also those who remembered him as an "uplifting spirit."

Needless to say, the road to murder is almost always a long one, and people who knew the killer just weren't aware of what was really going on within his mind and psyche. Otherwise they would have been alerted to the horrible feelings and thoughts lurking within this young man—feelings of rage, vengeance, and betrayal that led him to unleash his premeditated deadly assault against unsuspecting victims.

But many analysts of this horrible crime will say that the young man was very "angry." Nonsense. Anger had nothing to do with the killings. His horrific desires were nurtured over a long period of time by a penchant for firearms, images of violence surrounding his everyday life, a national backdrop of terror and warfare, and a society schooled in the art of repressing normal emotions.

We can also thank Jack Valenti, the outgoing president of the Motion Picture Association of America, for being in the camp of the Hollywood movie producers who have turned out a steady diet of sick violence that has been replicated in the minds and actions of a legion of immature and repressed individuals, like the young man who went on that killing spree in Seattle. This former aide to presidents Kennedy and Johnson should hang his head in shame for his personal contribution to this mentality of violence and killing. In a sane and moral society, he would be condemned as an insensitive, reckless criminal.

You might think that my statement about Jack Valenti is rash. After all, he has such a strong public image, what with being on the inside during the grandiose Camelot years in Washington, when America looked upon the Kennedy clan as shining heros, and later when he became the spokesperson for the elite of Hollywood producers.

Notwithstanding Valenti's public persona as president of the Motion Picture Association of America, he was in a position to attempt to reshape the direction of the industry and promote healthier content, but instead he further contributed to the general mentality of Hollywood producers who offer the public the lowest form of trash and violence available in the northern hemisphere.

Smiling Jack Valenti has stood by these smut-makers and purveyors of brute force in Hollywood while they pawn off their violence-ridden garbage and foster a climate of rape, murder, and hatred. These screen and television depictions, very much a part of our sick culture, exert enormous influence on hundreds of thousands of individuals who are susceptible to this form of "entertainment."

I came across a typical example on TV the other night: The scene was a middle-class home, where a raging father threatened his eight-year-old daughter, warning her to obey his commands or suffer untold punishment. To prove his intentions, he chases the young girl into her room, searching for her puppy, telling her that he will dispatch the pup. Desperate, the girl grabs the puppy and runs out of the house, quickly followed by her crazed father, who jumps into his SUV and chases after the girl. He pulls the car up in front of his terrified daughter, grabs the pup from her arms, wraps a towel around it, runs over to a railing above a river some 70 feet below, and throws the helpless pup into the water. The daughter immediately climbs over the protective rail and jumps into the river to save her dog.

I couldn't watch any more—it was so sick. And I could feel the anger swelling inside of me—how I wished I had Jack Valenti in front of me at that moment. I wish he could suffer the pain of tens of thousands of innocent people whose lives have been degraded and destroyed by the gratuitous violence presented on our movie and TV screens. He might then have some sense of how he has aided and abetted all the unnecessary and harmful productions spawned amidst his cartel of mindless Hollywood producers. These movie moguls don't give a damn about the socially destructive effects of their movies—as long as they're making big bucks. That's all that matters to them.

To add to their maladjusted behavior, these Tinseltown scions have the nerve to justify their marauding pull on the public's thirst for violence by denying that their product has any affect on behavior and morals. For them, cause-and-effect does not exist, and no one has suffered. It's all the whacky notions of deluded people who are too "sensitive," or jealous of those who make a success of their lives.

Just like the gunmakers who tell us that "guns don't kill, people do," these big shot producers, hobnobbing with the likes of Jack Valenti, wearing tuxedos and toasting one another at award ceremonies, go about their business and ignore all outcries against their factories of violence.

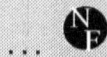

What most people don't realize about onscreen violence is that it's the easiest of all things to portray; sympathy, pathos, heartbreak, light humor, high comedy, and zaniness require various levels of acting skill. Hostility and violence, however, is a cinch for actors. In fact, I can take anyone from the street, put them on stage or in front of a camera—and I'll have them make Jack Nicholson look like an amateur! If you doubt this, you may recall that I taught acting (one of my students is an Academy-Award winner), and no one, but no one, man or woman, child or senior citizen, has any problem letting loose with profanities, threatening people, or blowing someone's brains out—it's less than child's play.

Strange things happen when you put a gun in the hands of individuals (especially men) with such aggressive impulses that they are not able to express or vent them in a safe way. I remember having such impulses when I was a teenager. However, I was fortunate enough to be a member of the Explorer Scouts, and as part of our Scout program, we joined the American Rifle Association (ARA) and participated in target practice with .22-caliber rifles. It was fun, competitive, and helped control my combative temperament. But you have to understand that this was taking place under supervised conditions and within the framework of a positive scouting program.

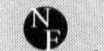

On February 13, 2005, Robert Bonelli, Jr. walked through the Hudson Valley Mall in upstate New York with a semiautomatic weapon and calmly shot off dozens of rounds, wounding two people before he ran out of ammunition. Bonelli, who was eventually sentenced to 32 years in prison for the crime, said he wasn't himself that day because of lack of sleep and drug and alcohol abuse.

"I'm sorry that all this happened. This is not the kind of person that I am," he said before sentencing.

No doubt, that's probably not the kind of person Robert Bonelli, Jr. was meant to be. But he more than likely witnessed enough violence in movie theaters and television screens to leave an indelible mark on his immature mind. And coupled with drugs and alcohol, he took out his hostility on innocent victims.

The ARA's indiscriminate support of Second Amendment rights, which allows gun makers to provide firearms to those who want to act out their violent thoughts, just as that young man in Seattle and the aforementioned person in Hudson Valley did, is an American tragedy and a travesty. Unfortunately, the ARA contributes big bucks to politicians who continue to place the ARA's interests above those of the citizens who want an end to violence.

Acting out rage and hostility is not that different from actual warfare—which is likewise easily acted out with skill by misguided soldiers led by an illiterate who loves to think of himself as "the commander-in-chief," especially when he steps out of a helicopter to strut in front of his troops.

What I'm getting at is that violence feeds off itself with hardly a nudge from any creative source. Indeed it has a sick and pathological life of its own. So movie producers have a field day showing it off to the American public, garnering accolades and awards for it, as well as millions in profit. And the American public should be chastised for their willingness to be fed this violence. *And none of it has anything to do with normal human anger.*

Note: In the process of lumping together anger and hostility, we train the public to fail to distinguish between a normal, healthy emotion and one that teeters on the brink of violence and destruction.

Again—we don't need anger management. **We need to deal with our hostile actions and control violence.**

The conglomerate would have you believe otherwise because it has a huge investment in proving that anger needs management, just as it wants you to believe that stress kills.

You must understand that the conglomerate is basically an industry that thrives on business deals, just like the military-industrial complex. And like all industry, it advertises and promotes its wares, aiming to sell the public on the need to buy these goods. When it comes to selling "anger management," they have an easy time of it, because the public is willing to accept the idea that anger is a bad thing. Once that concept is established and it becomes a mindset, the conglomerate's marketing of its products is as simple as getting kids to try chewing gum.

At that point, the big guns—the "A" teams—take over. In this case, we're talking about the psychiatrists and psychologists who amplify supposed anger with calculated success, for both themselves and the rest of the conglomerate scoundrels. And they are aided and abetted by the media, who do little more than report all the fabricated medical studies that indiscriminately buttress conglomerate missions.

Here's a typical example:

16 MILLION AMERICANS MAY HAVE ANGER AILMENT
It's intermittent explosive disorder

Lindsey Tanner, The Associated Press—June 6, 2006

To you, that angry, horn-blasting tailgater is suffering from road rage. But doctors have another name for it—intermittent explosive disorder—and a new study suggests that it is far more common than they realized, affecting up to 16 million Americans.

"People think it's bad behavior and that you just need an attitude adjustment, but what they don't know ... is that there's a biology and cognitive science to this," said Dr. Emil Coccaro, chairman of psychiatry at the University of Chicago's medical school. ...

Just read those words—"intermittent explosive disorder"—and "there's a biology and cognitive science to this," and you can see the game plan in operation. First make it sound like a clinically significant mental illness, add biology and cognitive science to the prevarication, and the public buys into it. Then you're easy pickings for the pharmaceutical team that follows on the heels of the medical mumbo-jumbo studies.

Guess what follows? As our medical expert Dr. Coccaro explains it, the disorder involves inadequate production or functioning of serotonin, a mood-regulating and behavioral-inhibiting brain chemical.

And wouldn't you know it—treatment with antidepressants, including those that target serotonin receptors in the brain, is often helpful, along with behavior therapy akin to anger management, Coccaro said.

What a crock from beginning to end! These liars, frauds, and schemers pull you right into the muck of their deceitful practices, using medical terminology to support their mindless claims, and because it's backed by the sick medical fraternity and all its conglomerate henchmen, it's an easy sell.

Instead of dealing with America's unbridled affliction with violence in all its ugly forms, whether it be road rage, domestic abuse, street gangs, outright warfare, or torturing prisoners, we target a natural human emotion and medicate millions of confused and ignorant people. The net results are predictable: Hostility and violence continues to escalate,[19] and America's drug fixation grows more out of control with each passing hour.

In an overall sense, the conglomerate has sold the American public on the idea that normal emotions are a source of illness that needs drug therapy and long-range maintanence. What insanity! The conglomerate's diabolical characters have turned anger into hostility, transformed human pain into depression, and transmuted fear into panic and paranoia. They have made normal human emotions *(which are part of our immune system)* into diseases, and turned tens of millions of people into drug-taking hypochondriacs.

What about depression?

I could go off on quite a tangent here, and take more shots at the lot of psychiatric madness that has resulted in millions of people being treated with drugs instead of conscientious therapy and counseling. But I'm going to simplify it with a story that typifies what's going on in the world of psychiatry. A woman who is suffering from a serious personal loss visits a psychiatrist who promptly tells her, "You're suffering from depression." The woman responds, "No, I'm not suffering from depression—my husband of 40 years just died and I'm in great pain."

Certainly there are people who truly suffer from serious depression, who *may*

---

[19] According to FBI data releases on June 12, 2006, murders, robberies, and aggravated assault increased last year, resulting in an overall rise in crime for the first time since 2001.

need medication. BUT the conglomerate doesn't distinguish between these extreme cases and those relatively ordinary human problems that can be effectively dealt with through various forms of nondrug therapeutic treatment and a goodly amount of concern and patience. Instead it continues to support the development of more and more drugs, so that it can maintain a never-ending multiple drug treatment program for millions of people in need of relief. When one pill fails, there's always another. The merry-go-round goes round and round and round....

> ### *What about anxiety disorders?*

If ever there was a con game run on the American public—this is it! Those people, groups, and organizations—many of which are nonprofits—have built a huge industry around a growing list of anxiety disorders **they've created for profit.** Their fictitious list includes generalized anxiety, obsessive-compulsive disorder, panic, post-traumatic stress, social anxiety, and specific phobias.

For each disorder they have developed an array of symptoms, descriptions, and, of course, drug treatment to facilitate their annuity ambitions. I mean, they have the public so cowed that it's pathetic.

Except for very extreme cases, most anxiety disorders can be successfully treated with psychomotor techniques (I have treated many such cases) that require no drugs.

Along the same lines as the anxiety-disorder racket, one of the most successful medical con games is to label certain disorders as "brain ailments." Dramatizing the disorder removes it from the realm of simpler therapeutic treatment and drops it right into the lap of the conglomerate.

You must accept that the conglomerate operates on the principle that more money can be milked from every human problem—providing that you intensify the problem to the extent that it becomes an actual disease. By labeling most commonplace human problems as diseases, the conglomerate essentially rounds up and corrals the public as if they were cattle being prepared for the slaughterhouse.

To demonstrate just how far the conglomerate goes in maneuvering the general public into believing that a relatively ordinary human problem is really a very serious one, I recently saw a TV ad that identified acid reflux as a disease! You bet! And I can guarantee that millions of Americans will now relate to it as a disease worthy of high-cost drug treatment. Can surgery be far behind? It's at hand!

Called the Stretta Procedure, it is used to treat Gastroesophageal Reflux Disease (GERD). Using an endoscope, a physician delivers radio frequency energy to create thermal lesions in the lower esophageal sphincter (LES) and gastric cardia (uppermost part of the stomach). This constricts the tissue and improves the thickness of the muscle wall in these areas. The result reduces acid reflux because the occurrence of LES relaxations is also decreased while LES pressure is increased. This in turn lessens refluxed acid into the esophagus. That's what they tell us.

And what about athlete's foot (easily curable with baby powder containing aloe), dandruff, or dirt under the fingernails? Certainly these are also diseases. And I can't imagine why the conglomerate hasn't yet labeled them as such.

While I'm on the subject, here's a list of newly discovered diseases—and you can be sure that the hundreds of drugs needed to treat them will soon be approved by the FDA and made available to the public:

- Obsessive Proletarian Fever
- Caddoan Freeze Complex
- Impulsive Elbow Niche
- Diabolic Dandruff Thrush
- Lock-knee Pork Collapse
- Compulsive Argonaut Tremor
- Conniving Toenail Syndrome
- Disabling Hip Flex Burn
- Multiple Tie-Down Disorder
- Multilateral Twixt Polarity
- Irreversible Ardwolf Pox
- Venetian Aberration Seizure
- Swarming Peacock's Disease

If any of you believe that the aforementioned new diseases actually exist—you're as gullible as the people who have accepted acid reflux as a disease!

To show you how efficient the conglomerate is with its follow-up promotion of drugs and medical procedures, just months after TV advertisements began portraying acid reflux as a disease, this report appeared:

STUDY COMPARES ACID REFLUX TREATMENTS
Drugs just as effective as surgery in managing it

Lee Bowman, Scripps Howard News Service—December 15, 2005

The first of a new series of federal reports intended to guide Medicare patients and their doctors in treating complex diseases concludes that drugs are as effective as surgery in managing gastroesophageal reflux disease. ...

This new series of reports goes on to say that the condition is caused when stomach acid enters the esophagus, causing heartburn and possibly long-term damage to the passageway linking the throat to the stomach. It also mentions that reflux disease is estimated to affect from 7 to 10 percent of all American adults, becomes more frequent with aging, is likely to require lifelong management, and found that, for most patients, a class of drugs called proton pump inhibitors, or PPIs, can be as effective in relieving symptoms and improving the quality of life as surgery that wraps part of the stomach around the esophagus to control acid.

Let's take a good look at what's really going on:

1. Heartburn has been around for a long time and was easily treated with simple over-the-counter remedies. *Now it has mutated into a serious disease.*

2. Out of nowhere, it's likely to require *lifelong management.* That means drugs and surgery.

3. The acid-fighting medicines you take may lead to far worse problems, including severe diarrhea and intestinal inflammation (colitis).

4. The conglomerate has gone into full battle array to *manage* this serious disease.

5. The government, using Medicare to spread the word, will encourage treatment on all levels.

You know what? There's truth in one thing about this acid reflux ascension: It's becoming more prevalent and much worse than old-fashioned heartburn. And guess why? There's something in the air (and possibly the water and our food) that's causing it. And that's not accidental. It's man-made and controlled (in the factories, refineries, and drug laboratories) by our oil industry and the conglomerate who are making fortunes as a result.

Another truth: Although researchers can't explain why it's happening, esophageal cancer is increasing at an alarming rate—and there's a direct association between this type of cancer and acid reflux. Need I say more?

> *Any tips for acid reflux sufferers?*

Try Bob Barefoot's Coral Calcium Supreme, which is 100 percent pure marine coral from Okinawa, Japan (but be certain that it's the real McCoy). If you drink a lot of juices, avoid the more acidic ones like orange and grapefruit juice, and replace them with apple juice. Chew your food thoroughly (at least 30 times), which increases the secretion of protective elements in saliva and other chemicals that help decrease acidity in the lower esophagus and protect those tissues. Also, use bricks or books to raise the head of your bed three to four inches (you won't notice the slight elevation that employs gravity to keep acid from refluxing into the esophagus). Finally, do a detoxifying cleanse—it can work wonders!

> *Are you accusing the conglomerate of creating disease only to profit from it by developing drug treatments and other medical procedures?*

Absolutely! It's no different than our government creating an enemy, starting a war against it, and handing the arms manufacturers and other conglomerates hundreds of billions in profit (without opposition from anyone but one senator from Minneapolis, who soon thereafter died in a mysterious plane crash). The more suffering and death, the more profits! The conglomerate are experts at this deadly game.

For example, creating more cancer by not putting more focus on prevention leads to the development of more expensive drugs to treat it, adding billions in profit to the conglomerate war chest. (In turn, the conglomerate places huge contributions into the hands of the politicians who are obliged to look the other way when cancer prevention is mentioned.)

The same system was employed to create the depression industry. Ordinary pain and sorrow has become a disease so that doctors, psychiatrists, and drug manufacturers have another cash cow.

Attention-deficit disorders follow the same game plan. Typical childhood problems have become labeled diseases that need medical attention and medication. (I know I'm being redundant—but I have no other way of driving this into your heads!)

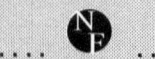

Then there's bulimia. The conglomerate invented it! The word "bu-limia" was unheard of by the general public until the 1980s, when the media started to portray it as a disease. Of course it needed treatment. With the media's wholehearted support, the public went for the game (as it always does), became afflicted, and paid through the nose for treatment that didn't work.

In fact, the obesity crisis as a whole has been dramatized to sell drugs! The conglomerate followed its tried-and-true equation: Sign up noted medical experts and researchers, arrange backing from the drug industry, redefine the problem as a "disease" needing drug treatment, and then get the doctors to prescribe the junk. The results: Drugs like Fen-Phen and Redux were billed as lifesavers but are now remembered as killers.

And when the truth finally comes out, all the experts who pushed the drugs into prominence (most were on the payroll of drug companies for decades) will get away with this human treason and murder because many years will pass before those lawsuits are heard. During the interim, the conglomerate will perform a few more end runs by designing new obesity drugs and hiring (paying off) more experts to endorse them.

It's a never-ending game plan. And it always works—because the public buys into all these media-supported games.

Amazing as it sounds, the American public actually turns to its agents of destruction for help. What could be more foolproof?

Just to show you that I'm not alone in believing the premise that the conglomerate literally creates diseases for profit, here's another take on this deadly enterprise:

DRUG COMPANIES
"INVENTING" DISEASES TO BOOST THEIR PROFITS
Mark Henderson, *The Times*—April 11, 2006

Pharmaceutical companies are systematically creating diseases in order to sell more of their products, turning healthy people into patients and placing many at risk of harm, a special edition of a leading medical journal claims today.

The practice of "diseasemongering" by the drug industry is promoting non-existent illnesses or exaggerating minor ones for the sake of profits, according to a set of essays published by the open-access journal Public Library of Science Medicine. ...

The article goes on to say that conditions such as female sexual dysfunction, attention deficit hyperactivity disorder (ADHD), and restless legs syndrome (can you believe it!) have been promoted by companies hoping to sell more of their drugs.

It's reassuring to know that others are aware of what should be obvious to the public, were it not for the lock that the conglomerate (especially doctors) has on people's minds.

The World News report goes on to say that other minor problems that are a normal part of life, such as menopause symptoms, are increasingly "medicalized," while risk factors such as high cholesterol levels or osteoporosis are being presented as diseases in their own right. **Even ordinary shyness is routinely presented as a social anxiety disorder to be treated with antidepressants.**

To be perfectly redundant, in the face of the calculated spins put on these medical issues, one would think that people would see through these simple manipulations and react with common sense and (at least) wariness—but it doesn't happen. If the conglomerate tells us it's best that we put on blindfolds and jump into a river—we'll seriously consider it!

❋ ❋ ❋

To cap off this question of creating disease, I must go into an area of American history that has had inestimable impact on every single one of us over the course of our lives.

The Harrison Narcotics Tax Act of 1914 was the single most important piece of drug legislation ever enacted in the United States. It required those who dispensed narcotics to register with the Bureau of Internal Revenue (predecessor to the IRS), pay a tax, and keep records of the drugs they dispensed. (Even then, doctors were dispensing drugs illegally for profit.)

The Act gave physicians the right to prescribe narcotics to patients, but the courts interpreted this to mean that physicians could prescribe narcotics to patients in the course of normal treatment, but not for the actual treatment of their addiction to narcotics. (Ass-backwards if you ask me).

Although the Harrison Narcotics Act was essentially a law for the orderly marketing of narcotics, in giving physicians the right to prescribe narcotics, *it unleashed the floodgates forevermore!*

The consequences of the Harrison Act are staggering. Over most of the 20th century in America, it created an ever-expanding commerce in illegal drugs, fostered drug abuse and addiction among millions of people, filled our prisons with hundreds of thousands of addicts and small-time dealers, established a climate of drug abuse acceptance among middle- and upper-class Americans, and allowed the medical profession to turn away from its traditional duties and become essentially drug dealers.

This went hand-in-hand with the aims and motives of the pharmaceutical industry, who soon parlayed the addicts' suffering and drug law enforcement into a means of escaping its own culpability in the growing national drug disease.

And while our government has spent billions of dollars on its useless "War On Drugs" campaign, **all but ignoring prevention and treatment,** the equation of supply and demand has made it totally impossible to control the amount of illegal drugs entering this country, as well as the amount of methamphetamine and other illegal drugs manufactured independently in America.

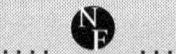

. . . .

With everyone's attention on the fictitious "War On Drugs" and the imprisonment of hundreds of thousands of addicts and dealers, the conglomerate is free to manufacture, prescribe, and market hundreds of billions of dollars in prescription and over-the-counter drugs.

It goes without saying that the conglomerate not only creates new diseases for which it will create scores of new drugs and surgical procedures, but it will also continue to support the "War On Drugs" to keep everyone off-track and maintain that status quo that allows it to abuse and murder at will.

❋ ❋ ❋

Adding a kicker to this **creation of disease for power and profit:** As I'm constantly harangued by supposedly intelligent people who take exception to my remarks about "the ignorance of people in general," I hereby submit the following short list of news stories and facts that have somehow been treated as isolated situations by the masses as well as the media. Instead of conjecturing the truth about these otherwise separate realities and conditions, I'm asking you, the reader, to expand your mind to see if it's possible to come up with a plausible answer (or two) to this riddle. Here goes:

1. President Bush proposes a plan (passed by Congress in 2005) to open Alaskan preserves to mining and oil exploration.

2. President Bush states that opening the Alaskan preserves to oil exploitation will lead to less dependence on foreign oil.

3. The Senate defeats a proposal by Senator Maria Cantwell to put the nation on the path toward reducing its dependence on foreign oil supplies by 40 percent over the next 20 years.

4. The cost of gasoline fluctuates wildly but generally upward, with no end in sight.

5. The nation's petroleum reserves are nearly full for the first time since their creation 30 years ago.

6. Reports appear that American oil companies are adding various new additives to gasoline.

7. An Environmental Protection Agency paper links gas additive with cancer.

8. A flu fiasco occurs in 2004–5, due to a supposed shortage of flu vaccine.

9. A strange—unreported by the media—viral infection strikes tens of thousands of people in Seattle (and more than likely other major American cities) in the late winter of 2005. Everywhere I went, for the months of March through May, people were suffering from the same dry cough, congestion, and flu-like symptoms, though it was not the flu. Among the hundreds of people I spoke to who had this infection, their comments were almost identical: "I've never had anything like this before." "This 'thing' doesn't go away, like the flu or a common cold." "It's almost like an allergy."

10. Warnings continue about a bird flu pandemic, and the fact that we're in no way prepared for such an epidemic.

11. President Bush's plan to take away free speech rights from 20 million public employees.

Without giving you the answer—I say **BINGO!** Now **YOU** put it together and see what you come up with. I dare you!

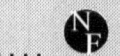

Should you question my veracity in alluding to some mysterious infamy, you don't have to go much further back than the Watergate scandal to see and understand just how things are plotted out and executed. You must also remember that the Watergate investigation would never have happened had it not been for the dogged determination of two American reporters, Bob Woodward and Carl Bernstein of *The Washington Post*. Without their persistence and the inside facts provided by Woodward's celebrated source "Deep Throat," Watergate would never have been revealed, and President Nixon would not have been forced out of office.

Why is it so difficult for otherwise intelligent people to believe that government leaders are capable of conspiring to destroy human life for profit and vainglory? It's been going on for centuries throughout history, and it's going on today. George W. Bush is currently prepared to use the first veto of his presidency on a defense bill to fund further military operations in Iraq and Afghanistan so that he can maintain the right to subject detainees to cruel and inhuman punishment. In other words, *torture*. Essentially, he will declare to the entire world his administration's utter moral bankruptcy. And there's no way to stop him.

The illiterate one in the White House, who has all but declared himself Emperor, does not even bother to veto bills he doesn't approve of. **He's gotten around that presidential option by reserving the right to disregard any part of a bill he considers an infringement on his sacred authority.**

Case in point: In December, 2005, President Bush signed a military spending bill (alluded to in the previous paragraph) that included an amendment banning the cruel, inhumane, or degrading treatment of foreign prisoners. However, he quickly put a statement in the Federal Register asserting his right to ignore the ban when

necessary, in his judgment, to protect Americans from terrorism.
President Bush has claimed the authority to disobey more
than 750 laws enacted since he took office. Only potentates do this!
America—where are you?!

So don't be quick to think that I'm paranoid and a lunatic for my line of thinking. Instead, consider the details, use your imagination (Einstein believed that the imagination was more important than science), and add up the facts. And when you finally see the obvious picture—***don't be fool enough to deny it.*** These conspiracies and worse continue every day all over the world.

Note: Had we paid attention to details and used our imaginations, 9/11 would have been avoided.

> ***Do you have a particular issue***
> ***with oil companies?***

Doesn't everyone? Unless you live in a cave or on a private island with your own renewable source of energy, you, like the rest of the common folk, are at the mercy of the energy suppliers. These "utilities" not only run herd over us to the tune of trillions of dollars, but as partners in crime with the Bush clan, they subjugate the American people to a never-ending display of criminal behavior of an extraordinary nature.

Let's begin with the news of January 30, 2006, which revealed that Exxon Mobil reported a profit of $36.13 billion in 2005.

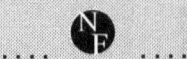

Two days later, President Bush not only defended the huge profit
of Exxon Mobil Corporation, but let it be known that billions more
would be needed for the war efforts in Iraq and Afghanistan.
Meanwhile Congress also approved a drastic cut in Medicaid and
Medicare benefits—just what the President ordered up.

Speaking of Exxon Mobil, here's something that further testifies to its already seedy (I'm being polite!) reputation: It has been more than 18 years since the day that the *Exxon Valdez* tanker ran aground on Bligh Reef and dumped 11 million gallons of crude oil into Alaska's Prince William Sound, and more than 13 years since an Anchorage jury awarded the fishermen and affected communities $5 billion in punitive damages. Guess what? Exxon still hasn't paid up—even with profits exceeding $36 billion last year.

While I'm on the subject of Exxon, I can't help but address the issue of periodic hikes in gas prices.[20] This isn't just a matter of economics—it's very much a health issue as well. How so? Everyone from the middle- and working classes to those in low-income and poverty situations suffer not only added financial pressures but emotional, psychological, and physical problems as well.

In many cases, people have been forced to abandon their normal lifestyles because they cannot pay their home heating and electric bills, much less afford to drive their cars to their places of livelihood. And for those with meager wages, we're creating a new lower class.

Once again, we witness how easy it is for the various conglomerates to take advantage of the public's inability to stand up and fight the good fight against the tyranny of the wealthy and the scheming intentions of both political parties. In this case, the public damns itself day in and day out by accepting price gouging on a grand scale—and not even raising its voice in outcry.

How do the conglomerates, guided by the present administration in Washington, get away with it? They have a foolproof game plan that they've worked on the public for decades, one which is so simple and yet unimaginative that it frightens me to realize just how gullible the average person is.

It goes like this:

- *Raise fuel prices and blame it on things that are not in our nation's control, such as rising crude-oil prices, fears about Iran's nuclear ambitions, dwindling oil supplies, and disruptions caused by the hurricane season in the Gulf of Mexico.*

- *Keep raising fuel prices until it hurts and then some. And make everyone bear the burden; the public, business sector, airlines, hospitals, schools, you name it.*

- *When it looks as if it will never level off, lower prices just a bit,*

---

[20] Besides registering at the gas pumps, higher fuel prices increase the cost of food and other commodities because they are often shipped by trucks, so the added fuel price is passed on to the consumer.

enough to provide a breather from the daily encroachment.

- *Hold those prices down long enough to make people feel hopeful, then gradually lower them a bit more, giving people a measure of new-found security and assurance that the worst is over.*

- *Maintain this level of pricing just long enough for people to get used to the status quo—and then START THE ENTIRE CYCLE ALL OVER AGAIN!*

- *And when the public begins to complain and the media pays some attention, the Bush administration pulls out one of its oil-infested stratagems from its game-bag—once again—by proposing the opening of the Arctic National Wildlife Refuge to oil drilling and production. It promises that this will provide America with more oil, decrease oil imports, and lead to lower gas prices—all of which is absolute hokum!*

It's gonna get you one way or the other!

To further the deceit, the president will enlist the support of the Environmental Protection Agency (EPA) to issue a tactical directive saying that it will consider fuel waivers on a case-by-case basis. What this seemingly innocuous statement really means is that clean air rules will be set aside—supposedly because such safeguards contributed to gas shortages.

You gotta love these bums!

Throughout this course of "tactical fuel economics," the press generally performs its most basic style of reporting, registering complaints more as statistics than as a serious national problem to be investigated and confronted. And the politicians in both parties—bless their corrupt hearts—go along with this treachery and treat it as just another sign of the times that must be swallowed without strong objection—in the hope that it will, like all problems, dissipate with time and be forgotten.

One must remember that our no-account Senate (including the newly elected one in November 2006) knows where its bread is buttered.

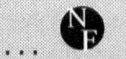

. . . .

On April 25, 2006, amid growing anxiety and anger about the rising

> cost of gas, the Senate refused to consider legislation by Senator Maria Cantwell, D-Wash., to make price gouging at the pump a federal crime.

All the while, the oil barons, conglomerates, and associated political cronies, along with our seemingly oblivious president, ignored the plight of the people, turning their backs on everyone but the rich and powerful.

If you think that t his form of economic warfare doesn't affect our well-being—you're greatly mistaken. It plays into every aspect of healthcare. Nick's solution: Next time they jack up the prices—a gas strike! No, I'm not kidding.

> *Even considering all your attitudes,*
> *as well as your documentation,*
> *don't you think you've exaggerated this thing*
> *you call the conglomerate?*

Oh, how I wish I were exaggerating … but the truth is … as bad as I've made the conglomerate out to be—**it's actually a lot worse.** Allow me to further clarify my position:

I recently watched a TV documentary that showed how chickens are dispatched by the poultry companies. As much as I think that I have witnessed all manner of inhuman and grotesque behavior, watching men slit the throats of these creatures and then hang them on hooks, leaving the chickens to undergo unimaginable death throes for up to a minute, was as repulsive as anything I have ever seen. Absolutely barbaric.

I quickly changed the channel to avoid seeing any more of this carnage, and it occurred to me that if aliens from outer space were to circle our planet and begin to capture and "harvest" our civilization (as in H. G. Wells's *War of the Worlds*), they might do so with the same indifference and aplomb as those individuals killing the chickens.

What does this have to do with the conglomerate? **Everything!** How can you be so blind to the incontrovertible fact that the people who have conspired to drug the masses for profit and power and plan, guide, and carry out the destruction of America's healthcare system look upon their "clients"—that's you and me—as no more than NEXT IN LINE ON THE FOOD CHAIN, right behind the poultry, fish, and cattle we consume? No manner of defense or denial can obscure this reality.

We are at its mercy, but it shows no mercy because *we're just statistics and numbers to be placed in the proper order for its assembly-line disposition and final settlement. Like chickens.*

Beyond this processing and arithmetic, the conglomerate is no better than the butchers of Auschwitz, who excused and rationalized their inhuman behavior with nationalistic fervor and Third-Reich ideology.

Throughout history, the bottom line of all the atrocities perpetrated against humanity is always the same: Huge numbers of people are killed for the sake of land, money, power, and some concept of higher order or mentality.

And no matter how you pretend that killing in one form is different than killing in another form, the pain and suffering that each human being and creature endures is very real, equal to the pain and suffering of every other human and animal. In this regard, we are all the same. *One dead body is just as dead as the next.*

So all of you apologists should stop ignoring the indisputable facts regarding the deaths of millions of human beings at the conglomerate's hands and face the fact that YOU ARE NEXT IN LINE!

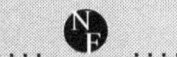

Many European nations have laws against Holocaust denial. These laws were enacted after World War II, and were meant to prevent any resurgence of Nazi activities. For the most part, they have been effective, and serve as a constant reminder of the horrendous reality of genocide. It should also be noted that America is dotted with Holocaust museums and memorials.

But there are no laws in America against genocide committed by the conglomerate, and there are no museums or memorials to commemorate the deaths of millions of people at the hands of these killers. And regrettably, Americans would deny this genocide, just as they refuse to accept their collective responsibility for allowing 43,000 road deaths, 200,000 drug-related deaths, 195,000 hospital deaths, 25,000 firearms deaths, and hundreds of thousands of smoking-related deaths—every year! We would not deny the World War II Holocaust—but we deny our own yearly holocaust. With this denial, we protect mass killers and allow the conglomerate members to make hundreds of billions of dollars in profit from their victims.

One must ask, what qualifies as genocide? Most dictionaries define it as "The systematic annihilation of a political, racial, or cultural group."

But what numbers must be involved? At what point do you go from mass killing to genocide? Is 500 too low? What about 10,000? Does that do it? And how about millions? Certainly millions makes the grade.

On that basis, the conglomerate more than registers on the depth chart with Hitler, Stalin, and all other genocidal maniacs. Then how do we, as supposedly intelligent and caring human beings, turn away from this gruesome reality, and pretend that it's not happening here? What will it take to make us come to our senses and put a stop to the killing? And to recognize the killers? **Why do you think I'm cursing mad? You should be, too!**

Never one to miss a chance to add a "kicker" to my message, there's much truth in the saying, "There's honor among thieves." That includes all the gangsters, lawyers, politicians, priests, doctors, insurance agents, repo artists, and pill-pushers who defend one another. Condemn them all! That's the only way to open the door to truth and hope.

That may be our only chance.

Before moving on, I must tell you a story that resounds in my mind whenever I think of the full dimensions of the conglomerate and our death-dealing healthcare industry.

In 1967, while having lunch in Little Italy (just a block from the headquarters of Encounter) with a current girlfriend, she introduced me to a strikingly handsome, well-dressed, executive-type young man, and we invited him to join us for a drink. Although he could only stay for a few minutes and didn't divulge anything about himself, this Adonis-like individual impressed me with his intellect and charm, and I couldn't wait to have my female companion fill me in on the details of his background, which I felt must include a very prominent vocation.

She looked around to make certain that no one was listening, then told me that her old friend was a hit man for the mob, and that he had been contracted for at least 40 killings.

About a year later, while having lunch alone in the same restaurant, the young hit man walked up to me and asked if he could join me, explaining that he regretted having to hasten away at our earlier meeting. I willingly agreed, and over a good Italian meal and a fine red wine, he questioned me about my work with

Encounter, expressing a great interest in our drug prevention program. In fact, he promised to make a donation.

When I questioned him about his own line of work, he didn't hesitate to tell me that he was indeed a professional hit man for the mob. As this was a very open conversation, I asked him about his feelings regarding this "work." He was blunt in telling me that it was no different than what the corporate gangsters did.

Although at the time I regarded his response as a rationale, 36 years later I am forced to admit that his reasoning—although barely an excuse to commit murder—is no less a matter of fact than all the typical defenses in one form or another of our corporate killers. Why? **Because the young man in question and the conglomerate both kill for profit.** In actuality, the conglomerate does it on a much greater scale than all the mobsters in the world.

And going back to my earlier question, why is one dead body less or more important than another? **And why is one form of murder looked upon as a capital crime and the other as a legitimate business?** Will anyone in his right mind please explain this?

> *You mentioned Americas collective responsibility for allowing 43,000 road deaths; can you elaborate on that?*

Let's start with some perspective: Forty-three thousand Americans were killed on American roads in 2005; more than three million men, women, and children died on American roads and highways in the 20th century, while five times as many Americans lost their lives on U.S. highways as were killed in all the wars ever fought since the U.S. Constitution was ratified. It should also be noted that the death toll on our highways makes driving the number-one cause of death and injury for young people ages 5 to 27. Get the picture?

According to the National Roads Authority, the main contributing factor to the extraordinary number of road fatalities in this country is the behavior of the road user.

To be more specific:

- The behavior of drivers contributes to 88 percent of road fatalities.

- The behavior of pedestrians contributes to 8 percent of road fatalities.

- Road factors contribute to 2 percent of road fatalities.

- Environmental factors contribute to 1.5 percent of road fatalities.

- Vehicle factors contribute to 0.5 percent of road fatalities.

To be even more specific, these are the main behaviors causing death and injury:

- Excessive and inappropriate speed.

- Driving while intoxicated.

- Failure to wear seatbelts and failure of parents to restrain their children properly.

- As pedestrians, cyclists, and motorcyclists, our failure to recognize our vulnerability and ensure our visibility to motorists.

- Driving while fatigued.

There are other mitigating factors that are not taken into account because there is no way to accurately access their damage:

1. **Road rage,** which is caused by numerous human problems, including impatience and repressed emotions that we bottle up during the course of the day and vent when we get behind the wheel—because it's relatively safe—especially if we're driving a big sports-utility vehicle (SUV). We also act out our rage toward drivers who behave like subhuman creatures (refusing to allow drivers to move into their lane, abrogating the responsibility to signal when changing lanes or making turns, and driving recklessly). Poor driving conditions (antiquated access and exit lanes, poor signage, and potholes) also add to the hazards of driving.

2. **Cell phones** not only add to the carnage but also illustrate just how dumb Americans really are. We should just as well pass a driving regulation that states "The law requires that you drive with ONLY one hand, that you focus less on driving and more on talking on your cell phone, and that you ignore the perils associated with distractions." These laws would also be posted on huge signs in every motor vehicle department, especially where people are registering to obtain a drivers license.

    If you think I'm being facetious—No! I'm being honest about something that any civilized human being would find inexcusable—were it not for the fact that the American public is willing to accept whatever is stuffed down its throat by lobbyists and special-interest groups—like cell phone manufacturers—in place of common sense and concern for human life.

3. **A sense of false security created by airbags**—which do not meet two basics standards—efficacy and safety. Note: The United States is the only country in the world where it is illegal to purchase a new automobile without an airbag that is known to increase harm in women and risk of fatality in children. Note: This is not to say I'm against the use of airbags, only to put it in a broader perspective.

4. **Television commercials** showing vehicles being driven at high speed, doing maneuvers that would be dangerous on racetracks, and crashing through stores and buildings. Of course, at the end of these commercials, the sponsor displays a small warning that the drivers are professionals and that others should not engage in these actions. That's as good as the warning labels on cigarettes and drugs.

If you don't think that these commercials (as well as dramatic presentations that show backroad drag-racing and shootouts) encourage similar behavior in tens of thousands of immature people and borderline criminals—you're among the ranks of ignorant people who refuse to believe in any cause-and-effect relationship.

There is no way to ascertain how many people actually die as a result of these commercials and presentations any more than we can estimate the number of deaths caused by road rage. What we can determine—beyond a shadow of a doubt—is that millions of people are subjected to pain, suffering, and cruelty at the hands of people who sometimes regard their vehicles as weapons and a means of netting out punishment.

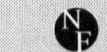

. . . .

I have to take aim at SUVs (as well as the automakers who manufacture these gas-guzzlers and death traps) ... because these vehicles are four times more likely to roll over than passenger cars in high-speed maneuvers and are six times more likely to kill occupants of the smaller vehicle when compared to a normal car-to-car collision.

> I also have to take special aim at SUV drivers… because the greater percentage of these people are not buying and using four-wheel-drive pickup trucks and SUVs for work, hauling, and off-road purpose—as much as they are using them to act out their hostility, venom, and egos.

If you think that this is just my opinion, you're not only failing to recognize an everyday reality that's happening on every street and road in America—you're also in complete denial about all those nitwits who spend their driving time trying to prove just how strong and tough they are. I watch these baboons burn rubber to show off, turn into your lane at the last moment without signaling, and lord over people in smaller, less-protected cars; I want to give them a dose of their own medicine. These are would-be killers. They belong in jails, not on roads.

Overall, it can be said that WE ARE LOUSY DRIVERS, DON'T PAY ENOUGH ATTENTION TO WHAT WE'RE DOING, AND OFTEN DON'T GIVE A DAMN. This, too, is part of our emotional, mental, physical, and spiritual state of being, and it certainly is a collective responsibility. Forty-three thousand lives taken yearly….

Appropo of this collective responsibility:

GREGOIRE SIGNS TOUGHER DUI LAW

By Curt Woodward, The Associated Press—March 16, 2006

Gov. Christine Gregoire signed a bundle of bills into law on Wednesday, including a long-standing effort to toughen punishment for repeat drunken drivers.

The measure would make a fifth DUI conviction in 10 years a felony. A DUI charge would also be a felony for drivers with previous convictions for vehicular homicide while impaired.

"This is a very important pubic safety bill to get incorrigible drunken drivers off our roads," Gregoire said before signing the measure. …

Pardon me, Governor, but in all my 70 years of existence, seldom have I come across such a piece of dribble. This supposed public safety bill is a surefire way to excuse drunken driving and slaughter on our roads—by passing an insignificant law that is a mockery to common sense and intelligence. Furthermore, Governor, your longstanding effort to toughen punishment for repeat drunken drivers IS NOT A VERY IMPORTANT PUBLIC SAFETY BILL. HELL NO!!!

Then why all the hype about this new law? It's good press for a first-term governor looking to impress her supporters and neutralize her opposition. To the politically uninitiated (which takes in at least 75 percent of the population), it sounds like a progressive piece of legislation—when in reality it is little more than a political ploy that "looks good." Similarly, Governor Gregoire initiated a new medical malpractice bill that is more image than substance but received plaudits for the effort nonetheless.

> *Why are you so angry?*
>
> *Wouldn't you be better off*
> *if you were more moderate?*

America has been thoroughly bamboozled by moderate thinkers, apologists, and frightened ninnies who will never deal with problems in a responsible way, and that includes being "responsibly angry." For instance, while I'm a great fan of former news anchormen like Douglas Edwards, Harry Reasoner, Eric Sevareid, Howard K. Smith, Chet Huntley, David Brinkley, Peter Jennings, and Walter Cronkite, I loathe their political correctness, wishing that they would have risen to the occasion to get goddamned angry instead of presenting their views in carefully measured tones.

We need people to act more like the passionate anchorman in Paddy Chayefsky's *Network* and shout from the rooftops, *"I'm mad as hell—and I'm not going to take this any more!"* That's the only thing that will get us off our asses and start us on the way to some genuine change for the better.

We need American Indians to really get angry, march in Washington, and get tens of millions of people behind them; we need the poor to stand up and fight the fight of the ages against the rich and powerful (start by demanding a $20-an-hour minimum wage); we need women to finally take the lead and pass the Equal Rights Amendment; we need the press and the public to condemn the U.S. gulag in Guantanamo Bay;[21] and we need the entire country to rise up against both political parties and get angry at what's going on in the name of fighting terrorism.

We need workable plans, not slogans from political hacks in both the Democratic and Republican parties or further polarization. We need strong medicine to cure what ails us.

---

[21] If any one person is held without rights, without legal recourse, it puts our entire society at risk.

We need a new political order that will unite America.

We're in the hands of madmen working in all branches of the U.S. government, who continue to support the environmental destruction of the planet; a military establishment that has lost its last two wars (and has been suckered into another losing conflict); and numerous conglomerates who place profit above human life. All these entities will join together and not just set up concentration camps like Guantanamo Bay and foster a climate of hatred that will result in the deaths of millions of people, but *will also—if not stopped within our lifetime—destroy all life on our planet!!! We are talking about apocalypse.*

Remember, all our meaningful scientific evidence points to the existence of global warming[22] and massive pollution of the environment, and now there may be no turning back from the ultimate consequences.

There is also the reality that large quantities of fissionable material and bio-weapon-grade smallpox virus from the former Soviet Union are unaccounted for. *Whether these materials were stolen or sold to extremist groups, this mysterious absence constitutes the most alarming possibility of all doomsday scenarios.* Putting together an atomic bomb is no longer such a classified secret. And with all the anti-American sentiment throughout the world mounting against us (and deservedly so), if you think that our enemies wouldn't use an atomic weapon against us—wake up! They'd be dancing in the streets!

Because of these factors, this planet could well be destroyed by a chain of disasters caused by biological weapons, global warming, and the continued desecration of all natural resources, or incinerated by a nuclear conflagration involving many countries and combatants throughout the world.

Hiroshima, Nagasaki, 9/11, and Hurricane Katrina will amount to little in comparison to what might happen. We are truly talking about *apocalypse.* BEWARE—the biggest weapon of mass destruction sits in the White House. Its name is George W. Bush—and it controls enough lethal material (both weapons and mentality) to destroy the world. Better believe it!

So don't tell me about being moderate. To quote from Tennyson:

> *Ring out old shapes of foul disease;*
> *Ring out the narrowing lust of gold;*
> *Ring out the thousand wars of old;*
> *Ring in the thousand years of peace.*

---

[22] Greenhouse gases reached record high levels in the atmosphere in 2004, according to the Geneva-based World Meteorological Organization. And a growing number of scientific studies support the theory that increased levels of carbon dioxide, methane, and other gases are accumulating in the atmosphere, trapping heat and raising the earth's average temperature.

> *Using your own terminology,*
> *will you at least "give it the barest"*
> *that you're an extremist?*

The powers that be (who are experts at controlling the public's mind and imagination) would have you believe that I'm an extremist. The truth is that the profoundly ignorant public is the real extremist. In a manner that makes any intelligent person shake his head in disbelief, the public refuses to accept what's right before its eyes, served up day after day.

The public's tens of millions of extremists in temperate clothing play it safe at the expense of those few who are willing to expose themselves to the barbs, threats, and attempts to portray them in turn as extremists and therefore dangerous.

The net result is that the supposed extremist has to do the work of countless people who remain deaf and dumb to what's right in front of their noses. In the process, the overwhelming number of "moderates" make it easy for all the conglomerates to steal and murder with impunity. I mean, it's a cakewalk for all these gangsters. They are the true terrorists.

> *Why does the will of the people—*
> *the "common" man and woman—go unheard?*
>
> *Doesn't anyone speak for them?*

There are so-called consumer advocates who do a piss-poor job of addressing the public's fundamental needs. These whiz kids have their own private agendas that have little to do with serving the public need and a great deal to do with building reputations, earning big bucks, and acquiring a power base from which to launch political careers. The whole lot of them haven't put a small dent into the armor of the conglomerate, and never will. Elitist prigs!

Then we have the media, who are supposed to guard free speech and democracy, but do little more than play-act at being reporters, analysts, and journalists. They are workers who do the bidding of their respective publishers and bosses like Rupert Murdoch (and there are fewer and fewer of these people, allowing for the concentration of vast power and influence). Most of them are addicted to power and vainglory pursuits, spreading their own rigidly defined social, economic, and political views.

Consequently, the media has been neutralized and plays little part in educating or awakening the public to the dangers that exist. If anything, **they are the primary promotional arm of the conglomerate.**

When you partake of the media, you must recognize that almost all of them depend on their advertisers for revenue, and the conglomerate is a heavy spender when it promotes its wares, especially drugs. Don't think for a minute that it will tolerate strong interference in its promotional campaigns.

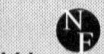

When I was growing up, the only medical commercials on radio and in the early years of television were for Bromo-Seltzer, Alka-Seltzer, Pepto-Bismol, and Bayer aspirin. That was it.

Now take a look at what we have—hunting grounds for the conglomerate: thousands of TV commercials and slick magazine ads every day, feeding our already vastly over-medicated society the pills, therapies, and medical gobbledygook that will put another hundred million people in early graves, while the conglomerate lolls in its thick cesspool of greed.

What is even more ludicrous, although most people never bother to think as such, is the frequent ending to most of these advertisements: "Ask your doctor about it." That's almost as absurd as "side effects may include headaches, nausea, possible infection, and diarrhea." Pardon my French, but FUCK YOUR DOCTOR! He couldn't care less about the junk he's helping to peddle or if it's going to turn you into a helpless, hapless, hopeless human wreck.

Back in 1904, many doctors advised black people to be X-rayed—**so that they could turn whiter**. That was their solution to racial problems! If you think physicians' current spoken and unspoken endorsement of these thousands of drug commercials is any better than their former advocacy of X-rays for blacks, you don't get it.

Speaking of commercials, Dr. Matthew F. Hollon, an internist at the University of Washington Medical Center, responded in an April 27, 2005 *Journal of the American Medical Association* editorial to a recent study that suggested that drug companies' advertisements affect what doctors prescribe:

> *Relying on emotional appeals, most advertisements provide a minimal amount of health information, describe the benefits in*

vague, qualitative terms and rarely offer evidence to support claims ... Because the safety of a new drug cannot be known with certainty until it has been on the market for several years, and since the drug withdrawals occur more than two-thirds of the time within three years of release, the FDA should consider a moratorium on advertisement of drugs directly to consumers for three years after initial market release.

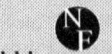

Not a bad idea. But it will never happen. More often than not, the FDA and the FCC will act only against alternative medical programs and naturopathic nutrients that are highly beneficial and not part of the conglomerate.

The wisest thing that all television viewers can do to protect themselves from the clutches of the conglomerate is to **stop watching all the commercials about drugs, medical treatments, insurance plans, and so on.** I mean—go beyond the Air Force motto by not giving these bums the benefit of the doubt. In fact, I wish there were a way to delete these commercials even before they rear their ugly heads. We need to be able to click a button and end their rule forever. That's one concrete way to stop the killings.

Another force that should be actively engaged as public spokespeople are the famous personalities and celebrities who are in a position to move the will of the public to center stage. Much to our great misfortune, these celebrities and sports figures have gone over to the enemy camp in droves. Why? For one thing, they are among the biggest drug abusers in the country themselves and can hardly speak out against the conglomerate that supplies their goodies.

Above and beyond this reality, the conglomerate is wise enough to know how to use and manipulate these people for its own benefit. How does it do this? Let me give you some examples.

A famous sports figure announces to the press that he has prostate cancer and that he will immediately undergo surgery and follow-up chemotherapy. So what happens? The press lunges for the big story, and thus the public is led to believe that surgery and chemo are automatically the way to go if you have prostate cancer.

A year later, the sports figure establishes a foundation to help educate the public about prostate cancer. Sound good? It does to the ignorant public. But in truth, and unbeknownst to the famous and honorable gentleman, he has become a shill for the conglomerate, who will benefit enormously from his name, reputation, and foundation.

Meanwhile, the public, including tens of thousands of men who will be diagnosed with prostate cancer each year, will be deprived of the chance to learn about other nonintrusive, nondrug-related treatment for prostate cancer. Consequently, other viable forms of treatment go unheard, neglected because they cannot provide the profits that are derived from surgery, chemotherapy, and radiation.

Then there's the famous cyclist, Lance Armstrong, who has won seven Grand Prix races (and has frequently been accused of doping), and openly shills for the companies that supplied his drugs when he had cancer. Listening to this guy on his television commercials promoting these drugs, one would think that the pharmaceutical manufacturer deserves a Nobel Prize.

He's a perfect example of someone who has gone over to the dark side. Whether he knows it or not, he has become a charter member of the conglomerate and profits from the suffering of all those who will be led to believe that his drugs are the best and only answer to cancer. THEY MOST CERTAINLY ARE NOT! There are organizations such as People Against Cancer in Otho, Iowa, as well as many others who have effectively combated cancer without drugs.

In numerous cases that I could cite, the famous people who might otherwise be supporting the public need for educational information (and who might trigger an awakening to the inherent dangers of conglomerate thinking and acceptance) are engaged in activities that openly support America's decaying healthcare system.

All the famous figures and personalities who act on behalf of the drug companies become part of the conglomerate's overall scheme to medicate the world for profit, promoting a drug culture that is extreme and dangerous.

In fairness to these famous people, many have agreed to act as spokespeople for drug companies because the products they advertise actually benefited them personally (in some cases they were cured of cancer). But they fail to realize that their advocacy of drugs or medical procedures creates far-ranging side effects.

They also fail to realize that they have reaped the benefit of the best medical treatment that money can buy. So they are in a very select group, which is not at all the case of the average American—who stands absolutely no chance of obtaining such privileged treatment. (Remember what happened in New Orleans after Hurricane Katrina!) This inequity contributes mightily to the horrendous disparity in medical treatment that exists in America.

On another level, although the personage is helping promote only one specific drug, the overall effect of the commercial in which s/he appears is that it does more to promote the drug company and its hundreds of wares than anything else. It's synergy in its most deadly form. Therein lies the rub; the well-intentioned public figure ends up promoting products s/he knows nothing about, as well as the entire drug culture. That's part of the conglomerate's scheme. And it works—to the tune of hundreds of billions in sales and tens of thousands of added casualties annually.

There are famous people who are exceptions to the general practice of celebrities promoting conglomerate wares. Two of the more renowned examples who deserve public acclaim for their magnificent service to humanity are the late Christopher Reeve, who devoted so much of his energy to his Christopher Reeve Paralysis Foundation (CRPF), and Michael J. Fox, who has done a fantastic job publicizing Parkinson's disease. Both of these "stars" (in the truest sense of the word) presented themselves in public with their disabilities, and they didn't do it to sell drugs.

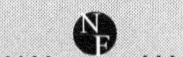

Another painful and infuriating example of how the Bush juggernaut treats all progressive healthcare measures; if enacted, its 2007 budget would kill the entire budget of the Christopher and Dana Reeve Paralysis Resource Center.

As I'm known to go off on a tangent, I can't let myself skip by the question of famous people acting as spokespersons for the conglomerate without covering the brouhaha between actor Tom Cruise and actress Brooke Shields. It centered around Cruise publicly attacking Brooke Shields for taking the antidepressant Paxil for postpartum depression.

Then he confronted *The Today Show* anchor Matt Lauer for not doing his research on psychiatric drugs like Ritalin and Adderall, which are often prescribed to children diagnosed with attention-deficit disorder.

The situation escalated when the American Psychiatric Association (APA) president Dr. Steven Sharfstein called the actor's comments dangerous. Sharstein went on to say that "It is irresponsible for Mr. Cruise to use his movie publicity tour to promote his own ideological views and deter people with mental illness from getting the care they need."

As if that weren't a sufficiently defensive posture on the APA's part, the organization's vice-president, Dr. Nada Stotland, came down even harder on Tom, who is a devout member of the controversial Church of Scientology, claiming that "We shouldn't be getting medical advice from people who don't have any training." (One of Scientology's lines of thinking is that people should avoid drug treatment and instead use higher doses of vitamins and minerals instead to cure many ailments.)

If you're wondering what the public thought of the conflict, a June 2005 MSNBC survey found that 69 percent believed that Cruise was "just plain wrong."

Now it's time for me to add my two cents worth:

1. Although I'm not a fan of Scientology, Tom Cruise doesn't need permission from the likes of the APA to voice his objections to the use of drugs. And the fact that he's an actor, not a quack psychiatrist, doesn't change that. In fact, I wish every responsible person in America would voice their opposition to indiscriminate drug use.

2. Brooke Shields has every right (but common sense) to use Paxil. However, I draw the line at any well-known person knowingly or unknowingly acting as a shill for the conglomerate. If she wants to go to hell on a rocket ship, that's her right. But she shouldn't be recommending others to go along for the deadly ride.[23] She should also realize that if she gets hooked on some junk, prescribed or otherwise, she can afford to check into the Betty Ford clinic— but those who are less well-heeled will end up most likely without rehab.

3. As for the APA, its disregard for conscientious patient treatment is directly responsible for the sick state of psychiatry in America. It has degenerated into little more than a massive drug dealership. That's not what its psychiatrists' training was for. (Or was it?)

4. I join Mr. Cruise and all other responsible and conscientious citizens who take a stand against the drug pushers.

5. It's unfortunate that the public's view and understanding of drug issues, including the ignorant support of an actress who doesn't know enough to use her junk and keep her mouth shut, is tantamount to the blind following the blind down the path to drug abuse and destruction. It's America's most crip-

---

[23] On May 13, 2006, both the FDA and GlaxoSmithKline, the maker of antidepressant Paxil, warned that the drug may raise the risk of suicidal behavior in young adults.

pling disease (a true "cancer"), and you don't need much intelligence or training to understand that.

✳ ✳ ✳

Then there are the whistleblowers. Thank God for this small band of courageous people who still believe in something and are willing to put their jobs, reputations, and lives on the line. Without them, very little hope for the future of our healthcare system or, for that matter, our ailing planet, would remain. Unfortunately, their revelations about corruption, neglect, massive schemes, or cover-ups (not to mention criminal behavior resulting in death) usually go unheeded.

It's also no secret that the majority of these goodniks suffer for their earnest concern for the public's well-being. They are penalized for revealing the truth, scorned and threatened by fellow workers, treated as informants and tattlers, cashiered out of their professions, and even beaten and murdered. But every now and then their will and determination succeeds over the conglomerate's hacks and pissants.

As if government whistleblowers don't have enough to contend with, Washington's menacing force in the White House is pushing the Supreme Court for a ruling that would make winning lawsuits claiming retaliation more difficult. This is a matter of First Amendment rights versus concealing government misconduct. (And an enormous amount of misconduct is going on in the Bush administration, as well as the opposition Democratic Party.)

✳ ✳ ✳

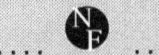

Dear reader, "Out of X" happened the very day I wrote the previous text dealing with government whistleblowers. I'm referring to the Supreme Court decision handed down on May 30, 2006, in which the Justices, in a 5 to 4 decision (with President Bush's recently appointed Justice Samuel Alito casting the deciding vote), scaled back protection for government workers who blow the whistle on official misconduct.

In practical terms, this means that 20 million public employees do not have free-speech protections for what they say as part of their jobs. This ruling is a victory for every crooked politician in America, one that will have sweeping impacts on the entire nation, and basically muzzle every worker who wants to reveal problems within government, whether it be about healthcare issues, hurricane preparedness, or terrorist-related security.

All along, I've denounced the tyrant in the White House, labeling him an illiterate psychotic, and if this doesn't show every American exactly what this demigod is up to, nothing will.

Next we have the FDA. Needless to say, this government agency (part of the Health and Human Services Department) should be at the forefront of addressing the will and well-being of the people. But judging from its actions (as indicated throughout this book), it appears that it sooner represents the politicians and the conglomerate, with little time for the medical concerns of the common man, woman, and child.

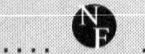

It's not surprising that the FDA continues to be confronted and attacked from all directions. Look at its recent track record: On August 31, 2005, Susan Wood, the women's health chief of the FDA, abruptly resigned in protest of her agency's refusal to allow over-the-counter sales of emergency contraception.

Five months later, she was quoted as saying, "The Food and Drug Administration has been 'hijacked.' " Speaking at the University of Washington, she also said, "The FDA seems to have lost its independence and lost its ability to make decisions based on scientific and medical evidence."

And less than four weeks after the resignation of Susan Wood, FDA Commissioner Lester Crawford also abruptly resigned. This came only two months after the Senate elevated Crawford to the top job.

The public cannot depend on the FDA to protect it from the conglomerate, because this agency is neither free nor independent of the administration's political and social agenda. To the contrary, our nation's medical and pharmaceutical decisions emanate from the Oval Office in the White House, all with the consent of the weak-minded in both political parties.

Even the American Medical Association has called for wholesale reforms of the FDA. If that doesn't tell you something—nothing will!

A final critical word about the FDA: On April 21, 2006, the FDA said that "no sound scientific studies" supported the medical use of marijuana, which contradicted other major studies, including a 1999 review by a panel of highly regarded scientists.

In March 1999, the National Academy of Sciences' Institute of Medicine (IOM) completed a review of the medical use of marijuana and related issues. The report, *Marijuana and Medicine: Assessing the Science Base*, was commissioned by the Office of National Drug Control Policy, after the people of California and Arizona voted for medical marijuana in 1996. The Institute of Medicine is widely considered the gold standard of American medicine. The IOM report recognized the therapeutic benefits of medical marijuana, urged that marijuana be made available to individual patients, and research continue on developing new drugs from marijuana.

Once again we witness how a government agency responsible for the public's well-being becomes a political tool of the Bush administration. Its support of the demoniac aims of the mindless one in Washington matches its willingness to align itself with the conglomerate's deadly profiteering and nationwide genocide.

❈ ❈ ❈

Last but not least, we have the Environmental Protection Agency (EPA). Judging from its recent track record, the word *protection* seems to be a misnomer. Actually, the current appropriate acronym of this agency should be *BPA*, for *Bush Protection Agency*, because the EPA is currently just another arm of all the big-time conglomerates that are locked in step with Big Brother's ambitions.

If you doubt this, read the following report.

**EPA TAKING 75% FEWER POLLUTERS
TO COURT, MAJOR POLLUTER CASES DOWN 90%
Utilities and Oil Companies Now On "Extended Vacation"
From EPA Enforcement; Lack of Action Reflects Cases Put
on Ice and Consistent Undermining of Staff Efforts**

Environmental Integrity Project Website—October 12, 2004

Polluters in the United States are breathing easier under the Bush administration's Environmental Protection Agency (EPA), which has engineered a 75 percent reduction in civil lawsuits filed against polluters, according to a new report released today by the Environmental Integrity Project (EIP). The steep fall-off reflects the decline in the number of lawsuits brought by the EPA after companies refuse to voluntarily settle Clean Air Act or Clean Water Act violations or fail to clean up pollution caused by their violations. ...

Key Report Findings

- *Clean Air Act enforcement is at a near stand still. Only nine such lawsuits were filed by the EPA from January 19, 2001 through January 18, 2004, compared to 61 in the three years prior to January 19, 2001.*

- *Clean Water Act enforcement is off sharply. This category of lawsuits declined from 56 between 1998 and mid-January, 2001, to only 22 between 2001 and mid-January, 2004.*

- *Hazardous waste law cases are way down. Lawsuits for violation of federal hazardous waste law (the Resource Conservation and Recovery Act) dropped from 19 to only five over the comparable three-year time periods.*

- *The nation's largest energy companies (and biggest polluters) are on an "extended vacation" from EPA enforcement actions. While the Justice Department has continued to litigate the cases it inherited from the previous administration, it has filed new lawsuits against only three energy companies between January 19, 2001, and January 18, 2004. That represents about a 90 percent decline when compared to the 28 lawsuits filed against power companies, oil companies, and pipelines in the three years leading up to January 19, 2001. ...*

- *The enforcement pipeline is running dry. In fact, many of the most significant settlements that EPA has celebrated either in press releases or in its annual enforcement reports resulted from lawsuits filed by the previous administration, according to the new report. ...*

- *What is behind the sharp drop in EPA enforcement? The EIP report concludes that it is "the logical result of a series of policy decisions that have effectively muzzled EPA's dedicated career staff." Among the examples cited of this muzzling are the following:*

  - *Power companies. Last November, the Agency's enforcement staff was told to "set aside" investigations against more than 70 power companies that are some of the biggest sources of air pollution in the U.S. The Agency had earlier referred 14 cases against power companies to the Justice Department for prosecution, but the Department has filed only one new case since January of 2001.*

  - *New Source Review. EPA's Office of Air and Radiation has effectively eliminated clean air "New Source Review" laws that forced power plants, refineries, and other manufacturers to clean up their oldest and dirtiest combustion or process units whenever they were physically modified. Those changes are being challenged in federal court, and the D.C. Circuit Court of Appeals has ordered the Agency not to implement the most significant rollback in rules after finding it might lead to irreversible harm to the environment, and may well be illegal. But the rule changes have had their intended effect in freezing any new Clean Air Act lawsuits.*

  - *Factory farms. EPA staff was ordered to cease investigations of industrial scale "factory farms" that house tens of thousands of animals, and make the air in surrounding communities unfit to breathe. Instead, the Agency has wasted the past three years offering amnesty for a voluntary emissions monitoring program that has yet to materialize. Clean Water Act rules were rewritten to relieve large corporate owners from liability for illegal wastewater discharges at their contract farms.*

- *Shackling the staff. The White House lost no time in trying to cut EPA's enforcement office, proposing in March of 2001 to eliminate more than 13 percent of the Agency's civil enforcement staff. Although Congress rejected these budget cuts, EPA delayed filling positions and "transferred" enforcement resources to Homeland Security functions that had already been fully funded by Congress.*

- *Emission standards. Just this year, EPA voluntarily abandoned its authority to tighten emission monitoring requirements in individual permits. This step backward ignores advice from the General Accounting Office and the EPA's own Inspector General, which have issued stinging reports about how inaccurate and unenforceable monitoring undermines emission standards.*

Here's further news on the dismantling of the environment:

ENVIRONMENTAL REVIEWS WAIVED IN PUSH FOR OIL

John Heilprin, The Associated Press—October 19, 2005

In an aggressive push by the Bush administration to open more public land to oil and gas production, the Interior Department has quit conducting environmental reviews and seeking comments from local residents every time drilling companies propose new wells.

Field officials have been told to begin looking at issuing permits based on past studies of an entire project, even though some of those assessments may be outdated. The instructions are in a directive from the department's Bureau of Land Management expected to cover hundreds of anticipated new drilling applications. ...

What this essentially translates into is that our environment's all up for grabs now. **Our parks, streams,[24] forests, and wildlife preserves are all legitimate targets.** And make no mistake about it: Under the guise of fighting terrorism and providing the U.S. with more oil, President George W. Bush, the world's great assassin, will strip it all away, piece by piece, acre by acre, and feed the trillions of dollars of profit to all his henchmen.

---

[24] Fireproof salmon, fish dosed with antidepressants, and shellfish tainted with amnesia-causing toxins can be found in the Pacific Northwest's Puget Sound.

Never one to beat a dead horse:

EPA TO BAR DATA FROM PESTICIDE STUDIES
INVOLVING CHILDREN AND PREGNANT WOMEN

Michael Janofsky, *The New York Times*—September 7, 2005

Researchers will no longer be allowed to include children and pregnant women in studies examining the effects of pesticides to help set federal standards, according to the first regulations for human testing of pesticides that the Environmental Protection Agency plans to propose. The regulations, to be proposed today, would also establish an independent oversight panel to ensure that all studies submitted to the agency were conducted ethically and followed internationally accepted protocols for human testing. ...

... The proposed regulations would take effect in January after a public comment period. ...

I'll bet there are some of you who will say, "That sounds good." That's because you're well-trained; you accept the spin and go about your business as if nothing is wrong. Well, excuse me if I clue you in: What this report really says—if you take the time to reread it—is that *the EPA had no regulations that protected children and pregnant women who have been guinea pigs for the government.*

And that patented BS about an oversight panel is another red flag that should tell any intelligent person what's really going on. Namely, someone blew a cover, and now the EPA (married to George W. Bush's ambition to destroy this planet from top to bottom), is putting out this "end run" to try to protect itself from flak.

Just to show you how little respect the EPA now has for the American public:

PESTICIDE TESTS MAY USE PREGNANT WOMEN, KIDS

Michael Doyle, McClatchy Newspapers—January 24, 2006

The Bush administration would allow some limited pesticide testing on children and pregnant women under controversial rules set to be made final as early as this week. ...

The illiterate one is at his game plan again! What makes this even more deadly than might appear to the average person is that he does these things so blatantly—as if he were a Roman emperor—and knows he can get away with it at every turn.

That's because all the major players—in this case including the EPA—are in his corner. God help us all! Especially the poor children and pregnant women, who will of course be the chosen ones for these atrocious experiments.

These guinea pigs will be used in much the same manner our unsuspecting troops were used time and again to witness atomic and hydrogen bomb explosions in nearby small Pacific atolls and never told of the dangers of radiation. Likewise, our troops in the Gulf War were exposed to various chemical and biological agents without knowing how badly their health would be affected.

While we're talking about the EPA and pesticides, here's another example of how the American public is treated like fools, accepting the designation without as much as a whimper:

PESTICIDES REACH MOST RIVERS

John Heilprin, The Associated Press—March 4, 2006

Most of the nation's rivers and streams—and the fish in them—are contaminated with pesticides linked to cancer, birth defects and neurological disorders, but not at levels that can harm humans. ...

This study, released by the U.S. Geological Survey, is the same kind of filthy lie that has been pawned off on the American public since the early days of mining and clearcutting of forests. The dirty job is done, to the detriment of the public and the environment, and the guilty parties, supported by government studies, claim that *no harm is being done*. Asbestos is okay, radiation levels aren't too high, pesticides in our water can't hurt us, and eating fish that are contaminated won't make us ill. And don't forget that mercury in the blood, brain, and body are not harmful, and smoking doesn't cause cancer or other diseases.

What's equally maddening is that our leaders in both political parties, who are totally aware of what's going on, won't do a damn thing to protect us. How can they—when they are dependent on corporate contributions and huge lobbying campaigns to keep them in office. It's one big rat race, always has been, and always will be—because the public won't stand up and fight against it.

On a similar level, millions of American schoolchildren and their teachers are being exposed to high concentrations of lead in their drinking water, as well as other environmental toxins such as arsenic that leave them sick and endangered. In her latest crusade, Erin Brockovich charges that fumes from active oil wells under the campus of Beverly Hills High School have caused inordinate levels of cancer and other disorders among the school's graduates. But these health issues and others, like mold on the walls, are often left in the bureaucratic hands of school officials who are unwilling to move beyond the status quo—a system that lacks accountability and oversight.

As if we didn't have enough pollutants to contend with, America has yet to face the ever-growing pile of electronic waste that the public discards indiscriminately. These electronic devices (TVs, computers, cell phones, etc.) contain permanent toxins such as lead, mercury, cadmium, chromium, and barium. Disposing of this electronic refuse will soon become as big a problem as getting rid of nuclear waste.

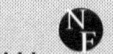

There are many American nuclear waste horror stories, and although a number of inventive ideas for the safe disposal of the deadly material have been put forth, of the 30,000 metric tons of spent fuel rods and 380,000 cubic meters of high-level radioactive waste produced so far, none of these materials have found anything more than interim accommodation.

No wonder. The cost to build a waste treatment plant at the highly contaminated Hanford Nuclear Reservation in south-central Washington has risen from $4.3 billion in 2000 to $12.2 billion in September, 2006. And this new estimate (which does not include the contractor's fee) also extends the projected start of operations to 2019, eight years past the date legally required under a cleanup pact signed by the state, the Energy Department, and the EPA.

In spite of this, more nuclear power stations will be built. Talk about beating a dead horse!

As if the EPA weren't doing enough damage to our environment and health, it is allowing soot pollution to continue unabated without any new long-term limits. Health and environmental groups have sued the government to force it to tighten its limits, but all the EPA says is that it will review new scientific findings before issuing another ruling.

More hogwash and madness! The diesel exhausts from trucks, ships, buses, and trains are silently poisoning millions of Americans. The EPA's current position is based on a 1997 standard that wasn't good enough then and is certainly not good enough now.

Without tightening the permissible concentration of fine particles in the air, we will cause an untold number of additional premature deaths from heart attacks, lung cancer, esophageal cancer, asthma, and other illnesses. And, once again, if you think that all that supposed acid reflux and esophageal cancer is primarily caused by acid in your stomach and other natural causes—wake up!

To show you just how far the EPA has removed itself from being an agency that protects the public, when an independent scientific review panel advised the EPA that a chemical used in the manufacture of Teflon (produced by DuPont) and other products should be considered a "likely" carcinogen, it countered the EPA's determination that there was only "suggestive evidence" of potential human carcinogens.

Of course, the EPA position supports the position of the DuPont Company, which is the second largest chemical company in the world (behind Dow Chemical) and very much a part of the conglomerate—most definitely an original charter member.

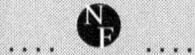

We must also realize that various other government agencies are in cahoots with the EPA when it comes to covering up for the chieftain in Washington, D.C. For instance, we have the Energy Department, which deals with nuclear waste dumped in Nevada; apparently they acknowledged that U.S. Geological Survey hydrologists made up facts, deleted inconvenient data, and kept one set of pertinent facts for themselves and another for quality assurance officials. But instead of confronting these federal workers, the Energy Department stated that the work was sound—**although it will be redone to comply with quality assurance rules.**

This type of cover-up is standard operating procedure for government agencies—and feeds into the almost unrestricted imperial powers of the Bush administration.

To put EPA matters in clear perspective, six former EPA heads (including five Republicans) recently accused the Bush administration of neglecting global warming and other environmental problems. I beg to differ: He's not neglecting them—**he's going all-out to destroy the environment.** He's doing everything in his endlessly growing power to see to it that our grandchildren will have to wear protective breathing devices before daring to walk on the streets. And he's doing it without any resistance from the so-called Democratic Party.

. . . .

On October 30, 2006, Prime Minister Tony Blair, President Bush's number-one ally, his main man in Europe, who has supported Bush's Iraq war—and suffered the political consequences in his own country—appeared at a news conference in London, where he took great exception with President Bush's climate policy. In fact, Britain issued a sweeping warning that the Earth faces a calamity on the scale of the world wars unless urgent action is taken.

Bravo Tony! Never too late to join the good guys.

The British government also said that former Vice-President Al Gore has agreed to provide advice on climate change. Now get this: Tony Blair is taking up with the likes of Al Gore! What does that say about the prime minister's attitude about George Bush's environmental policy?

A warning to the British people (and all Americans): While Al Gore may have some pertinent things to say about environmental matters, beware of the hypocrite—who went into hiding to lick his wounds after he lost his presidential bid to George Bush—and didn't reappear until 2005. Greenhouse gas emissions were rising during that critical period, and we didn't hear a peep from Al Gore until it was time for him to play his political card, hoping to reemerge from obscurity and regain prominence in the Democratic Party.

Shame on Al Gore—another environmental phony.

Here's but another example of how poorly America is served by the EPA:

COURT BLOCKS ATTEMPT TO EASE CLEAN AIR RULES

Mark Johnson, The Associated Press—March 18, 2006

A federal appeals court Friday blocked the Environmental Protection Agency from easing clean air rules on aging power plants, refineries

*and factories, one of the regulatory changes that had been among
the top environmental priorities of the White House. ...*

At this point in time, we must realize that the EPA is not only in George Bush's back pocket, but it will acquiesce to anything he wants, regardless of how much damage it does to the environment and the health of Americans. **In truth, this is a license to murder.**

A final note on EPA madness: With all of the things that the government failed to get right in the aftermath of Hurricane Katrina, one of its biggest and most immediate decisions was to relax (and put aside) environmental regulations—resulting in massive water and air pollution. These waivers took place without any public participation, and you can bet your bottom dollar that oil companies have taken full advantage of the situation and not only added considerably to the pollution but pocketed hundreds of millions of fast bucks.

Without going into details—because it would take another hundred pages to even skim the surface of my charges—as much as the EPA is directly responsible for handing over the reins of environmental leadership to the homicidal maniac in the White House, I must point my finger at the true villains of the looming environmental disasters. This will shock you and no doubt infuriate many who will take immediate exception to my accusations. But nonetheless, it must be said: *I blame all of the major environmental groups, both in America and throughout the world, for the current decimation and the upcoming total destruction of the environment.*

Why? Because they have used most of their time, money, energy, and reputations on themselves! They have consistently and utterly refused to join together in universal concord and solidarity to fight the battle of the ages against those who would defile and destroy the earth for profit and power.

These supposedly idealistic organizations are private institutions that consist of vainglory seekers who are more interested in their personal achievements than they are in truly saving this embattled planet.

The lot of them are on ego trips that I characterize as *loving themselves in the environment—not the environment in themselves.*

While they have been so actively engaged in looking after their own reputations at the expense of the environment they're supposed to be protecting, the George W. Bushes of the world, aided and abetted by the submissive politicians of most political forces, have been running amok—with little in the way of interference or opposition to concern themselves with. That's why one illiterate president has been able to destroy almost everything in his path. There's been no one to stand against him. Certainly not the environmentalists! Shame on all of you. You have not fought the good fight.

One last thing for the environmentalists to look at: Instead of wasting time defending yourselves against my accusations and denunciation, I implore you to consider one all-encompassing reality: **We are losing the war for the environment on all fronts.** We cannot regain the lost rainforests; hundreds of tons of pollutants are being pumped into our water, air, and soil every day; global warming is here to stay; ozone depletion is on the increase; America continues to consume more and more of the earth's limited resources without concern for the rest of the world's population; energy conservation is a mock joke (solar and wind power, like the electric car, are history and the idea of sustained energy is ignored); and the mentality that supports the environment's destruction grows more blatant and power-hungry with every passing moment. WAKE UP ALREADY!!!

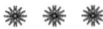

I have to add one more name to the list of those who should be speaking for the public good—our Congress. It has been said, "With friends like that—we don't need enemies!" Ditto for Congress! Our elected representatives on both sides of the aisle have shown an utter disregard for the public's well-being that seriously borders on treason. They might just as well have proclaimed President Bush their one and only leader and chief conspirator, and passed an amendment to the Constitution granting him unrestricted imperial powers. Never before in American history has there been such an example of one-man, one-party rule.

Former Minnesota Governor Jesse Ventura once remarked that Soviet Russia's one-party system wasn't that much different than America's two-party system in that we only have one more choice than they had. Well, that's all changed now. With the acquiescence of the (former) Democratic Party, America has, for all intents and purposes, been reduced to one-party rule. In effect, we are forced to go along with whatever the Bush administration dictates. Here's one example:

HOUSE ACTS TO END SOME FOOD LABEL WARNINGS

Zachary Coile, *San Francisco Chronicle*—March 9, 2006

The House approved a bill Wednesday night that would wipe out state laws on safety labeling of food, potentially affecting alerts about carcinogenic ingredients, lead in candy and allergy-causing sulfites.

The vote was a victory for the food industry, which has lobbied for years for national standards for food labeling and contributed millions of dollars to lawmakers' campaigns. But consumer groups and state regulators warned that the bill would undo more than 200

*state laws, including California's 1986 landmark Proposition 65,
that protect public health.*

*"The purpose of this legislation is to keep the public from
knowing about the harm they may be exposed to in food," said Rep.
Henry Waxman, D-Calif., a chief critic of the measure. ...*

Once again, power politics, engineered by highly paid lobbyists who have been
granted carte blanche by our bribed politicians, take precedent over the will of
the people.

> ***How does the conglomerate maintain such
> widespread control over almost all aspects
> of the American healthcare system?***
>
> ***Don't federal regulations govern the
> actions of many organizations and agencies?***

You would think laws would govern much of what goes on in the system, but you
have to understand that the powers that be have great political savvy and wield
enormous power in the halls of Congress. As an example of how things work:

EX-REP. TAUZIN TO BE LOBBYIST FOR DRUG FIRMS
Robert Pear, *The New York Times*—December 9, 2004

*Rep. Billy Tauzin, R-La., a principal author of the new Medicare
drug law, will become president of the Pharmaceutical Research
and Manufacturers of America, the chief lobby for brand-name drug
companies, the trade group said yesterday. ...*

*... Miles White, chairman of Abbot Laboratories and of the
trade association, sitting next to Tauzin, said he agreed that the
industry had lost the trust of patients.*

*... Tauzin, a one-time Democrat who became a Republican in
1995, has a wealth of connections in Congress, where he has served
for 24 years.*

*Drug makers said that the job was not a reward for Tauzin's work
on the Medicare bill, which followed the industry's specifications in
many respects. The law was signed by President Bush on Dec. 8,
2003, a few weeks before a lawyer for Tauzin began talks with the
drug trade group.*

Tauzin, 61, was the latest policy-maker to move from government to industry. "It's a classic example of the revolving door," said Lawrence Noble, executive director of the Center for Responsive Politics, a nonprofit group that studies money and politics.

Thomas Scully, the administration's main negotiator with Congress on the drug bill, got a waiver of federal ethics rules that permitted him to negotiate with potential employers while he was still running the Medicare program. Since he joined a law firm last December, Scully has registered as a lobbyist for drug companies, including Abbot and Aventis.

Tauzin and White refused to discuss Tauzin's new salary, except to say it was comparable to the pay at other large trade associations. People at other trade groups believed that Tauzin was receiving $2 million a year or more.

Rep. Pete Stark of California, the senior Democrat on the House Ways and Means Subcommittee on Health said: "As a member of Congress, Billy negotiated a large payout to the pharmaceutical industry by the federal government. He's now about to receive one of the largest salaries ever paid to any advocate by an industry."

Tauzin wrote large parts of the new Medicare law as chairman of the Energy and Commerce Committee and as a member of the conference committee that hashed out differences between the House and Senate in four months of intense negotiations last year.

The law steers clear of price controls and price regulation, which are anathema to drug companies. The law forbids the government to negotiate with drug manufacturers to secure lower prices for Medicare beneficiaries.

Federal law prohibits a former member of Congress from lobbying the House or Senate for one year after the lawmaker leaves office. In that "cooling off period," Tauzin cannot directly lobby Congress himself, but can legally tell other people how to lobby. In addition, he can make campaign contributions, attend fund-raisers and "interact socially" with people in Congress.

Rep. Henry Waxman, D-Calif., who has focused on health policy for 30 years, did not question the legality of Tauzin's move. But Waxman said: "The appearance is terrible. A chief architect of the Medicare prescription drug legislation is now going to represent the chief beneficiary of the bill. This will only reinforce the public's disillusionment with Congress." ...

... In his last election campaign, Tauzin received $174,000 in

contributions from health professionals and $119,750 from makers of drugs and other health products.

Well ain't that just dandy! This entire sick episode smacks of a conflict of interest on every conceivable level, and yet absolutely nothing can be done about it. Once again, the conglomerate writes its own laws. As always, the public be damned!

Here's another winner:

LOBBYIST ACCUSED OF BILKING TRIBE
**Abramoff, partner may have siphoned
millions from Choctaw, senator says**

Suzanne Gamboa, The Associated Press—June 23, 2005

Lobbyist Jack Abramoff and his partner created tax-exempt groups to funnel money to themselves from Indian tribes trying to build political support for their casinos, according to documents released at a Senate hearing yesterday.

Sen. John McCain, R-Ariz., chairman of the Senate Indian Affairs Committee, described it as a scheme to bilk millions of dollars from the tribes.

"Today's hearing is about more than contempt, even more than greed," he said. "It is simply and sadly a tale of betrayal." ...

This scandal is of particular importance because it is easily one of the most devious and far-reaching acts of corruption to hit Capitol Hill in many years—and that says a lot!

It involves congressional bribery, illegal campaign contributions (which lawmakers in both parties are now scrambling to donate to charities to save face), money laundering, shady plea-bargaining, and a host of typical political machinations that harkens back to the days of Tammany Hall,[25] Watergate, and worse.

It's a classic example of how deeply rooted corruption can become when it is supported by most of the powers that be in Washington. And make no mistake about it, many hands reached out to take part in this lobbyist racketeering.

As of December 2005, the full story of this investigation has yet to be concluded. Much more remains to be revealed. So stay tuned.

---

[25] Tammany Hall: The Democratic political machine that dominated New York City politics from 1854 through 1934. Although it offered a source of hope and a means to survival for many immigrants, it symbolized political patronage and became a bastion of corruption.

ABRAMOFF GUILTY PLEA SHAKES CAPITOL HILL

Scott Shepard, Cox News Service—January 4, 2006

Former Lobbyist Jack Abramoff, a longtime associate of top Republican leaders, pleaded guilty Tuesday to conspiracy, fraud and tax evasion and agreed to cooperate with federal officials investigating political corruption in the nation's capital. ...

The next day, Abramoff completed his plea deal by admitting to conspiracy and wire fraud charges. *And that's still only the beginning! Much more to come....*

And here it is: In spite of the fact that the Abramoff affair threatens to be the most far-reaching example of power-politics and corruption since the Watergate scandal, Congress will do nothing about it! No investigation into misconduct on the part of lawmakers will be carried out, no commitment will be made on the part of the congressional ethics committee to uncover the truth, and no need for pardons will be required because no one will be reprimanded. This is what happens under one-party rule.

However, our Congress *is* clever enough to know that it must make some attempt to cover its tracks ... and on March 9, 2006, they pulled a classic end run to escape the accusation of not being serious about breaking the bond between Capitol Hill and the lobby racket. It was a beaut! Textbook stuff, right out of all the two-bit political maneuvers that have ever been perpetrated on the American public. They decided to bar members of Congress from accepting gifts and meals from lobbyists.

On the surface of things, government watchdog groups have been given a reason to believe that this ban on giving gifts and meals will actually accomplish something, as if it were a commitment to reform. That's ludicrous, because this bill merely acts as a caveat, signaling the lobbyists to take other approaches to their bribing and solicitations (as if they don't already know how to do that).

And if you think that our politicians will be able to resist the keen temptations of big lobbying contributions, you're off your rocker. The entire system is too entrenched in the minds, hearts, and pocketbooks of our governmental felons (the entire lot of them!), and it would take nothing short of a Constitutional amendment to break the back of this corrupt institution.

Abramoff will get his deal, everyone else will cover their tracks (any rush to reform lobbying will get lost in the shuffle), and the public will swallow the whole affair and chalk it up to business as usual in Washington.

Once again, it's a prime example of the American caste system at work: a free pass for the big shots who commit massive crimes, while the ordinary citizen is brought to task at the drop of a hat.

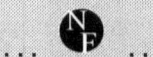

The key fact surrounding these reports and all others dealing with lobbyists is that anyone dumb enough to think that lobbying is an honorable institution of government should have his head examined! Lobbying constitutes the single most illicit and sinful practice known to any democratic-minded government.

Commonly referred to as "influence peddling," lobbying is built on the premise that big business, special interests, and powerbrokers are granted the right to take advantage of the public, creating their own set of rules and devices to satisfy the greedy bastards that control this country.

Note: On November 15, 2006, Jack Abramoff reported to federal prison to begin serving a nearly six-year prison sentence as federal inmate No. 27593-112.

Here's more of the same:

STATE'S FIRMS PUMP MILLIONS INTO FEDERAL LOBBYING

Charles Pope, *Seattle Post-Intelligencer*—April 9, 2005

According to an exhaustive study released Thursday, by The Center for Public Integrity, a Washington, D.C.-based nonpartisan group that monitors ethics and money in government, special interests have spent $13 billion since 1998 to lobby Congress, the White House, and federal agencies.

And, researchers say, the total is only going to rise.

"Today, federal lobbying is an industry in its own right," said Roberta Baskin, the center's executive director. "It employs almost 14,000 people who are paid to influence the decisions of Congress, the White House, and officials at more than 200 federal agencies." ...

NEY ADMITS GUILT IN LOBBY SCANDAL

Philip Shenon, *The New York Times*—September 16, 2006

Rep. Bob Ney of Ohio admitted Friday that he had effectively put his office up for sale to corrupt Washington lobbyists. ...

And guess who's up there with the biggest lobbyists?

MEDICARE LAW PROMPTS A RUSH FOR LOBBYISTS
Robert Pear, *The New York Times*—August 23, 2005

The new Medicare law has touched off explosive growth in lobbying by the health care industry, whose spending on advocacy here far exceeds that of consumer groups and other industries like defense and banking. ...

... With hundreds of billions of dollars at stake, health care providers, insurers, drug makers and pharmacies are continually trying to influence rules for the drug benefit and other initiatives authorized by the law. ...

Last year alone, the health care industry spent $325 million—more than any other sector—in its efforts to influence Congress and federal agencies, according to Political Money Line, a nonpartisan group that studies reports filed with Congress by lobbyists and their clients.

Drug companies led the way. They reported spending $86.9 million on lobbying last year, followed by hospitals with $55 million and doctors with $35.4 million. ...

... "Every health care interest has a voice on Capitol Hill," said Elizabeth J. Fowler, a lawyer who recently left the Democratic staff of the Senate Finance Committee to join a consulting firm. "What you lose in the process is consumer and beneficiary voices. We heard a lot more from industry interests than from beneficiaries." ...

We lose a lot more than that, Elizabeth. We are so overwhelmed by the conglomerate that we lose hope. We accept each defeat. We give up. Unconditional surrender.

The victors are the cronies and powerbrokers concerned with special interests that favor the rich and powerful. The rest of us are left to trust that the governing principles of our society can be adequately served by merely empowering individuals to turn to the ballot box every few years.

What utter nonsense! The control of our nation is not in our hands. We are not a country of "We the People." No *democratia* remains in our corrupt form of government.

Pardon me while I beat a dead horse once again, but here's another example of how things work:

HEALTH CARE INQUIRY CASH MISDIRECTED

Robert Pear, *The New York Times*—**May 16, 2005**

Money earmarked by Congress for investigating health care fraud appears to have been shifted improperly to other purposes, like fighting terrorism, congressional auditors say in a new report.

The report, to be issued this week by the Government Accountability Office, says health care cases got short shrift from the FBI, which was supposed to use the money exclusively to investigate fraud against Medicare, Medicaid and other health programs. The money came from an account in the Medicare trust fund.

The FBI was unable to show that it had used the money for the intended purpose, the report said, noting that FBI agents "previously devoted to health care fraud investigations were shifted to counterterrorism activities" in the past three years. ...

... Senator Charles Grassley, R-Iowa, who requested the study, said, "It's inexcusable that the government cannot account for millions of dollars set aside to fight health care fraud." ...

Joseph Ford, the bureau's chief financial officer, said the attacks of Sept. 11, 2001, "demanded an instant, 100 percent commitment toward counterterrorism," and he said "almost every FBI agent in the world" had been required to work on those cases. ...

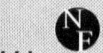

The following should also be pointed out to Senator Charles Grassley: The government not only cannot account for millions of dollars earmarked to fight healthcare fraud, but the FBI also uses September 11th as its rationale for its lack of financial accountability.

For the sake of argument, let's say we accept that the FBI had to "demand an instant, 100 percent commitment toward counterterrorism." What in hell's name does that have to do with financial accountability? It merely sounds like a grand excuse (opportunity) to steal money from the Medicare trust fund. Furthermore, within this same report about money being misdirected from its intended purposes by the FBI, we find the following statement:

"Medicare, the insurance program for the elderly and disabled, paid more than 1 billion claims a year. The Bush administration says that last year, 9.3 percent of the claims were paid in error, resulting in overpayments of $19.9 billion to doctors, hospitals and other health care providers."

Does that mean that $19.9 billion in errors was returned to the government, or is this a case of the conglomerate skimming off the top?

＊ ＊ ＊

What's the story with Medicare and Medicaid?

It's a gruesome story of bureaucratic ineptitude, greed, and outright stupidity that has yet to be played out to its rock-bottom level. Just give the illiterate one in the White House the balance of his term in office, and he'll show you what he's still got up his sleeve.

President Johnson signed the Medicare law into effect in 1965. It's basically an insurance policy funded by the government. The Medicaid portion of the program is supposed to provide health insurance to low-income families and others with limited resources, while Medicare is an insurance program for eligible individuals over the age of 65 and those with disabilities.

As to how it actually works, there are more than 100,000 pages of regulations—which mandates that the entire system remain in a chaotic state for all those involved, including patients, doctors, hospitals, caregivers, and health insurance companies.

Even worse, its provisions and regulations are always subject to revision, recall, and manipulation at every turn of the political screw, resulting in unimaginable confusion and buck-passing on the part of administrative personnel on all levels.

In other words—it's a total mess from top to bottom. It doesn't just need fixing (that's impossible!), it needs to be trashed—because it was bad to begin with, got a lot worse when Congress passed the HMO Act of 1973 (which imposed regulations and tax rules that forced most large companies to use HMOs for employee health plans), and has become the antithesis of what it was meant to be.

To take it a step further, the conglomerate has taken the Medicare program under its wing and parlayed its drug schemes into a nest egg of ever-hatching drug and insurance company plots and tactics, all aimed at profiteering on an-unheard of level and medicating as many Americans as possible. That's the real story.

As an example, here's a quote from the 2006 government handbook *Medicare & You*: "As we age, most people need prescription drugs to stay healthy." This statement is repeated again and again throughout the handbook. Can you imagine? Here we have Medicare openly schilling for the conglomerate!

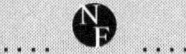

Medicare operates along similar lines as the insurance industry, only the language is different. For instance, the insurance industry uses "deductible," while Medicare calls it a "spenddown." What it really means is that if you can't meet the spenddown, you have no insurance. Plain and simple.

To show you just how far they go, as of January 1, 2006, a new Medicare prescription drug program went into effect. That is, it should have gone into effect—but no one seemed to know how it would operate. Senior citizens (myself included) were bombarded with letters and proposals from insurance companies, and pharmacists throughout the country didn't have a clue as to what was going on! It was an absolute fiasco—as only the American government can entangle itself in.

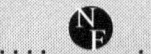

The new prescription drug plan of 2006 was ballyhooed as a great savings for people in need of drugs. In actuality, some people have realized savings. But that might only last as long as your insurance holds out. Then you'll be left out in the cold, wondering who you can turn to for your meds. You know what? You might be better off—because you might just have to start cleansing your drug-worn body of all the junk (toxins) you've been feeding it. That includes painkillers that will eventually destroy your vital organs.

What this drug plan is really about—if you bother to think about it—is a conglomerate smokescreen of unbelievable proportions—because what it basically accomplishes is to promote drug use as the essential form of medical treatment for everything under the sun.

Using Medicare as its primary shill, the conglomerate is getting billions of dollars of free publicity for its junk heap. The net results over the next few decades will include hundreds of millions of more addicted souls going to early graves, prescription in hand.

Meanwhile, millions of low-income people will have to pay more for healthcare under a budget bill worked out by Congress. And many of them will have to drop out of the Medicaid system entirely. The Senate has already approved the bill. Note: Guns instead of butter (and healthcare) is the rule of the day.

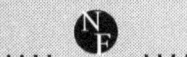

By its very nature, the Medicare program exemplifies the American caste system in its most insidious form. It separates the haves (those with Medicare coverage) from the have-nots (those with Medicaid coverage).

More and more Americans will be left at the very end of the health help-line with nowhere to turn, no place to appeal. Like victims of Hurricane Katrina, they will sit alone and wonder what ever happened to America. The only answer they will get is, "The rich get richer, the middle-class protects its flanks, the poor get poorer, and don't expect it to change—unless something drastic should intervene. In fact, prepare for the very worst—and keep a set of eyes in the back of your head."

Just to show you that I'm personally affected by this outrageous and dehumanizing Medicare madness, I just received a letter which reads, "Your Medicare benefits have been reduced by Congress due to increases in your deductibles and Part A co-insurance payment. Now, Medicare pays less of your health care cost and you are responsible for the unpaid balance."

What the aforementioned letter amounts to is ... *Nickolas Vassili, Korean War veteran, 70 years of age, no longer has any medical coverage.* No surprise: Like the infamous Captain Hook—Bush wants his war!

When I get right down to it, every time I witness tens of thousands of baseball fans standing during their seventh-inning stretch and singing "God Bless America," I want to scream at the top of my lungs, "What are you singing about?! America? God? Or are you unknowingly just heaping more praise on the millionaire ballplayers and on the conglomerates that don't give a damn about the ordinary folk who can't afford to pay for a visit to a doctor, much less buy a ticket to a ballgame!

Save your singing for an America that really gives a damn! So much for Medicare and Medicaid. ...

> ### What about nongovernmental organizations like the American Cancer Society?
>
> ### Can they be trusted?

While I can't accuse them or many other well-known charitable and humanitarian agencies of being in bed with the conglomerate, I can safely say that they are on the wrong track when it comes to helping to cure cancer. To support this contention, here is an article by Samuel S. Epstein, M.D., professor emeritus of Environmental and Occupational Medicine at the Illinois School of Public Health and author of *Cancer-Gate: How to Win the Losing Cancer War.*

CANCER WAR SHOULD FOCUS ON PREVENTION

Samuel Epstein, Guest Columnist, *Seattle Post-Intelligencer*—April 27, 2005

Today, there are generals waging a war that continues to take a massive toll of Americans' health and life. These generals are asking for billions of dollars—on top of the more than $50 billion already spent—to defeat the enemy's scourge. But increasingly, independent experts are reporting that the generals' intelligence and strategies are patently wrong, and that they consciously misrepresent critical facts in order to paint false, rosy scenarios.

In all likelihood, you must suspect that I am referring to the Iraq war. But there is actually another war being handled with startling ham-handedness and deception. It's a war that claims far more victims than the war against terror. It is the war against cancer.

In 1971, President Nixon declared war against cancer and Congress passed the National Cancer Act. These actions ushered in the new battle, spurring a 30-fold increase in the budget of the government's National Cancer Institute—to a tune of $5 billion this year. The new war also helped the nation's leading cancer charity, the American Cancer Society, raise tens of millions in public donations.

With the wind at their backs, and locked at the hip, leaders of the NCI and ACS became the generals in the new war, and have spent billions of tax and public dollars in waging it over ensuing years.

But after three decades of highly publicized and misleading promises of progress, the sad reality has finally dawned: We are in fact losing the cancer war, in what can only be described as a rout. The incidence of cancers—notably breast, testes, thyroid, myeloma, lymphomas and childhood—all unrelated to smoking—has escalated to epidemic proportions, now striking nearly one in every two men, and more than one in every three women. Meanwhile, overall mortality rates—the indicator of our ability to survive cancer once it strikes—have remained unchanged for decades.

There is strong scientific evidence that this epidemic is due to avoidable exposures to industrial carcinogens in the totality of the environment—air, water, soil, workplaces as well as consumer products—and even some common prescription drugs.

But our ongoing defeat in this war is attributable to two important factors.

First, NCI and ACS have focused their abundant resources and institutional mindsets not on preventing cancer, but on attempting to treat it once it strikes. The NCI, for instance, allocates less than an estimated three percent of its budget to environmental causes of cancer, while the ACS allocates less than 0.1 percent toward this goal. As recently admitted by the president of one of NCI's leading cancer centers, most NCI resources are spent on "promoting ineffective drugs" for terminal disease.

By forsaking prevention—the basic principle that medicine has taught us over the centuries, and the need for which science again underscores in the war against cancer—our cancer generals have embraced a "damage-control" strategy, akin to treating wounded soldiers, rather than trying to halt further advance of the enemy.

The simple fact—the more cancer is prevented, the less there is to treat—continues to elude the generals' master plan.

Another reason why our cancer generals are so disserving is that they have become far too chummy with special interests who either oppose cancer prevention policies or who trivialize cancer prevention. The ACS heavily depends on their "Excalibur donors"— a gallery of chemical industries opposed to regulating carcinogens, and pharmaceutical companies seeking approval of their highly touted miracle drugs—drugs that have shown limited if any success over decades.

Similarly the NCI has also developed incestuous relationships with cancer drug companies. Indeed, a former director candidly admitted that the NCI "has become what amounts to a governmental pharmaceutical company."

In order to change course, drastic reforms are needed in the cancer war high command and strategies. Both the NCI and ACS must be required to devote at least equal priority and resources to prevent as to treat cancer. The NCI and ACS must also be required to inform the public, Congress and regulatory agencies of substantial scientific evidence on industrial, and other avoidable causes of cancer. Congress should also ensure that companies that pollute our environment and consumer products with industrial carcinogens are held to the highest standards of accountability and disclosure.

Nearly every American knows the pain to family and friends caused by cancer. The crime is that so much of it is avoidable.

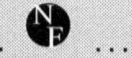

Bless your heart, Dr. Epstein, for having the courage to speak out so forcefully. However, any hope of seeing a change is a pipe-dream for lots of reasons. With 700,000 tons of industrial pollutants pumped into the air, soils, and our water **DAILY**, the concept of prevention becomes increasingly out of reach with every passing moment. Only the roaches will survive!

You must also remember that the conglomerate is well-prepared for any opposition plan that would sabotage its prescribed course—*the ongoing development of more drug treatment for the ever-growing number of cancer patients.*

From my viewpoint, it's safe to say that... were it not for the conglomerate's all-out dedication to profit-taking from drug treatment, and the support of the bribe-takers in both political parties, **most forms of cancer would have been cured 25 years ago.** The same goes for many other killer diseases.

In fact, we should recognize that the flip side of cure and prevention is almost always drug treatment and surgery because that's where the market exists.

It's similar to the prison system; there's no money in prevention. The same holds true for drug prevention and most social problems—people (officials, leaders, etc.) don't want to solve problems—they want to treat them and use them for profit and career advancement.

These people want to maintain their salary lines and perpetuate their positions. Don't you get it? Solve the common cold, crime, drug addiction, cancer, poverty, and so on, and all the big shots lose out.

And as always, ego plays its part in preventing prevention. I recall a doctor I met at Kings County Hospital in Brooklyn back in 1951, when my father was dying of Hodgkin's disease. I asked him why they couldn't cure cancer. His answer was, "There are people all over the world working on a cure—but they won't come together and cooperate to find the cure." He was dead right.

So there is little reason to have faith in miracle cures, much less basic prevention programs. It can't happen under present conditions because the unaware and unsuspecting public is fed a daily dosage of media propaganda that supports the conglomerate's course of action.

As an example:

NEW CANCER DRUGS 'MULTITASK'

Marilynn Marchione, The Associated Press—May 14, 2005

A new generation of experimental cancer drugs is poised to upstage current hotshots by attacking the multiple methods tumors use to grow and spread, instead of just one.

These drugs are like a repairman who brings an entire toolbox to a job instead of just a wrench or hammer. ...

... Doctors hope the new generation of cancer drugs will do just that by blocking cancer's multiple pathways, such as cutting off the blood supply to a tumor or jamming the "switchboard" it uses to send messages to grow and spread. ...

... For these and others with advanced cancers, the new multitasking drugs might at least make cancer a stable, chronic condition. So far, tumors eventually find ways to defeat even new drugs like Avastin that shut down one process. ...

... Other scientists are trying to get the same multitasking approach by combining single-target drugs like Avastin and Erbitux.

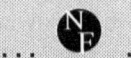

Sounds good, doesn't it? An entire toolbox of drugs—instead of a miserly one or two! How can you go wrong? You should take advantage of the fire sale and order a couple of those babies!

You can bet that the average hopeful person will look upon such drugs as a new advance against cancer. Even with that drug regimen running $40,000 to $60,000 a month, it will find broad acceptance and become a staple feature of our war on cancer.

Let's take it a step further: Genentech (another conglomerate entity) plans to charge about $100,000 a year for a drug already widely used for colon cancer called Avastin, which will be used as a new treatment for breast and lung cancer. With people willing to pay big bucks to extend their lives for a few months, do you think anyone is going to take interest in preventing or curing cancer?

Incidentally, Genentech, the manufacturer of Avastin, revealed that the **average wholesale price for a dose of the drug is $3,779.** Note: By the time the drug passes through a distributor and to the individual hospital, the markup approaches 300 percent!

Here's another classic example of how the conglomerate, aided by the media—and the political hacks in Washington—fools the public into thinking something good is happening:

$100 MILLION PROJECT TO GET TO THE ROOT OF CANCER
Lauran Neergaard, The Associated Press—December 14, 2005

Cancer is a disease of genes run amok, and scientists have found only a fraction of the bad actors. Tuesday, the government unveiled a $100 million project to speed discovery of culprits and cures, the first step toward a comprehensive map of cancer's genetic makeup.

It's an audacious project—the technology to even try it wasn't available just a few years ago. ...

The article goes on to highlight cancer statistics, how a Cancer Genome Atlas will "tackle the cancer problem like it's never been tackled before," and how the project will bring together researchers who now work independently to hunt not just specific cancerous gene mutations, but chromosome rearrangements, faulty on/off switches, and other abnormalities.

All of this sounds progressive, imaginative, and hopeful. HOWEVER...toward the end of the article, the true nature of the project is revealed: The payoff could be huge. A handful of so-called targeted drugs—Herceptin, Gleevec, Iressa, Tarceva—are proving very effective in battling certain cancers in patients with specific faulty genes.

That's only a small portion of patients: About 20 percent of breast cancer patients have the genetic aberration that Herceptin targets, and just 10 percent of lung cancer sufferers harbor the mutation that Iressa and Tarceva target.

After reading through all my documentation and accusations, let's see how smart you've become: Can you figure out what this $100 million project is really about?

If you're still in the dark—**this is a $100 million gift to the conglomerate!** Under the guise of "tackling the cancer problem like it's never been tackled before," the project experts will do enough research to provide the drug companies with new genetic codes—which will be used to develop new drugs. Yeah...more and more drugs...more and more billions in profit for the conglomerate. **And 20 years down the line, we'll still be losing the cancer war.**

One of the saddest things about our dedication to drug research is that other forms of research in many vital areas (including cancer) does not receive appropriate funding. As an example: Unlike the many Hollywood stars and well-known personalities that peddle drugs on television advertisements, both the late Christopher Reeve and Michael J. Fox used their time, resources, and energy championing the cause of stem cell research. On September 14, 2000, testifying before Congress on stem cell research, Michael J. Fox had this to say: "... The consistent and inescapable conclusion is that this research offers the potential to eliminate diseases—literally save millions of lives... It's time to act on what we've learned. Sadly, we've already lost two years' progress toward a cure. Further delay could come at a high price. ... I see in these cells a chance for a miracle cure. Release our tax dollars so that scientists can do their work."

Those words were spoken more than six years ago—and while our tax dollars are going toward funding an illegal war, and most research is still focused on creating more drugs, we're no closer to releasing funds for stem cell research than we were in the year 2000. And if the lunatic in the White House and his supporters in both political parties have their way, there will be no meaningful stem cell research for many years to come.

Another way of looking at this issue is that the battle isn't just against disease—it must be fought against the conglomerate that will continue to stand squarely in the way of prevention and cure. As long as they are in the driver's seat, they will only support the creation of more drugs—and hundreds of billions of more profit.

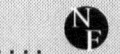

Whenever anyone talks about health research in America, they're basically talking about creating more drugs—primarily for the sake of profits. That's really what it's all about. Don't be fool enough to think otherwise.

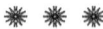

And in the intervening years, you will read countless reports on new therapies for various forms of cancers; the latest deals with ovarian cancer, which is the deadliest of all reproductive cancers in women. This report highlights supposed survival increases of more than a year, which is a meaningful survival increase for any type of cancer—if it provided a year of *quality* life—which it rarely does.

So what it really comes down to—as always—is that we're talking about a new drug that barely lengthens the life expectancy of the cancer patient, who will undoubtedly spend most of his or her remaining days *under care*. Is that well and good? Except for the conglomerate—absolutely not!

Once again, we're putting our time, energy, money, and research efforts into creating more drugs—instead of prevention and cure.

Doctors often add to these problems by not warning female patients that the drug treatment that may save their lives may also destroy their fertility. They also neglect to inform them of various options that will enable them to have children, providing that they act before treatment. This only adds to the multitude of health-care problems in America, including malpractice suites against doctors who fail to adequately carry out their responsibilities.

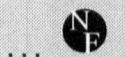

As an added disadvantage to the drug scheme of treating cancer, a large percentage of cancer patients cannot tolerate the chemotherapy or radiation that routinely follows surgery. And those that are willing to tolerate the treatments suffer from a wide range of side effects, which hardly enhances the quality of their lives during those additional months they live.

> The tradeoff is not a positive one. And the drug treatment fo-
> cus goes almost 100 percent of the way in keeping us on the same
> nonpreventive course.

The media also plays a big part in shortchanging prevention programs. For instance, the federal government has a national breast and cervical cancer early-
detection program, run by the Centers for Disease Control and Prevention, which
provides screening and other services to low-income women who do not have
health insurance or are underinsured.

Wouldn't you know it... our president—in need of more money for his war in
Iraq—proposed a cut in this vital program—which would mean that 4,000 fewer
women would have access to early detection. Was there any media outcry against
this proposed cut? Of course not. There's no big advertising bucks involved for
them. Likewise, the media pays little attention when the president cuts other cancer prevention programs.

Meanwhile, our environmental pollutants will increase, causing millions more
cancers, and the conglomerate will continue to thrive in the midst of this carnage.
Fat chance we have against them. And nary a word of opposition will be heard
from the NCI or ACS, much less our political leadership.

✳ ✳ ✳

To take the general issue of prevention one step further and for the sake of showing you just how weird a society we really live in... here is a scenario that I have
witnessed in many forms throughout my lifetime:

Picture a seriously depressed neighborhood, with rampant unemployment,
crime, drugs, roach-infested housing, and little in the way of hope for change.
No one wants to invest in this neighborhood, and government agencies refuse
to appropriate funds for its redevelopment, even though it would take only $10
million to deal with the squalor and hopelessness and set things in motion for a
turnaround.

One morning a seven-year-old girl is walking through a field when she suddenly falls into an exposed well. She lands some 30 feet below and begins to scream
for help. Several hours later, someone walks by and hears her faint screams, and
within minutes police and emergency units from the fire department arrive on the
scene.

Over the next 24 hours, while the rescue team tries repeatedly to reach the
helpless and possibly dying girl, the incident attracts widespread media attention.

Thousands of people surround the area and pray for the girl, and that vigil turns into a major news story that focuses the attention of millions of people on that field in that depressed neighborhood.

Rescuers finally reach the girl and pull her out alive, and millions of television onlookers cry out for joy, as if they had personally been saved.

Now here's the thing: Just one day earlier, no one had interest in coming into that neighborhood and resurrecting it. No agency gave a damn about what was happening there. And the public certainly wasn't moved to deal with the problem. But when one individual was trapped in a life-and-death situation, suddenly the police and fire departments, all sorts of emergency rescue teams, the media, and the public all rise to the occasion and are willing to do whatever is necessary to save this one person—even if the rescue mission costs more than $10 million. What does that tell you?

It tells me that we sit on our haunches and do nothing about a serious blight in our midst until we are emotionally moved to take action in order to pacify our guilt and neglect. It tells me that we should care about the thousands of people who live in that neighborhood, instead of just showing our concern for one imperiled person. It tells me that we will not spend the money necessary to prevent poverty and suffering unless it gives us a personal charge, then we'll spend any amount of money necessary to deal with the emergency.

We won't do the right thing—but we will take extraordinary action to make ourselves feel good. (We'll spend thousands of dollars to rescue a cat from a tree!) Social workers!

So whether we ignore prevention because it doesn't pay well enough or because we don't have the vision that should move us to action, it still comes down to poor thinking and lack of humanity. We shouldn't have to wait until a young child falls into a well or a Hurricane Katrina lays waste to a city. We should always think *PREVENTION*.

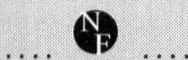

The earth provides cures for diseases. But at the rate that we're destroying the rainforests—they'll be gone before we can use them.

＊ ＊ ＊

Once again, forgive me for beating a dead horse BUT... on Tuesday, January 3, 2006, the entire country was riveted to its television news stations, watching the grim events taking place near a coal mine in Tallmansville, West Virginia. After 12 of the miners trapped in a coal mine explosion were reported alive, it turned out that all but one of 13 miners were found dead.

Needless to say, it was another classic example of how prepared Americans are to involve themselves emotionally when lives are at stake, and how much time, energy, and money we will spend to save those who are entrapped in a well or mine. These real-life scenarios bring out the social worker in all of us. We desperately want things to work out, and we cling to the slightest hope that a miracle will take place—so that we can share in the rewarding experience of beating death. It's as good as any Hollywood script, and just as phony.

Those miners died because the mining company didn't fully abide by the laws and regulations that apply to its safety responsibilities. In simple terms, the disaster could have and should have been *prevented.*

As for all the heartfelt drama (and make no mistake about it—millions of Americans felt a great deal—including me), when the miracle was taken away, we felt as if something in each of us died.

The major problem with this great American drama is that people won't stop to realize that millions of fellow Americans living in poverty, dying from diseases that should have been prevented, lying up in prisons, and going without any hope of getting a fair share in the American dream, will also go without the miracle. Only there will be no TV cameras focused on them, no media circus, no national attention, no outpouring of sympathy or concern. They will just go their doomed ways, with no one coming to their rescue.

If you still refuse to accept that as a nation we turn our backs on suffering, just look at Hurricane Katrina victims—so long after the devastating event.

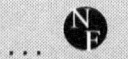

As if the poor and bedraggled victims of Hurricane Katrina hadn't been put through enough, on the one-year anniversary of the deadly event, New Orleans residents had to suffer the added ignominious experience of witnessing the appearance of our infamous president on their ravaged soil. Smiling like a Cheshire cat, the illiterate one, who a year earlier would only look down at the massive destruction from the safety of his helicopter (never daring to venture on land), came to make political hay—at the expense of those who had been abandoned by the political mob in the White

House. Watching the President go through his sickening act, I could only wonder why the good citizens of this gutted community didn't attempt to lynch him! It would have been a deserving finale.

> *Do you have some choice words about nonprofits? You've alluded to negative feelings about them.*

You read me well! The good folks with the 501c3 status are, by and large, profit-making in intention and reality—which makes the whole deal one big, bogus fraud from top to bottom.

Let's take a look at the simple truths about these organizations:

1. Generally speaking, they spend anywhere from 50 to 85 percent of all donated funds (whether from individual donations, corporate donations, grants, etc.) on administrative costs. So 50 to 85 cents on the dollar doesn't get spent on the cause for which the organization was supposedly established. Another way of seeing the nonprofit for what it really is—a tax haven—is that these institutions are not required to give more than 5 percent of their funds away in a given year. That certainly makes for a high-profit business.

2. Among the larger and more prominent nonprofits, it is common for their CEOs to receive extraordinary salaries and perks. As an example, Marsha Evans, former CEO of the Red Cross, received $651,957 a year. You call that nonprofit? Hell—I'm not about to donate money to the Red Cross knowing that so much of my buck is going to provide more personal luxuries for the head of that institution.

3. Nor am I going to donate to environmental groups that pay their CEOs big bucks. For instance:

   - Greenpeace USA $65,000
   - National Wildlife Federation $180,000
   - The Nature Conservancy $196,000
   - National Resource Defense Council $200,000
   - Environmental Defense Fund $262,000

Get outta here!

4.   The usual excuse for such salaries is that the company wants to attract quality leaders. Hah! Are you telling me that there are no good people out there who wouldn't work for a lot less? Hell—there are millions of well-educated Americans whose jobs don't pay a living wage.

If our government weren't so steeped in corruption, nonprofit agencies would not be allowed to plunder at will. A true nonprofit would spend all their income on taking care of the work it was meant to do. No one would take a salary above the bare minimum. And all its administrative expenses would be paid for by government funds.

As it now stands, the nonprofit situation is nothing but a racket for most of those involved. And I am quite correct in cursing them out. They are !*@* thieves and liars.

Before closing my comments about nonprofits, on July 21, 2006, *The Washington Post* reported the following:

> *Health and Human Services Secretary Mike Leavitt and his relatives have claimed millions of dollars in tax deductions through a type of charitable foundation that until recently paid out little in actual charity, tax records show. ...*
>
> *... The Leavitts used nearly $9 million of their assets to set up the foundation in 2000 under an obscure provision of the federal tax code. But unlike standard private foundations, which are required to give away at least 5 percent of their assets to charitable causes, the Leavitt organization donated less than 1 percent of its assets in 2002, 2003 and 2004. ...*
>
> *... The tax structure used to create the foundation is called a Type III supporting organization. The Internal Revenue Service has said the category is rife with abuse, designating "supporting organizations" this year as one of its "Dirty Dozen" top tax scams, along with Internet identity theft and offshore banks. ...*
>
> *... "They're basically sitting on all this money, getting a charitable write-off and doing nothing with it," said Rick Cohen, executive director of the National Committee for Responsive Philanthropy. ...*

This report is but another reason why I look upon most nonprofits as nothing more than legalized schemes to rip off the public. And not surprisingly, the ever-ignorant American public turns the other cheek and offers itself up for more abuse at the hands of these charlatans.

> ### *Is the entire country in denial?*

Bravo for asking! And the answer is FUCKING-A-ABSOLUTELY! Uncontrovertibly. In fact, we Americans don't know how to stop denying our wrongdoings. The immediate act of denial is in our blood, part of our DNA. Catch someone with his hand in your wallet and he'll not only deny it—he'll sue you for defamation of character! He might even bring criminal charges against you!

Nobody—but nobody—in America EVER does anything wrong. The only people who admit to any wrongdoing are some criminals brought to trial. The rest of the population consists of pure angels.

If you ask why, the answers are clear and obvious, beyond challenge.

Here's a beginner's list:

1. Our heads of state (whether they be Republicans or Democrats) lie through their eyeteeth. They face the nation and run every type of false story that will keep them in office long enough to ensure that they end their careers with a presidential library that will enshrine them in the hearts and minds of people forevermore. Small example: Bill Clinton telling the world that he didn't have sex with Monica Lewinsky. The semen is there to prove his guilt, but instead of admitting the truth, he does the "American thing." And of course there's today's archliar, George W. Bush, who wouldn't screw around in the White House but will fabricate false allegations that kill hundreds of thousands and endanger the world.

2. Church leaders cover up the criminal acts of thousands of priests who have exploited, molested, and raped tens of thousands of children. And over the years, they do nothing to expose the guilty ones, usually going out of their way to protect these common criminals and, when necessary, transfer them to another state or even country, where they can continue to sexually molest young children.

3. The conglomerate, who has laid waste to our health and supported untold schemes to get rich at the expense of millions of lives, and who has never in history told the truth when confronted.

4. The many other conglomerates, composed of industrialists, banking consortiums, mega-corporations, and foreign interests who have more say in the workings of our government than American citizens, all of whom conspire to maintain their control and dictate how we live and die. Like the rest, denial is their strong suit.

5. Many prison officials, who believe in nothing but cruelty and punishment, and neglect all human decency and concern for those found guilty of crimes. These people control the locks and keys of the prison system, using their positions to commit appalling crimes against inmates. And when someone blows the whistle on them, they turn it back on the prisoners.

    We also have our military prison system, with its hidden terrorist-detention camps (as well as its gulag in Guantanamo Bay), where torturing prisoners—to the point of driving them to suicide—who have not even been charged with a crime is a daily occurrence that's accepted as a means to an end. Of course we deny or rationalize this torture.

6. The court system, which is controlled by the legal profession and dispenses two different forms of justice: one for the rich and powerful, the other for the poor and downtrodden. Its true aims and ambitions are always skewed toward attaining greater power and prestige, and it takes more bribes than any common criminal.

7. The sports world, who, like all other conglomerates, thinks only of big bucks and power, and who ignores the lies, cheating, doping, and criminality of its stars and superstars. For the sports world, denial is an art form, almost always respected and accepted by the cowardly press.

8. The entertainment industry, whose rich and powerful moguls feed the public a steady diet of violence and stupidity and do more to lower common standards of behavior than any other group in existence. These people never consider the impact of their "creative decisions" any more than they consider the impact of their common denials.

9. The military, consumed with thoughts of victory and glory, no matter how many innocent people are killed by guns, bombs, missiles, and ordnance. These mindless leaders resort to a plethora of lies and defenses to explain their distorted body counts and acts of cruelty against innocent citizens.

10. The educational system, which distorts truth and justice and fails to enlighten and create a greater vision of life, love, and humanity. It does not educate, and it infiltrates young minds with deceitful tactics such as ignoring inter-

racial problems, pacifying national policies like the war in Iraq and what happened during and after Hurricane Katrina, and does not debate issues such as torture, all of which leads to an ever-increasing lack of fundamental human skills. In the process, children learn to shy away from truth and lie like everyone else.

11. The media, which no longer reports the truth, but places news events in the context of what their bosses and advertisers want the public to be told. To add to the absence of a balanced system of reporting news and events, an astounding lack of quality reporting exists because there are few independent journalists. There's no longer any room for such people.

12. The corporate world, which has, with few exceptions, become the trading ground for lies, deceit, fraud, and acts of cruelty that would make most despots and dictators flush with envy. Whether you're talking about phone companies or credit card processors, from A to Z they are always in full denial. They are the models for the rest to follow, supplying the gangsters of all the conglomerates—medical, social, political—with their hired hands.

13. The ordinary Joe and Jane, who think of themselves as good people. There are tens of millions of them who work hard, pay their taxes, don't commit crimes, have a sense of right or wrong, and believe in more than the buck. The only problem with them is that they're addicted to common behavior and common thinking. These same good folk will look you in the eye and tell you that they voted for George W. Bush and would do it again without blinking an eye. They recite lots of reasons for believing in the Iraq war, opposing gun controls, and supporting measures that pollute the air and water and cause untold damage to our health and the entire planet. In spite of their basic human goodness, they refuse to look beyond their entrenched values and beliefs, will go to their graves sticking to the same rules, and will never consider any alternatives to their way of thinking. These people, along with all the rest, are in complete denial because they refuse to THINK and use their IMAGINATION.

* * *

All these powers that be set examples for the rest, to the extent that most of us are incapable of accepting responsibility for our actions. *And why should we be willing to admit to anything when no one else does?*

Behind all the lies and denials is our common fear—more like terror—of what might happen if we revealed the truth about ourselves. We would look terrible and be regarded as unworthy of trust, respect, and love. In reality, the opposite is true.

As Thakur said, "Just confess your own faults in anguish before you are accused by others. You shall remain blemished, an object of affection to the world."

The other component of denial is ego. When we are accused of any wrongdoing, the ego often takes command and we close the pathways to truth and conciliation. Once again, Thakur had it right. "That which, when opposed, seeks to assert itself, is ego. When the ego dissolves, then and there the soul becomes possessor of all qualities—the absolute."

I weep for those of you, especially the young, who will remain in a personal purgatory as long as you pretend to be self-righteous and indignant in the face of your lies and deceit. Fools. You can do no greater harm to yourselves than when you give in to your denial. A lifelong Achilles heel and an albatross around your neck—who needs either of them?

Denial and ego bound together prevent America from dealing with its problems, and this composite is tearing us asunder. It affects the individual, who practices it on him/herself in so many ways daily, all the way up to our leaders. It's a national disorder, a way of life, a hopeless pattern that bends and distorts everything, and prevents us from making the difficult choices that could still save this planet from extinction.

Is there no hope?

False hope is no hope at all. From 70 years of living I've learned repeatedly that those prophets of hope do nothing but recycle the same phony messages. They are guilty of denying any true basis of hope—in which case we are better off with no hope at all.

As long as we refuse to recognize just how hopeless things really are, there's no reason to believe that we will find true hope. That, in essence, is the major problem; we can't accept the veritable truth that should make us cringe in terror and disgust, because we will sooner hold out for some unforeseen miracle or pill than look at what we must do to finally begin to change.

As an example, I watched a television report on the massive national problem of foster children being neglected, beaten, molested, and even killed because the various agencies responsible for these children are simply not doing their jobs. At the program's conclusion, a foster-care official was asked to assess the overall situation. She answered, "It will get better...because it has to get better."

This social worker's mentality (wanting to feel good about herself in her work and believing in her agency in spite of its obvious failures) is one of the root causes of all these national problems. This blind hope is counterproductive to any genuine hope for change because it fails to acknowledge just how bad the problem really is, and that it will take concrete planning and action—not baseless statements like "It will get better because it has to get better"—to move things forward and reform conditions.

Here's another example of false hope: On October 26, 2006, Senator Barack Obama, Illinois Democrat and a potential presidential candidate (an up-and-coming superstar), spoke to 2,500 people in Bellevue, Washington, saying, "We've got to have hope. We've got to have a belief in things not seen. We've got to have a belief in better days ahead."

The Senator's words, echoing the title of his new book, *The Audacity of Hope: Thoughts on Reclaiming the American Dream,* ring hollow and illustrate the kind of childishness that Americans are so willing to accept. Obama, like the rest of the big-name politicians in America, would offer you a fig leaf instead of clothing—and if the particular lawmaker has charisma and personality, you'll buy into it. That's because you're dumber than dumb.

Tell the poor, the uninsured, and the struggling lower-class to pay their fuel bills and their rents, and to scrabble for what little they have in terms of the necessities of life, with Obama's words of hope. Ask them to live on things not seen.

The rich and powerful want us to believe in their false hope—so that they can continue to ride the gravy train—while Katrina victims still languish in broken homes, while children go hungry, while people can't afford to visit a dentist when they've got a bad toothache.

Constantine Stanislavsky, the great Russian acting teacher who pioneered Method acting, once said, "One must work in order to be inspired." He was quite right, as any good actor can tell you. But the political actors who ask Americans to have hope in the face of a do-nothing Congress, are not looking to inspire as much as they're looking to trick people to vote for them. And once that's accomplished and they are elected, it's business as usual.

So much for the charming Senator from Illinois.

To be redundant, **we must first recognize that the present course is hopeless in order to get on another track.** That's our only hope. Our planet suffers from depletion of its natural resources, our environment is systematically being plundered and destroyed, our healthcare system is a monument to failure (**and a monumental failure**) that will ultimately implode, and hundreds of millions of people are impoverished, living without reason for hope.

And we are, whether we wish to believe it or not, on the brink of the worst possible terrorist attack imaginable.

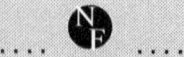

Common sense (and history) should tell you that Usama bin Laden and his radical network are planning more attacks on America and those countries viewed as their sworn enemies. In fact, in an audiotape aired on January 19, 2006, Usama bin Laden warned that his fighters are preparing new attacks in the United States but offered America a "long-term truce." Needless to say, and as I'm sure Usama bin Laden expected, the truce offer was ridiculed by the White House and the rest of the political establishment in both parties.

I would categorically state that Usama bin Laden—no matter how you view him—can be taken on his word. He will hit us hard—and we will not be prepared for the consequences.

In the 2006 CNN TV documentary aired nationally, "In the Footsteps of bin Laden," it was acknowledged that before Usama began planning 9/11, he first received approval for the attack on both the civilian and military targets from the chief cleric of his Islamic movement, Ayman al-Zawahiri. It was further acknowledged that bin Laden has since received approval for a nuclear attack and upwards of ten million lives being taken. Coupled with bin Laden's warning in January 2006, we have good reason to regard such an attack as viable, if not probable.

There's also every likelihood that bin Laden and his network paid strict attention to our lack of preparedness before, during, and after Hurricane Katrina in the fall of 2005. So we have good reason to expect the worst. And when it comes, perhaps in the form of a nuclear attack on a major American city, we will pay an incalculable price in lives and devastation—and all the hope in the world won't change that.

Former Minnesota governor Jesse Ventura (who I believe is one of the smartest people in America) hit upon another potential scenario, which involves only a small number of combatants: Considering the alarm and terror that was spread in 2002, when John Allen Muhammad and his young protégé Lee Boyd Malvo killed 10 people and wounded three others in Virginia, Maryland, and Washington, D.C. in a string of sniper shootings, can you imagine what could happen if just five crack teams of snipers were to carry out a similar series of attacks?

Speaking of Jesse Ventura, he also said in a 2005 television interview that Usama bin Laden "is going to hit us hard." Better believe it.

And all the hope in the world won't change that. No doubt our present administration in Washington will continue to issue hopeful claims that fly in the face of what would be obvious to most intelligent people, were it not for the fact that our press no longer reports the true extent of our unpreparedness against attack or natural disaster.

As an example, a few months ago a truck overturned in a Seattle tunnel, causing gridlock throughout the area for the better part of the evening. Everything within a radius of five miles was at a standstill. Over the next two days, I searched Seattle's two daily newspapers for some report of this accident, hoping to find some indication that the press had been alerted to this example of just how little it takes to stop us in our tracks—with only one truck accident. But no report was published of the accident or its implications.

That's how unprepared we are for any natural disaster or adversarial attack. Not only will we be caught flat-footed, but to be sure, our illiterate and mindlessly preoccupied President and his henchmen—as well as the newly-elected Democratic senators and congressmen who now control both house of Congress—will be at a loss for what to do. Again, hope alone will not solve the problem.

Hurtling headfirst into cataclysm and catastrophe, America has lost touch with its soul, the latest living proof of the decline of a once-powerful and well-intentioned nation. We will go the way of all past civilizations that refused to recognize and confront their problems. Just read history.

This is no doomsday prophesy of old. Its reality is right under your nose, close enough to smell and touch. And it's closing in faster than anyone cares to admit. In that regard, we're all guilty of aiding and abetting all the evil conglomerates. We refuse to stand up and fight the true enemy, the ungodly lunatics who preach and kill at the same time.

We turn our back on the suffering and destitution of our planet, concerned only with our own selfish needs, not realizing that we are destroying our own lives as well as any hope of salvation. In the end, our earth will survive through whatever we put it through, but WE and other forms of life (except for the roaches) won't.

The conglomerate, along with an equally destructive political-military-industrial complex and religious factions that pretend to be of a spiritual order, has all coalesced into an America of the rich and powerful who don't give a damn about common folk. There's no one currently on our side. And those that pretend to be are as bad as the rest because their hypocrisy defeats any possibility of progressive movement, leaving the ordinary man, woman, and child with little in the way of hope for something better.

And our beloved doctors, with their sworn oath to "First, do no harm" are among the worst of the elitist characters that stand in the way of possible change before it is too late. Their pen-and-prescription-pad mentality has wreaked harm and destruction on legions of unknowing patients.

While they're rich, bloated, and sicker than most of their patients, they receive awards and testimonials, while the public hardly takes notice of their true credo.

Therefore, we must forge a new hope from an entirely different set of principles and realities, totally apart from the sleazy Big Brother system of cronyism and corruption, and all the conglomerates that now control our destiny.

If you can go as far as to *give it the barest,* yours truly has an idea—which came upon me through some alien force—that could finally offer a challenging hope for redemption. I will reveal this "cosmic idea" before I pen my last words in this book.

In the meantime, I have one last thought about hope to share with you: Beware of the prophets of hope who are shielded with middle- and upper-class backgrounds. These people constitute a legion of social-worker types who love to portray themselves as do-gooders and champions of the poor and downtrodden. Most of them really love no more than themselves in all their charitable work and hopeful claims.

How can I be so sure? Well, the last time I looked, I didn't see any hordes of hopeful, liberal-minded intellectuals condemning what's going on in Guantanamo Bay, Iraq, many parts of Africa, or in New Orleans. And I certainly haven't heard any voices raised in favor of a $20-an-hour minimum wage for all workers. Perhaps this is a classic example of life imitating politics.

In fact, relatively few people are attempting to fight the good fight. Among them, Senator Robert Byrd (D-W.Va.), Senator Dick Durbin (D-Ill.), Representative Charles Rangel (D-N.Y.), Representative John P. Murtha, Representative James Moran, (D-Vi.), NAACP Chairman Julian Bond, singer Linda Rondstadt, and documentary filmmaker Michael Moore have issued strong statements against the reigning Bush.

And except for Harry Belafonte, who calls Bush a terrorist; singer Natalie Maines of the Dixie Chicks, who said the group was ashamed that Bush was from Texas; Cindy Sheehan, whose son died in the Iraq war; and Michael Berg, whose son was beheaded in Iraq, there has been little outcry against the evils of our present regime in Washington.

Not that the conservatives or those in the center are any better at facing up to the frightful goings-on in America. Like the so-called liberals, they offer no reason for hope.

> ### *What are we left to believe?*

I must fall back on the answer I've given since my first day of military basic training: "Believe nothing that you hear and only half of what you see." Yes, that Air Force motto still holds true in this world of madness and deceit, especially in the face of the conglomerate, which cares not for truth or human compassion. As long as it remains in the driver's seat of America's healthcare (and declining health)—don't trust anything it says.

Keep a set of eyes in the back of your head, and stay away from drugs, doctors, or hospitals. You'll live a lot longer and have a shot at a quality life, as opposed to being one step removed from the grave at the whim of the conglomerate.

> *Isn't there anything that can be done*
> *to move healthcare in the right direction?*
>
> *There must be some way....*

There are many things—but first we must fully acknowledge that THE ENTIRE SYSTEM IS A MONUMENT TO FAILURE THAT MUST BE DISMANTLED FROM TOP TO BOTTOM BEFORE ANYTHING CAN BE DONE. That's the bottom-line prerequisite for moving forward. Otherwise, the political powers that be will bamboozle the public over and over again with their false hope and corrupt schemes for supposed change and advancement.

We'll be led down the golden path with more studies, senate hearings, administrative proposals, compromising solutions, and a slew of claims and reports that indicate progress and revitalization. **Don't believe one single word of it.** Trust the Air Force motto instead: Believe nothing that you hear and only half of what you see. And remember the magician's saying: The hand is quicker than the eye.

If we fail to heed this warning, the path to our healthcare system will go from horrific to absolutely catastrophic—that's if we're able to avoid a pandemic or nuclear attack.

The rulers in public office will trick the American public with healthcare bills and enactments that will be nothing more than watered-down versions of watered-down versions of watered-down versions of proposals that barely scratch the surface of the healthcare problems faced by everyone but the rich and powerful.

Even then, they will tweak their meaningless measures, further debate and then compromise all issues, and serve up their calculated deceptions with great fanfare and hubris. And we'll be right back where we started and going nowhere faster than ever!

So you must accept the fundamental truth that healthcare reform is intrinsically linked to political reform. In other words, nothing will get better unless the political climate undergoes extreme change. That's a given. (Except for the hope-hucksters.)

> *If it were somehow possible to*
> *jump-start America's healthcare program*
> *from scratch, would you venture some*
> *perspective about what might happen?*

Unfortunately, as I see it, our chances of starting all over again are—under present circumstances—nonexistent because simply too many forces (both houses of Congress and a number of conglomerates) oppose any meaningful change. They are too comfortable with their riches, power, and control to yield any sovereignty or equal rights to the masses, and they would quickly challenge any such opposition before it could gain momentum.

The only way in which control can be returned to "We the People" would be either through revolutionary thinking: a cosmic idea that would unite the common public, or as a direct result of a catastrophic event such as a nuclear attack or a pandemic. That's the only way it will happen.

If we should be blessed with a peaceful, nondevastating event that would prompt the people to take back America, then all things would be possible. Returning to my earlier statement about our nation's capacity to rise to the occasion in the 20th century, we could indeed begin anew—providing we had the right starting point.

On that note, I venture the following two prerequisites for any significant launch:

1. **First clear away our outstanding national guilt by FINALLY dealing with the truth about the founding of the United States.** I'm obviously talking about the indisputable fact that we stole this land from the Native American Indians. From colonial times to the Wounded Knee massacre, we conquered the American Indian peoples and eventually relocated them to Indian reservations.

   We demand restitution from criminals, but we have never paid it for crimes (genocide) committed against American Indians.

   • What does this have to do with American healthcare? **EVERYTHING!** Truth and human compassion are the cornerstones of a nation's health. Until an American president stands before a joint session of Congress with the entire population witnessing the proceedings, and apologizes and asks forgiveness for what happened on behalf of all those

people collectively responsible for the complex historical
conflict that claimed so many lives and decimated the native
American Indian population, we shall always have a hole
in our soul and never be healthy. After all, we apologized
to the Japanese-Americans for interring them during WWII
and we've built many memorials for Jews murdered in the
Holocaust, but we have yet to truly show our sorrow and
contrition for what we did to American Indians. It's time we
face up to our guilt and culpability. **Doing this would be the
most liberating act of our time, enabling us to step forward
and start down the path of creating a healthcare system
that embodies all of the elements of spiritual, physical,
mental, and emotional health.**

2. **America must hold a new constitutional congress.** Our Constitution must
    be reevaluated to update 17th-century thinking to deal with 21st-century real-
    ities, and rewritten to reflect the needs of all Americans, so that everyone can
    have the right to life, liberty, and the pursuit of happiness—and that certainly
    includes the best in healthcare.

    - It will take a monumental movement (over a number of
      years) unlike any that has ever been seen in America to gain
      a foothold on a march toward rewriting our Constitution.
      But it must begin because the original document is archaic,
      boundlessly predisposed to unjust legal interpretation, and
      does not uphold existence in its current form. As an example,
      the Constitution states, "A well-regulated militia being
      necessary to the security of a free state, the right to bear arms
      shall not be infringed," has nothing to do with the rights of
      criminal gangs to posses and use semiautomatic weapons
      to kill rival gangs or for serial killers or mass murderers
      to threaten entire cities. Furthermore, in the United States,
      approximately 5,000 children under 15 years of age are
      killed every year due to guns (not to mention the many more
      children who are permanently disabled). The creators of the
      Constitution certainly didn't have this in mind.
          It should also be recognized that the framers of our
      Constitution could not envision that our country would
      remain divided on all of the major issues of our time—like
      abortion, gun control, capital punishment, and gay rights.

Without revisions, our Constitution—as interpreted by the legal profession—practically mandates that 50 percent of the people disagree on the issues and live in conflict with the other 50 percent of the population. That leaves our nation permanently polarized.

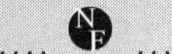

America must somehow find the ways to resolve the outstanding issues of our times. Unless we come to terms with abortion, gun control, capital punishment, women's rights, immigration, and all the other major challenges and conflicts that block progress, reform, and a higher set of values, we cannot endure as a nation for long.

As long as we remain polarized, with 50 percent of the people opposed to the will and needs of the other 50 percent, we can never stand united and face the future with hope and the determination to find peace and prosperity for all people.

Therefore, it must be the responsibility of the new constitutional congress to enact amendments to our Constitution that would enable us to take the aforementioned issues out of the hands of politicians controlled by special interests, removing them from the "contest" arena—so that the polarization will finally end.

Most importantly, it must wrest control of our nation out of the hands of the legal profession and give it back to the hands of the people. We cannot take back America until we dislodge it from the grip of lawyers, judges, legislators, and politicians, who will of course do everything in their great power to prevent a new constitutional congress. And they are backed by conglomerates, big business, the military, conservative America, and all those who cherish the Constitution as it is. Make no mistake, they will be formidable. But until these controllers are reined in, absolutely no hope remains of creating a healthcare system that will actually serve the needs of all Americans.

We are not talking about some international conspiracy, a communist takeover, or anarchy. We are talking about freedom, true equal rights under the Constitution, and a rebirth of ideals that could get America on the road to solving its issues and inequities and becoming a peaceful role model for the rest of the beleaguered world.

If we can accomplish these two primal objectives, then we can forge an alliance among all health givers, focusing our resources on lifesaving measures, such as preventing and curing cancer, AIDS, and all other diseases, and providing universal healthcare. And don't for a moment think that we don't have money to do this. Enough money exists for everything—providing that no self-serving conglomerates are present to divvy it up among themselves.

Having said this, I'm about to reveal how I plan to jump-start this peaceful revolution—with a cosmic idea that will forge a new hope to return America to "We the People."

Earlier in this book I stated, "The control of our nation is not in our hands. We are not a country of 'We the People.' No democratia remains in our corrupt form of government." A primary reason for the demise of our country's principles and values is that the greater majority of its citizens have shied away from direct involvement in decision making, relegating such responsibility to elected officials who first and foremost attend the bidding of the powerbrokers, lobbyists, and conglomerates that subjugate the will of the people.

In exchange for this sellout of human rights and liberty, we are given the opportunity to cast our votes in elections, a process that seemingly provides us with choices. That's what we've been told and trained to believe. But between you and me—the act of voting and $2.75 buys you a cup of coffee. "Am I being cynical?" you ask. NO! I'm calling it just like it is—a watered-down, cleverly packaged manipulation of supposed freedom of choices—which in reality amounts to little more than SELECTING BETWEEN ONE OF TWO SETS OF WEALTHY, CORRUPT LAWYERS AND SCHEMERS, who are all beholden to those who line their campaign chests with contributions that are no more than political payoffs (outright bribes) for favors to be received.

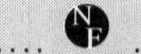

As for any of the independent parties or their candidates, whether it be Ralph Nader (should he make another run), Lyndon LaRouche (who ran for president on eight consecutive occasions), Ross Perot (who already garnered 19 percent of the popular vote in 1992), the American Independent Party, the Alaskan Independence Party, or any other unallied band, they do not hold the key to progressive change or liberation from the hands or hooks of the various conglomerates that control our country's destiny. They do not stand any chance against the might of powers that be because they will all stand alone rather than join together under one banner. This is not only self-serving but also candidate-driven rather than vision-driven. And it does not really offer America another choice. It merely advances the ambitions of yet another rich and power-hungry lawyer or public force.

As for the Democratic and Republican parties, you call this a choice?! You're telling me that by casting a vote for one of two dishonorable political hacks, I'm participating in true democracy? I've got news for you—that's not what the Greeks originally had in mind, or what our founding fathers envisioned. (Although there is some evidence that the founding fathers were riding on rather high horses themselves, playing to some double standards that haven't changed to this day. But they were probably closer to the ideal than the cesspool that is standard thinking now.)

So why do we accept this carload of unadulterated hogwash? Have we become so complacent that we no longer even know what our nation is supposed to stand for? Are we so disconnected from what's going on in America that we don't recognize how we've been conned by these sleazy politicians and the conglomerates that pull our strings like wooden puppets? How do we wake up and acknowledge our apathy, and begin to put the democratia back in democracy? What's the answer?

WE PROTEST AND REVOLT AGAINST WHAT'S GOING ON—BY NOT VOTING IN THE NEXT PRESIDENTIAL ELECTION IN 2008.

Your immediate reaction to this idea might be, "What good is that going to do?" How's this for starters:

1.   It will unite us in common cause.

2.   It will tell ALL the politicians that we're no longer going to be a party to sham democracy.

3.   It will give Americans the chance to regroup and start fresh, not along political lines, but on a new course of action that will free us from our decades-long malaise.

4.   It will allow us to forge new hope based on facing up to the challenge of sav-

ing our country, world, environment, and humanity from apocalyptical fates.

5. It will give us something we can truly believe in, and commit and devote our energy to.

6. It could become a national movement, giving rise to a genuine third party that will lay a new cornerstone for liberty, freedom, and prosperity for all people.

This vast undertaking will be called TBA—**TAKE BACK AMERICA.** And our party's first aim will be to deny the vote to the scoundrels who have stolen the country from the people.

For those of you who might point out that a group of well-known people, including prominent politicians like John Kerry, Hillary Clinton, Gary Hart, Howard Dean, and Senator Barack Obama, along with such notable public figures as Robert Redford, Reverend Jesse Jackson, Bill Moyers, and Ariana Huffington, are involved with another campaign to TAKE BACK AMERICA that is a project for America's progressive majority, I am well aware of it.

In order that you not be confused, let me state this categorical difference between the two programs: The so-called project for America's progressive majority has established typical political aims, such as making the economy work for working people, cleaning up government, fighting poverty, restoring America's leadership, and building a healthcare system that assures coverage for all. Fine words. Strong slogans. But here's the time to really believe in the Air Force motto "Believe nothing that you hear and only half of what you see."

Why? The politicians who are talking this talk have done nothing but sit on their laurels throughout the two Bush administrations, while they ignored the critical issues that were tearing this nation apart. None of them opposed the Iraq war; none of them are now calling for American withdrawal from Iraq; none of them mention our gulag in Guantanamo Bay; none of them have offered any plan for cleaning up our corrupt government, or fighting poverty, or drastically raising the hourly minimum wage, or challenging the conglomerate that is responsible for our country's backward healthcare system. And none of them would—in a million years!—ever come out for a new constitutional congress.

These same do-nothing political hacks are only after one thing—YOUR VOTE to take back America FOR THEMSELVES! They want to sit in the White House, pose as heads of state, make speeches, propose bills, act as if they're confronting issues, and retire from office with the full expectation of building their Presidential Library. And that's what they will do. AND NOTHING WILL CHANGE— because **these people don't have solutions to our country's problems** any more than the present bunch of politicians who sit in cabinet meetings pretending to have answers to our nation's and the world's conflicts.

You know why NONE of these political hacks can do what they promise? It takes many years to develop imaginative skills; it takes great energy to solve problems; it requires dedication to the long struggle to right America's course. And NONE of these politicians—in either party—possess these attributes. Why not? Because they spend their waking hours thinking about themselves in office, raising money (and taking bribes), running for election, and doing little else than preparing for the next election. That's what goes on—and that's why America's problems are not being dealt with.

On the other hand, my greatest ambitions center around having grandchildren, enjoying family and friends, sitting by a fireside with a glass of bubbly, listening to music, and conducting my imaginary symphony.

And because I have devoted so many years to imaginative pursuits and problem-solving, have enormous energy, and am absolutely dedicated to the cause of helping people take back America—I can truly guide things in that direction.

That's why I'm proposing that we turn away from the corrupt politicians in both parties by NOT VOTING IN 2008.

To those who would say "Wouldn't it be better to just vote the scoundrels out of office?" my (REDUNDANT!) answer is … NO! Because nothing would really change. The Democratic Party is no longer a viable opposition party. It has, for all intents and purposes, joined hands with the Republican Party, and suffers from the same corruption and willingness to compromise values and ideals. Don't you get it—they've sold out!

. . . .

On November 7, 2006, 79 million Americans went to the polls and swept the Democratic Party into a majority in the U.S. House and the Senate. This shift in power did not come about as a result of newfound faith in the Democratic agenda as much it was the voters turning away from the Republican Party.

Fed up with the Iraq war, corruption on Capitol Hill, a do-nothing Congress, and a president who has all but ignored the ideal of "We the people" in favor of one-man-one-party rule, the people have—FINALLY!—spoken.

However, to be quite blunt, after all the cheers for the winning candidates have died down, and the bows have been taken by the newly elected officials, all of the hoopla and $2.75 might just buy you a cup of your favorite latte.

True to form, the new Congress will do more than the outgoing collection of pests and pissants. There will be less strutting about (even on the part of Bush, who doesn't wish to be a lame-duck president for the next two years—so he will pretend to behave as if he gets along with the bipartisan program) and more down-to-earth congressional activity, all geared toward positioning the reigning political party for the big prize—the White House in 2008.

Democratic Party leaders will quickly establish priorities:

- A concerted effort—beginning with the Iraq Study Group proposals—will be made to change the course of the Iraq war and even to begin bringing our troops home. But it will be too little, too late, and many more Americans, as well as Iraqi citizens, will be killed before the war is ended.

- The minimum wage will be raised from $5.15 to $7.25, with the hope that it demonstrates a sincere desire to improve low-income people's living standards. But who can live on $7.25 an hour?

- Legislation will be advanced to reduce the number of uninsured Americans, and medical benefits for treating illness will be improved. But passing all this won't even begin to scratch the surface of what really needs to be done to provide adequate healthcare for all Americans.

All in all, the Democrats will—in the aftermath of the previous Republican-dominated Congress—"look good," and the American people will feel a sense of relief, and believe that THEIR VOTE COUNTED!

But it won't matter … because the real power in America will remain in the hands of the same people who designed and labored for the Bush era; the powerbrokers, lobbies, various conglomerates, coupled with the military-industrial complex, the utility barons, and all those who have a stake in maintaining control over the will of the people will still be in the driver's seat.

Consequently, our newly elected Congress will ultimately follow the dictates of these bosses:

- There will be no immediate closure of Guantanamo Bay or our secret hidden prisons, and we will continue to torture prisoners.

- America will maintain its one-sided position in support of Israel, and the Israeli-Palestinian situation will remain as volatile as ever, leaving our country vulnerable to attack.

- The threat from bin Laden will increase with every passing day.

- Our borders will remain insecure, in spite of any wall or fence that will be built. (It's ironic that in 1987 President Ronald Reagan stood in front of the Brandenburg Gate to address 20,000 Berliners and call upon General Secretary Gorbachev to "tear down this wall.")

- The minimum wage won't be raised to a realistic living standard.

- America's healthcare system will continue to erode.

- Cancer and all other deadly diseases will neither be prevented nor cured.

- Hurricane Katrina victims will still be left in the lurch.

- Climate warming will continue to increase.

- We will not apologize to American Indians.

- There will be no congressional Congress to revise and revitalize out archaic Constitution.

Whether they're a member of the Republican or Democratic Party, they will still be bought and sold by the highest bidders and will spend their time and energy reinventing themselves so that they can remain in office as long as possible.

The needs of the people will continue to be given short shrift in favor of the conglomerate's, and the rich and powerful. And if you think for one moment that exchanging the illiterate one in the White House for the likes of Hillary Clinton, Al Gore, Howard Dean, Barack Obama, or John McCain will alter our nation's present course of corruption in government, environmental suicide, and indifference to poverty—you're as deluded as those who voted George Bush into office.

Hillary Clinton would do little more than bask in the reflected glory of being the first woman President and go about her compromising ways, which might endear her to the centrist crowd (especially if her husband hangs around), but will accomplish no more than any other ordinary hack politician.

Al Gore, who recently reemerged after six years in political hibernation, will drag out his environmental credentials and undoubtedly play that card for as much as it's worth, but when it comes to dealing with critical issues, he'll be just "one of the boys."

As for Howard Dean, John McCain, or Barack Obama, they certainly show some character and energy, but so did a lot of other politicians over the last decades—which doesn't go very far when you're faced with a political system that will not support the needs of the vast majority of America's citizens.

The aforementioned political scenario won't be altered by any other presumed candidate, whether it be Bill Frist, Joe Biden, or Diane Feinstein. No matter who is named to seek the White House, s/he will follow in the footsteps of those that have gone before them over the last 40 years—which will not do enough for our beleaguered country or the world to save us from a cataclysmic destiny.

Another way of putting this (and quoting from Thakur): "What is the point of chasing out the lions, if only to bring on the jackals?"

Our only hope is to stop ourselves in our tracks, begin anew, and start on the journey we must take ... if we are to do what will otherwise be entirely impossible. We need a new breed of people in America!

President Franklin D. Roosevelt set out to right the course of America when it was mired in The Depression. He used extraordinary imaginative skill, creating a New Deal that encompassed relief, recovery, and reform, as well as the Works Progress Administration (WPA) a remarkably innovative program that actually created jobs for writers, painters, and thousands of jobless people. Even then, his efforts were not enough to do the job, and were it not for the advent of the Second World War, there's no telling what might have happened in America.

Roosevelt's successor, Harry S. Truman, was neither a lawyer nor a college graduate, and he faced seemingly insurmountable challenges, both on the home front and throughout the world. Although I didn't agree with everything he said and did, Truman had courage, took risks, and when he said "The buck stops here," he meant it.

Perhaps Truman's crowning achievement was the Marshall Plan, which rebuilt war-ravaged Europe. Under the plan, called The European Recovery Program (ERP), the United States offered up to $20 billion for recovery, providing the allied countries of Europe could agree about the use of the aid, which they did. The plan worked. By 1953, Europe was on its feet again.

I bring this up because America badly needs a Marshall Plan of its own if it is to fulfill a healthy destiny instead of self-destructing. And we can't do that unless we change our thinking and set our sights on a new vision of an America that truly serves the needs of all people, not just special interests. That's what TBA will do! And harkening to FDR, the American people need a "new deal."

So join the revolution! Make your next presidential vote a NO vote—against all that stands in the way of healthcare relief, recovery and reformation, saving the environment, eliminating poverty, and becoming a nonviolent, peace-loving, health-giving model for the rest of the world.

All of which means:

- We leave Iraq.

- We close our gulag in Guantanamo Bay, and all other prison camps.

- We apologize before the world for our treatment of the American Indians.

- We establish a minimum wage of $20 an hour for all workers.

- We begin the reform of the entire American healthcare industry.

- We hold a new constitutional Congress.

So if we don't vote, what happens then? Where do we go from there?

The one place WE MUST NOT GO is into the arena of debate with the forces that presently control the workings of our political and healthcare systems. We can't get into their ballpark. They want nothing more than to entangle us in their agenda of worn-out ideas and attitudes, and they will attempt to lure us into argument and polemics about a range of controversial topics, so that they can create comparisons as to what they will accomplish as opposed to what we represent. That's the time-honored game played between political parties—trying to look good at the other's expense.

Instead, we must focus on the need to purge ourselves of our national cancer of political corruption and denial on the part of the rich and powerful, and the cancer of ignorance and apathy rampant in the general public. We desperately need this cleansing before we can find solutions to our problems. **It's no different than cleansing your body of all its toxins—so that you can start clean and be fully prepared physically, mentally, and spiritually for healthy regeneration and longevity.**

However, we are not yet prepared to purge the toxins from our minds and souls. As examples, we have grown selfish and mindless, to the point that we use cell phones while driving, in complete disrespect for all those we endanger; we ignore national crimes such as the existence of our gulag/Devil's Island in Guantanamo Bay, unmindful of the ideal of justice and protection under the law for all people; and in spite of all the right words and promises, we have turned our backs on the victims of Hurricane Katrina.

Until we acknowledge that *we* are the major part of the problem, turn away from denial, and prepare our body, mind, and spirit for the work ahead—we will not be ready to move forward on the new agenda.

That's why we must first entrench ourselves with the one specific goal of getting the American people to realize that the hope for the future lies in turning away from the present corrupt standard, and that the ONLY way to do that effectively is to cast your vote as a NO vote in 2008. That's our message—and we're going to stick by it!

So let's proceed to get out the NO vote in 2008—and bring back choice to government.

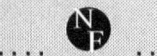

Dear reader, you have heard me use the term "Out of X" on numerous occasions, and indeed "Out of X" happened just a day after I wrote the previous paragraph. I'm referring to the Supreme Court decision of October 17, 2006. On that date, President Bush, without fanfare, signed a new law—the Military Commissions Act of 2006—which basically overrides the Supreme Court's sound imposition of limits on executive power.

On this dark day in American history, this Orwellian law gave Bush the right to decide what constitutes torture and allows him to set his own guidelines for interrogation of prisoners. It also permits withholding evidence from defendants in certain cases, and denies detainees the right to file *habeas corpus* petitions to challenge their detentions in federal courts. Note: The tradition of *habeas corpus* dates back almost 800 years to the Magna Carta, and has been a core value in America law.

But that's not all: Under this new law, Bush also has powers to designate who is an illegal enemy combatant, which potentially subjects American citizens as well as foreigners to indefinite detention WITH NO POWER TO APPEAL.

Want more? Our power-mad president can now interpret the Geneva Conventions on Human Treatment of Prisoners of War. Meanwhile, the CIA will keep on sending prisoners to hidden prisons around the world—and those Gestapo-like interrogators that torture prisons will have immunity from prosecution.

> And here's the "Out of X" that should make every American stop in his tracks and think about what has happened to their country: There was little opposition from the spineless Democratic lawmakers, who surrendered to the despot as they have done all along.
> The "opposition" played it safe. You bet!
> If you really want to TAKE BACK AMERICA—then start with a NO vote in 2008.

Withholding your vote in 2008 would not be a cop-out. Quite the contrary: If you believe in true democracy, then you must be willing to fight for it. Merely voting for one of two political hacks—and they ARE all political hacks—is the true cop-out—while opposing the sick regime of corruption, bribery, war, environmental destruction, dysfunctional healthcare, and injustice is going to be hard work all the way down the line. That's what your vote is really about—the choice between going in the right direction or keeping the depraved political system in tact. Think about it. ...

✳ ✳ ✳

A closing thought: After the Asian tsunami catastrophe of 2004, so much money was contributed that the various relief and rehabilitation agencies receiving donations asked the public to STOP making contributions! Can you imagine what we could do if we also freed up all the money going into war efforts? We could tackle any job and get it done! In the process, we would enrich not only our own lives, but billions of others throughout the world.

That's the legacy we should be preparing for our children and their children to come.

> *Is there any one thing you want*
> *to say to young people?*

Yeah ... get your health act together before you become a prime candidate for diabetes, cancer, heart attacks, stroke, or suicide. The conglomerate took aim at you before you were born and has been preparing you for the junk heap ever since.

Just like the tobacco merchants who got baby-boomers hooked before they were aware enough to protect themselves from the Marlboro Man's overtures, the conglomerate has carefully finessed you into the drug and medical traps that will destroy your ability to think, as well as your immune system, leaving you as help-less victims within a hopelessly lost society riddled with the poorest healthcare of all the industrialized nations.

Wake up! Break away! Throw the shit prescriptions out the window! Get a new medicine to fix your body and soul. It's out there for you but you need to start now. **Tomorrow may be one day too late.**

Never the one to miss a chance for a grand curtain call, here's the kicker to end all kickers (at least for now):

GLAXO CHIEF:
OUR DRUGS DO NOT WORK ON MOST PATIENTS
Steve Connor, *Independent/UK*—December 8, 2003

A senior executive with Britain's biggest drugs company has admitted that most prescription medicines do not work on most people who take them.

Allen Roses, worldwide vice-president of genetics at GlaxoSmithKline (GSK), said fewer than half of the patients prescribed some of the most expensive drugs actually derived any benefit from them.

It is an open secret within the drugs industry that most of its products are ineffective in most patients but this is the first time that such a senior drugs boss has gone public. ...

... Dr. Roses, an academic geneticist from Duke University in North Carolina, spoke at a recent scientific meeting in London where he cited figures on how well different classes of drugs work in real patients.

Drugs for Alzheimer's disease work in fewer than one in three patients, whereas those for cancer are only effective in a quarter of patients. Drugs for migraines, for osteoporosis, and arthritis work in about half the patients, Dr. Roses said. Most drugs work in fewer than one in two patients mainly because the recipients carry genes that interfere in some way with the medicine, he said.

"The vast majority of drugs—more than 90 percent—only work in 30 or 50 percent of the people," Dr. Roses said. "I wouldn't say that most drugs don't work. I would say that most drugs work in 30 to 50 percent of people. Drugs out there on the market work, but they don't work in everybody."

Some industry analysts said Dr. Roses's comments were reminiscent of the 1991 gaffe by Gerald Ratner, the jewelry boss, who famously said that his high street shops are successful because they sold "total crap." But others believe Dr. Roses deserves credit for being honest about a little-publicized fact known to the drugs industry for many years.

"Roses is a smart guy and what he is saying will surprise the public but not his colleagues," said one industry scientist. "He is a pioneer of a new culture within the drugs business based on using genes to test for who can benefit from a particular drug."

Dr. Roses has a formidable reputation in the field of "pharmacogenomics"—the application of human genetics to drug development—and his comments can be seen as an attempt to make the industry realize that its future rests on being able to target drugs to a smaller number of patients with specific genes.

The idea is to identify "responders"—people who benefit from the drug—with a simple and cheap genetic test that can be used to eliminate those non-responders who might benefit from another drug.

This goes against a marketing culture within the industry that has relied on selling as many drugs as possible to the widest number of patients—a culture that has made GSK one of the most profitable pharmaceuticals companies, but which has also meant that most of its drugs are at best useless, and even possibly dangerous, for many patients. ...

Response rates: Therapeutic area: drug efficacy rate in percent

* *Alzheimer's: 30*
* *Analgesics (Cox-2): 80*
* *Asthma: 60*
* *Depression (SSRI): 62*
* *Diabetes: 57*
* *Hepatitis C (HCV): 47*
* *Incontinence: 40*
* *Migraine (acute): 52*
* *Migraine (prophylaxis): 50*
* *Oncology: 25*
* *Rheumatoid arthritis: 50*
* *Schizophrenia: 60*

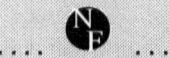

The aforementioned response rates are nothing more than that—
RESPONSES—**not cures.** And they do not reflect the true nature
of the patients' overall quality of life, nor do they indicate that the
people on these drugs would not have been better off not taking
them or seeking alternative treatment.

If this doesn't get the drug message across to you—at any age—then you're really a hopeless case. Don't you get it—no matter how clever the commercial is, or what your doctor tells you (yeah—ask your doctor about it!), the drug-medication-JUNK they're prescribing and selling you most likely DOESN'T WORK.

You're not only wasting your money, you're also destroying your immune system. And as that happens, you're inviting more illness, disease, and premature death. That's what the conglomerate got you into—and it's time you to walk away from their deathtrap and join the ranks of people dedicated to a healthy, long-lasting, drug-free existence. All it takes is your decision.

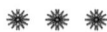

I said that this part of my book was not for the faint-hearted—and I meant it! But now that I've pretty much said my piece about America's healthcare system and what needs to be done to change it, I think it's time I drift back to my original theme (diet and exercise) and then conclude with a chapter dealing with Nick's Workout Plan.

Part II.
What Goes Around
Comes Around

What Goes Around Comes Around

I can't escape the fact that my life has, in many ways, been centered on food. It's not that I live to eat, but being as I'm Greek, one never knows. What's important is that I don't cop out on what I have to say about my way of dealing with my food love or addiction. So let's go right to it!

The way things are going, the number of American overweight children will increase significantly by the end of the decade, with profound impacts on public health. Looking at this painful reality, we can see what's in the future: more and more bloated bodies turning to the conglomerate for help. They'll receive prescriptions, surgery, and whatever newfangled gimmicks the conglomerate invents and return time and again for more quick fixes. That's the primary model being presented to them, all geared up to reap its deadly results.

As if this reality weren't enough, American children were dealt another blow when Bush administration budget cuts ended funding in 2005 for the government's VERB campaign, a program that was once touted as spurring a 30 percent increase in exercise among the preteens it reached. All this when one-fifth of U.S. children are projected as likely to be obese by the year 2010.

Meanwhile, despite my lifelong earlier obesity problems, my weight and metabolism remain what they should be. At the age of 70, I'm as good a model of health as you'll find.

As you initially started out to write a diet book (contained within the framework of your autobiography), would you say that diet and exercise are the main things to work on if we are to attain good health?

Although diet and exercise boost the immune system, it's not that simple because good health involves the total upholding of existence, which involves much more than just diet and exercise.

Look at it this way: If it were only a matter of eating the right foods, getting the proper amount of exercise, and staying in good shape, then how do you explain the early deaths of so many human beings who meet that criteria? Do you remember J. R. Rodale, the founder of *Prevention* magazine? He died suddenly of a heart attack and he wasn't an old man. Then there's Jim Fixx, the famous marathon runner who wrote bestselling books on health and dropped dead at an early age. And what better more recent example than the creator of the Atkins diet, who also died prematurely.

Millions of examples of apparently healthy people exist who ate right, exercised, and were in good shape—yet they succumbed to serious health problems and died at an early age. So what happened? Needless to say, it's different with each person, but—**something obviously went wrong**.

Was an emotional, mental, or spiritual element out of sync with the rest of the body? Was it behavioral or physical? Environmental or genetic? In any case, something besides the basic ingredients of diet and exercise had to be the culprit. Knowing that, we must examine ourselves in a total way, rather than fragmenting our lives into so many different compartments.

That's essentially the problem: We rarely, if ever, see ourselves as a total entity of body, mind, personality, character, and soul. With this mindset, we can't possibly get a clear sense of the full rhythm of our existence, and as a result of this only partial realization of self, we don't get our act together. We only react to matters of an immediate nature. Even then, we usually deal with our problems only superficially.

I recommend a holistic approach to living that includes a good diet and proper exercise, without which we certainly aren't going to survive our full number of allotted years. These factors will play a huge role in improving the quality of our lives.

> *Any final (for now) words on the problem*
> *of obesity and being overweight?*

As I've been dealing with it for 70 years, I've got a mouthful to say. (No—I didn't mean it as a pun!)

America's weight problem has reached humongous proportions and can only get **much worse**. In just seven years it's gone from back-page news to front-page headlines. As a nation, we're getting fatter and fatter, more and more sedentary, and less and less active, relying more and more on drugs and surgery to answer weight woes. We're suffering from greater occurrences of chronic illnesses associated with being overweight and obese, such as high blood pressure, heart disease, diabetes, and depression. Obesity has also replaced disability as the major problem for the elderly. It's an epidemic to hearten the lives and bank accounts of the conglomerate.

Recently I sat in an airline terminal in Seattle, waiting for my flight to be announced, and casually looked around at the 200-odd people who were also waiting there. I was amazed at what I saw. Eight out of every 10 people of all ages were obese. It was the most graphic description of this growing national illness that I have ever witnessed or imagined.

When I boarded the plane for my flight, all three of the flight stewardesses were also obese, a grim reminder of the fact that there's no getting away from the dimensions of the problem.

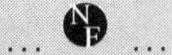

Roughly two-thirds of American adults are overweight or obese, with excess weight threatening to overtake tobacco as the number-one cause of preventable deaths in the United States, according to a study published in the March 10, 2004 issue of the *Journal of the American Medical Association* by researchers from the national Centers for Disease Control and Prevention.

Skyrocketing obesity rates are linked to an explosion in diabetes cases among children and adults. On November 11, 2005, Yale University researcher Derek Yach predicted that within two decades, obesity-related diabetes would become the leading cause of death in the country unless the increase in obesity is checked. For many known reasons, diabetes facts are appalling, and they will continue to worsen—perhaps at an even more accelerated level than the worst present-day scenarios indicate. In fact, it is expected that one in three children born in 2000 will develop diabetes.

Too much fat also increases the risk of an ever-growing list of health problems, including many different types of cancer. With excess fat comes elevated cholesterol levels, and conglomerate operatives have concocted all sorts of drugs to lower these levels. The major problem, besides the overall drug dependency and undermining of the immune system, is that serious side effects often result from using these drugs.

In any case, the true dimensions of America's weight problem are inestimable, and only the conglomerate benefits.

The reasons for our added bulk are all around us—in the cars we insist on using for every outing, in the giant mugs we fill with whipped-cream-topped mochas, in our poor eating habits, in a culture where everybody seems to be rushing around and yet sitting still most of the time.

What experts fail to note are the strong emotional factors that always lurk in the background, such as individual or group resentment and rage toward those who grow richer by the hour while the less fortunate can barely make ends meet. There is the pain and terror of young adults who discover that their prospects for a creative and rewarding life are much lower than what they had envisioned as young children growing up in an affluent society, the awareness of looming environmental disasters that our nation contributes to and refuses to deal with, and an ever-present fear of adversarial attack, war, and worse.

All these *feelings* are intrinsically woven into the fabric of our everyday life and have a direct bearing on our yearning to satisfy our emotionally starved lives, on the calories we then nervously consume, and on the pounds that refuse to be shed. So once again, we need to address a total picture that's bad, not just the weight factor.

We're also an unhappy society—no matter what polls and interviewers tell us or how much we lie to ourselves and others. You can measure it by the looks on most people's faces, by our growing impatience with everyone, and by the hostile ways we drive our cars.

I must also mention that our overall lack of physical activity is more noticeable than ever before. When I was growing up on the streets of New York City and Brooklyn, "street games" like slap-ball, punch-ball, stoop-ball, stick-ball, dodge-ball, ring-o-lee-veo, and Johnny on the Pony, to name a few, were the norm. They provided kids with a wide range of physical exercise, as well as social skills derived from these interactions. And school budgets provided funds for a greater range of extracurricular activity.

That age of games and socializing has fallen by the wayside, replaced by TV and computers, neither of which provides today's children with the physical and mental aliveness that their souls crave.

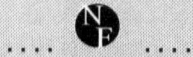

Children are tethered to technology as never before, with iPods, computers, and sophisticated cell phones extending the sitting-in-front-of-the-screen time to the point where it should be considered a public health issue, just like smoking and violence.

Although numerous health clubs are a part of most communities, we still don't get enough exercise to meet the minimum guidelines for physical activity—30 minutes of moderate activity five days a week.

"The level to which you can be physically inactive in a day is utterly amazing," says Dr. Brent Wisse, who treats overweight and obese patients at Harborview Medical Center's Weight Disorders Clinic in Seattle. "You're not going to fix that by going to the gym and spending half an hour on the treadmill."

So what should you do? Above all else—don't turn to drugs because they yield minimum results and come with a host of potentially dangerous side effects.

Don't consider stomach surgeries, including those that restrict food intake, as they can lead to serious complications and death. Not only are you playing with your life when you undergo one of these procedures, but you are also joining the conglomerate's chump-list, for which you will pay dearly in the years ahead. **Every time you have any physical problem, you will want to resort to drugs and surgery to relieve it.** So both your life expectancy and your quality of life will undoubtedly be diminished. *Out of touch with how you should be feeling, you'll accept infirmities as being normal for your age.*

The first thing you must do is take a good honest look at your entire lifestyle and evaluate what's causing your weight problem. Is it a lack of willpower or a biological problem? Whichever it is, one thing's for sure: Your general lifestyle contributes to the problem in numerous ways.

Although you may not be able to currently control your metabolism or your desire for candy bars, you most certainly can plot a course of general lifestyle changes that will enable you to get on a different road and gradually take back your life. Pardon the redundancy, but I want you to stop and think about those words—**"Take Back Your Life."**

Taking back your life won't be easy by any means because it might involve changing jobs; moving to another city, state or even country; or redefining your entire approach to life—all of which can be exciting and enriching. In a word, follow Thakur's theory and ask yourself (constantly), "What upholds my existence?" Once you know what those criteria are—you **must** follow them! Otherwise there's no hope of effectively dealing with the underlying causes of your being overweight or obese. You will surely fight an increasingly uphill battle with your weight, and the accompanying illnesses will mount accordingly.

All the aforementioned is my way of saying that **THE BEST DAMN DIET IS NO DIET AT ALL!** Except for a small percentage of extremely obese people, the rest of society can make do by following a basic program of careful nutrition, working out regularly, abstaining from drug use and trusting their immune systems, adjusting metabolic imbalances with natural remedies, not pampering yourself with rest and rehab every time you have a health problem, finding active and creative outlets, and developing lifestyles that truly uphold existence.

Simple? No. A lot of hard work? You bet. But this approach is practical, within range, and sustainable.

On that note, I strongly urge you to consider one of the safest and healthiest first moves on your road to taking back your life—a cleansing fast. In this case, I would recommend something that I ventured in June of 2006.

✳ ✳ ✳

I had battled and successfully beaten obesity, gambling, migraines, asthma, caffeine dependency, and numerous emotional hangups, and with June busting out all over, it was time to cap it off and fine-tune things. And this is how I decided to do it—with a nine-day cleansing program.

The Isagenix Health and Wellness System is designed to provide nutrition as it revitalizes and cleanses, while at the same time helping you lose unwanted body fat. (Note: This is not an arranged promotion or endorsement for the product. I chose it because it was highly recommended by my friend Dr. Randall Nozawa.)

Using liquid supplements, nutrient capsules, a snack made of a balanced blend of proteins, carbohydrates, and essential fats, and water, along with a nutritional liquid shake that tastes like the real thing, it was just what I needed to get into optimum condition.

For those of you who might decide to go on a cleansing program, the most important thing I can tell you is that 75 percent of what you must endure is mental and the rest is physical. If your mind is attuned to the experience as a health-giving, spiritually uplifting task, it will be an adventure; if it is fraught with worry and negative anticipation, it will be nerve-wracking and physically debilitating. So you would be wise to meditate and prepare your mind for the test.

As I am going to give you an abbreviated blow-by-blow description of my diets and fasts (see pages 336 to 340), I'm going to do the same with this cleansing.

Day 1: Feel surprisingly relaxed and unworried; after a lifetime of strenuous dieting and fasting, this should be a piece of cake! Although I'm not a big fan of ordinary water (if it's not made of grapes and doesn't have bubbles, it will never make my top 10 list), I can see how it would help flush out whatever toxins my body has maintained. So I went along with the regimen and swallowed the prescribed eight glasses of water—without any questioning or animosity. As for the supplements, no sweat. Easy and painless. And best of all, no hunger pangs. As for sleep, it wasn't the best. It was hard coming by, as it usually is the first days of any fast.

Day 2: Another cakewalk! No cravings for anything. Maybe that's because I'm too busy to think of my stomach. In any case, except for the absence of time spent preparing and eating food, it's a relatively ordinary day. Let's see—worked on this book, took care of some bills, had my Isagenix stuff, worked out, then had a boxing class (which is like boot camp!), and, oh yes, started a revolution called TBA (for Take Back America). No kidding! Sleep? About the same as Day 1.

Day 3: Nothing unusual or different to report. Went about my daily business in much the same way as ever. The great thing is that my phone has yet to turn into a hamburger, and my computer into a meatloaf. And there's no sense of persecution. I'm free to enjoy the fresh air, sun, good music, and a productive day on this book. Not bad. And sleep was a bit better.

Day 4: This is often the toughest day of any fast; perhaps it's because your body and mind have finally accepted the message that it's not business as usual, and that it may go on this way indefinitely. In any case, I was surprised to discover that it was the same as the previous three days. So it was "no sweat," and I just kept at things as if everything was normal. Even found that sleep was almost normal.

Day 5: Had a grueling workout this morning. For the most part, there were no signs of weakness. So there's no physical hurdle to get over, at least thus far. And with four days to go, which will include two more heavy workouts and two boxing classes, I have reason to believe that I can get through the entire nine-day fast without any noticeable change in physical strength or endurance. In fact, my work on the computer is more tiring than my workouts. Sleep pattern still not up to snuff, but I'm not surprised because older people don't usually sleep too well (part of the aging progress that no one has found a solution to), but there's always hope.

Day 6: One thing for sure: The cleansing process is working; I'm feeling it throughout my body AND mind. Also, feel lighter, from fat loss. Also more alert. Still no hunger pangs or cravings, and no "food" thoughts. Haven't even thought about the bubbly! Sleep was an on-and-off-again thing.

Day 7: The last third of the cleansing is greeted with sunshine and no food cravings. Actually looked forward to the shake. Filling enough, nutritious, and yummy. Can't wait for my boxing class tonight. Mind clear, alert, ready to tackle the world's problems. Why not? Nothing new in the sleep department. Although it is what it is, it hasn't hampered my alertness or activities during the day. In fact, there's little sign of a yawn.

Day 8: Stamina and mental alertness steady as they go. Feel like running most of the time, even after an arduous workout and boxing class last night. Likewise, no telltale signs of persecution, and no cravings. With only one more day to go, it's as good as it gets. All fasts should be like this! No change in sleep pattern.

Day 9: It's great knowing I've come through the fast and cleansing unscathed. Haven't had one serious moment or bout of restlessness, irritation, or bedevilment. Looking back on decades of fasting, this has been the easiest of all. Not surprisingly—for me—the fast has been done in conjunction with a heavy workout schedule. One might think that it would be less stressful to do as little as possible during a fast, but the exact opposite is true (at least for me). I crave activity. And after another heavy workout followed by a boxing class, I'm ready to tackle anything—including a somewhat restless sleep.

All Over: One always feels weird coming off an extended fast. You're cleansed, empty, uncraving, having gone without "real" food for so long. But questions immediately arise: Will you go back to old ways or retain the spirit and message of the cleansing? Will you maintain your new glamorous shape? (I lost nine pounds and looked better than ever.) And for how long? What will it have meant? In my case, I'm determined to stay the course, remain my new self, and move forward. I'm on my way!

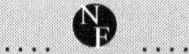

One of the added benefits of the nine-day cleansing was that it eliminated my acid reflux, which I had attributed to my intake of fruit juices, age, and whatever is in the unhealthy air we breathe. This was completely unexpected. A wonderful reward!

Returning to the question of overall health in America, I went to my high school's 50th-anniversary reunion in Las Vegas in 2004. If ever this was an opportunity to learn about health and the conglomerate, this was it. As you may recall (if you've read my autobiography) from my earlier stories about James Madison High School in Brooklyn, its students were mostly Jewish and from middle-class homes. A very high percentage went on to college, got degrees, opened businesses or got good jobs, and retired with plenty of money in the bank and all the insurance policies needed to keep them in good stead with their doctors and pharmacies. And 300 of these people gathered for our reunion in Las Vegas.

And what kind of physical shape were they in? By my standards, with all their retirement benefits, 50 years of uncommonly good living, and the best in medical care, almost all of them were in poor physical condition. The sad part about it was that almost all of them were actually proud to tell you about their by-pass surgeries, cancer treatments, diabetes, and drugs prescribed by their great doctors—whom they trust completely.

So many of the conversations began and ended with, "My doctor this... my doctor that... he prescribes this... he prescribes that." And like so many Americans, they wore their assorted illnesses like badges of honor. Whether they were doing this to gain attention or sympathy, or it's a matter of misery loves company, or they're just plain ignorant doesn't matter nearly as much as the fact that they're all aiding and abetting the wrong support system.

Instead of rallying behind good health and quality longevity, they're sitting in the same camp with their doctors, hospitals, and pill salesmen. And because they have all bought into the same batch of illnesses and treatments concocted by the conglomerate operatives, they identify with and totally support their privileged positions as next in line on the human food chain. And not one of them knows the REAL problem!

Listening to my old classmates talk about their physical deterioration as if it were a positive thing, while remembering how alive and vital they once were—and still could be—made me so angry that I wanted to grab each of them and shake them awake long enough to listen to my views. But I behaved and didn't confront anyone with my attitudes, as it was a reunion, not a seminar or lecture. When I was repeatedly asked how I had managed to stay in such great shape, I just said, "I work out regularly," and left it at that.

As an afterthought, ever since my early days at a therapeutic center, where I first learned that "there was no refuge from myself," I have regarded the typical "How are you?"—"I'm fine" opening dialogue between people as hokum and worse. Apropos of this, I am convinced that most people who automatically claim to be fine (like my old classmates) have systematically denied the truth to cover up and escape just how bad they really feel. If 4,000 therapy groups didn't prove that to me—nothing will.

But there's another reason for this individual and collective denial, closely related to a lifetime of physical neglect, emotional immaturity, and drug use. It's a form of distancing ourselves from what might have been. When we are asked "How are you?" and we automatically answer, "I'm fine," it's based on our general perspective of who we are—not who we should be.

IF it were possible for us to actually feel the way we would have, had we not been led down the garden path by the conglomerate and instead followed a course of drug-free living, consciousness-building, immune system support, and a holistic upholding of existence—and if we could juxtapose that feeling with how we now feel when we say "I'm fine"—what would we experience? I think we would feel unimaginable pain and sorrow about what we've made of our lives.

But because most of us cannot experience this role reversal, we remain blind, unaware of our living truth. We will never know what it feels like to truly be fine, because we're too far removed from it and we now have little reason to believe it's still attainable. That's where we are really lost. We could be youthful and healthy again, living drug-free lives and experiencing a full, rewarding existence well beyond the limited number of years that we foolishly allot ourselves.

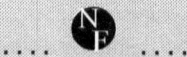

Apart from the relatively poor health of my high school compatriots, what was even worse was hearing them talk abut their children and grandchildren's health. They have "modeled" for their younger loved ones, leading them down the same drug-oriented medical paths. Hearing their stories about drug treatments prescribed to those children was enough to make me feel hostile.

What has been wrought on the minds and hearts of our ignorant society? Why is the human condition so devoid of hope? And why are greedy lunatics allowed to take command of our lives and destroy everything that is holy and beautiful?

As it stands, America's health is not only in great decline—it sucks! I can only urge you, the reader, to regain a sense of your own personal worth, the power you possess within that frame we call a body.

Regardless of your present physical condition and age, you can do many health-giving, strengthening things for yourself, the most important of which is WORKING OUT.

A week before I wrote this chapter, the manager of my health club asked me if I might participate in a videotaped advertisement for a senior's health club. As I'm always on the lookout for anything dealing with health and fitness (especially among senior citizens), I readily agreed.

Well, let me tell you... it was another colossal example of how misguided we are. The group consisted of 25-odd seniors in deteriorating health. The trainer, a gal who runs the grueling body-sculpting classes I take, led these people through a very mild exercise program consisting of simple physical activity conducted while *seated.*

None of these exercises could get within a mile of actually helping these people get on the road to recovering their physical health and well-being. Needless to say, the trainer could do no more, restricted as she is from taking any risk. The seniors themselves are, of course, under their doctors' care and would not exert themselves.

As much as I wanted to yank them out of their self-indulgent physical stupor, I knew too well that saying a word would be useless because these senior citizens would be unable to understand. They are members of the conglomerate's select club, and their life's course has been nurtured for many decades, leaving them no choice but to fulfill their deadly destinies.

How I would love to get them in my gym! Within four to six months I would have most of them doing the same kind of workouts I do. Although they would not be nearly at the same level or intensity as I am, they would nevertheless get off their present-day track to regain a youthful attitude and some physical tone, energy, and stamina. But that can't happen because I would need to do direct battle with their doctors and carry millions in liability insurance.

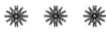

Before getting into the Best Damn Workout Ever, this is a good point to interject all of the relevant diet and obesity material referenced to in the preface of this book.

I hope you'll be ready for it!

Part III.
Roman Emperors of Old

Roman Emperors of Old

Dear reader, the following references are taken from the autobiographical precursor to this book, *So Much Pleasure, So Little Pain*.

As much as I would like to recreate the actual transitions to these accounts as they appear in the autobiography, I cannot do that without writing another book!

You will have to be satisfied with these bare accounts, which, as explained in the preface, will provide you with the essential links to *Monument to Failure*.

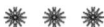

I observed my 40th birthday on October 10, 1976. I, my wife Nan, and our two young children, Billy and Jenny, lived in a large, comfortable farmhouse in East Quogue in Long Island, New York, with four other families and some single individuals. We were all members of Journey-Alert Incorporated, a nonprofit educational community with roots in the humanist movement of the 1960s.

What I remember most about that birthday was that everyone in the Journey community treated it as an honest-to-goodness milestone. Except for the infants, everyone found a way to ask, "How does it feel to be 40?"

I preferred to ignore the question because it raised the specter of middle age, something that hadn't weighed heavily on my mind. But with the event at hand, there was no avoiding the question. So, I tried to act nonchalant about the overblown affair, shrugging it off with, "No big deal, just another symbolic growing-of-age indicator, like 16, 21, and 30, just grist for the greeting card manufacturers."

Trouble was, with such intense focus on my milestone birthday, I no longer felt so casual about the number 40. Like it or not, Pandora's box was open, and I was on the defensive, trying to convince myself that there was nothing to it. After all, I'm exactly the same person I was yesterday at 39, I told myself as I inspected the scattering of gray hairs on my head, wondering if they would now multiply more rapidly.

That evening my friends and family carried in a gigantic buttercream birthday cake from the Lafayette Bakery in Greenwich Village, my all-time favorite sweetshop. Staring at the 40 bright candles, I wanted to shout, I'm not going through with this! I don't want to be 40! Why should I be 40? Instead, I looked at everyone's smiling face as they sang a robust "Happy Birthday" and decided to blow out the candles on cue. After all, I was happily married, the father of two great kids, in control of my life, and looking forward to a very promising future.

Within a matter of weeks, however, an identity crisis of enormous proportions, brought on by anxiety over the future and loss of self-esteem, assailed me. Panic-stricken, I feared a recurrence of severe migraine attacks, something that I hadn't suffered in 18 years. While the headaches remained a thing of the past, my other lifelong affliction, obesity, the true demon of my entire existence—rose up before me. I finished off the last of the freezer-stored birthday cake, and I was, for God knows the umpteenth time in my life, FAT. With Thanksgiving less than two weeks away, no less.

I prepared to go on one of my patented diets, a program established just before I was married in 1970, by downing a meal of three Dagwood-size bologna sandwiches, a double portion of french fries, two Greek cheese pies, half of a Sara Lee chocolate cream pie topped with a pint of orange sherbet, and a quart of Budweiser. Then I went to a movie, where I washed a giant bucket of butter-soaked popcorn down with several large containers of Coke. Not to be shortchanged before retiring for the night, I completed my diet preparations with a cold bottle of champagne and a bag of taco chips.

The next morning I felt ready to go, but when my wife Nan served me the bowl of brown rice and glass of water that would be my steady diet for two weeks—as prescribed years earlier by my guru Thakur—I felt sick to my stomach. Feeling loathing and disgust for the rice and water, I was completely thrown by this negative reaction. In 23 years of ritual dieting and cleansing, I had never before had such a problematic reaction; it had always been so easy.

Going over the situation in my mind, it seemed obvious that my "over 40" hang-up had wiped away my resolve. My only choice was to fall back on my ultimate weapon against encroaching obesity—starvation.

I made ready: Standing naked in front of a full-length mirror, I told myself, You're not a man. You're a pile of ugly flab. A fucking slob if ever there was one! This went on until I reached a satisfactory state of self-revulsion. Then I sat on a pillow and meditated, uttering my mantra over and over, all the while keeping the face of my guru, Thakur, in my mind's eye.

After reaching the proper level of inner calm and centeredness for starvation, I concluded my preabstinence countdown by drinking a magnum of champagne, consuming an extraordinary amount of popcorn saturated with butter and salt, and hauling myself to bed to sleep for 19 hours. Nothing could stop me now.

After nine days of total fasting, with absolutely no food or drink,[26] my weight

---

[26]   Most people in Western society pessimistically shake their heads in doubt whenever I speak of going without food or drink for nine days. They quickly play the expert, telling me that it's impossible to survive that long without any water. Nothing could be further from the truth. In India, this is hardly an exceptional feat of endurance. In fact, documented records show that Indian mystics have long survived without any sustenance for months. It is a matter of preparation and mind control. I

had fallen to within legal limits. I had triumphed over my life's adversary again. There was only one problem—I was on a collision course with Thanksgiving, the one day in the year that strikes terror in the heart of anyone with a serious weight problem. In no mood to break out the champagne, I felt that a stake had been driven through my stomach.

My ever-loving wife, who has endured many of my fasts over the years, tried to assure me that everything would be all right. She smiled at my wacky puns, listened patiently while I expressed pained outrage at the lifelong weight problem, and ministered to my every need. But it didn't help.

Never one to give up, Nan urged me to stay clear of the treacherous day by hightailing it out of the farmhouse while the gettin' was good.

"Take a bottle of wine and some chips and check into a motel for the day. You can watch the football games on television. You don't have to be here," she cautioned.

But I refused to consider parting from family and friends on Thanksgiving Day, no matter how severe the temptations and traps.

I came up with a battle plan: to act as if there was nothing to fear, pretend to be in a cavalier mood, to skip lightly through the day without any serious consequences.

As part of my act, I dressed to look thinner than I actually was, wearing trim slacks that would have fit perfectly had I just come off a slightly longer fast. The vanity, like the act-as-if strategy, was ill-conceived. I realized as much the moment that I strolled into the dining room on Thanksgiving morning, viewed the bountiful display of appetizers laid out on the 12-foot-long picnic table, and knew that I would not last the day without bursting a seam.

I might have attempted to control my desire for the cheeses, fruits, nuts, breads, spreads, and liquid refreshments, if I'd had someone to talk to me about my recent fast. Unfortunately, everyone was busy helping prepare the main courses, so no one could act as a buffer. Left to my own madness, I reached out for the first deadly piece of sharp provolone. Nan had been perfectly right; I had no business being there.

The medical scale in the bathroom confirmed my worst fears. After one meal, albeit stretched out over five hours, I had gained more than six pounds—and the day was still young.

I remained in the bathroom for a long time, staring down at the terrible numbers and feeling more self-pity than I could ever remember. Right then and there

---

was fortunate enough to learn these basic elements of fasting from close disciples of Thakur, who was, among many supernatural things, a spiritual adviser to none other than Mahatma Gandhi, who certainly knew a thing or two about fasting.

I knew that I had absolutely no intention of doing anything about the flash weight gain. No—I was through! Once and for all! I just couldn't hack it anymore. Since I was six months old, when my fat cells began to accumulate at an alarming rate to my mother's great satisfaction, I had suffered this cruel and unusual punishment, and now, after 40 years of constant struggle, I was finally quitting. Enough was enough. I couldn't bear the thought of another fast and I could no longer fight off the karma.

Looking out of the bathroom window, I focused my deadened mind on the open field behind the farmhouse, where people with full bellies and bright smiles were organizing the annual Thanksgiving Day football game. One thing was for sure, I wouldn't play this year. I'd be lucky to sneak into my bedroom unnoticed, undress, and hopefully fall asleep into some form of merciful oblivion.

Taking a last look out of the window, I saw my three-year-old son, Billy, glee-fully carrying the football, trying to run away from the grownups. Tripping over himself, he fell down rather hard and the ball tumbled out of his hands. An older boy swooped it up and ran from Billy. Jarred by the fall and annoyed at having lost possession of the football, Billy ignored his pain and embarrassment to chase after the older boy.

I suddenly started to cry uncontrollably. The hurt poured out in volumes. Turn-ing away from the window, I looked at myself in the mirror above the sink and watched the tears streaming down my face. Then I slowly lowered my head ... re-signed to my fate ... after 40 years of self-inflicted torture.

In the next few minutes, all the curious and outlandish features of my personal-ity—no doubt a result of my enduring bout with obesity—drew together in an em-pirical illusion as real as any dream or fantasy that I have ever experienced. I was transported through the gates of time, to a magical kingdom where there was no concern for how I looked, where rumor and insinuation had no place, and where I could do whatever the hell I wanted, as long as it did not hurt anyone else.

Dope-fiends, alcoholics, gamblers, and overeaters populated this supernatural domain. And there I was, in full-blown Greek regalia of princely shirt and tapered pants, as thin as a wisp, dancing the sirtaki, while eating all manner of delicacies from the luscious fingertips of waitressing nymphs.

As I watched myself dance and eat to my heart's content, purple clouds rolled by as the sun set and rose three times. In this span, I did not rest or digest, and yet I could not put on weight. It was a miracle—as if the food did not pass from my mouth to my stomach and to my bowels. The days simply passed and there were no longer any problems to deal with—because I was in Paradise!

Less than an hour later, I stood in the kitchen, one hand stroking Nan's hair and the other gingerly picking away at three varieties of stuffing. My wife, to-tally aware of how agonizing the day had been for me, couldn't understand why

I seemed so happy and relieved. She had no way of knowing that the battle was finally over. Minutes later, I went outside and joined in the football game.

Later that evening, after the Thanksgiving guests had long since departed and the entire Journey community had gone to sleep, I was still at work on the remains of the feast. First came the stuffing and turkey, then the hardened mashed potatoes with cold gravy, baked potatoes with some freshly melted butter, jellied cranberry sauce, and blueberry and pumpkin pie, followed by assorted leftover cheeses, nuts, fruits, and of course the bubbly.

As I stuffed myself to the gills, outdoing all previous bouts of such passion, I fantasized running throughout the house shouting, I did it! I did it! Look at me—I did it! But I was too busy foraging among the bones, scraps, pans, and jars—savoring the vast pleasure of that most memorable and glorious day of absolute gluttony.

At four in the morning, I stopped eating and drinking and walked up the stairs, feeling an emotional gratification that had escaped me over a lifetime of fatness. As I walked into the bathroom, I wanted to laugh loudly enough for the whole house to hear, knowing that the scale could no longer deprive me of sweet and complete victory.

Sometime later, I stopped to peek in at Billy, who was sleeping comfortably. Feeling a powerful need to share the important event, I bent over to carefully hug and kiss him. He barely stirred.

Then I went into my bedroom, quietly stood at the foot of the bed, and looked at the figures of my slumbering wife and our six-month-old daughter, Jenny. At that very instant, I desperately wanted to wake Nan. She would have been astonished that in less than 24 hours, I had consumed more than 30 pounds of assorted food and drink—some 38,000 calories in all—and weighed exactly the same amount as I did when I had started that fateful day!

In fact, I had lost about half a pound...

✱ ✱ ✱

At first, it was a real pain in the ass, or should I say in the throat? I stuck my fingers in my mouth three, four, often five times a day (as many times as I ate), trying to induce the food to leave my stomach before it did any harm. It also took too damn long, anywhere from 30 to 40 minutes at a crack. And it was painful, if not outright dangerous, as there was the very real possibility of choking. But all these problems were eliminated entirely when I chanced upon the hitherto unknown reality that I was *doing it all wrong*—which is the case with millions of bulimics worldwide.

All it took was a bit of common sense before realizing that correcting and solving the problem was ridiculously easy. In practical terms, it's as if these millions of long-suffering people with their fingers down their throats are trying to get from one side of the moat to the other by jumping into the muck and slowly plodding through it, when all they have to do is lower the drawbridge and walk across.

It defies imagination to think that no one else has figured it out, and it proves my axiom: *"It's not that I'm so smart—but that you're so dumb!"* This rude awakening is right on the bulls-eye because these legions of bulimics are still *doing it the wrong way,* when they could easily remedy their dire situations and make their lives a hell of a lot less painful and complicated.

So what's the secret? I give you the equation: $WC = M^3 - D$, which translates into, *"Weight control equals mass to the 3rd power minus dilution."* If you don't get it, the solution is **dilution**.

Allow me to illustrate. Take an empty quart-sized water bottle and fill half of it with pieces of chewed food: a sandwich, french fries, cake, pie, whatever. Now, turn the bottle on its side or nearly upside-down and see what happens. The food gets stuck in the neck of the bottle—right? Even if you shake it violently, it still acts like ketchup that refuses to come out.

Now fill the remaining space in the bottle with liquid. Again, turn the bottle on its side or nearly upside-down and see what happens, especially if you give it a light tap. Bingo! It spills out, sandwich and all.

That's the basic principle, and it works. It's a million times easier, safer, and faster. I have more than a sneaking suspicion that the Roman emperors who ate until their stomachs were about to pop and then purged probably knew as much.

When I realized that it was a matter of dilution, I simply drank more liquid or had soup with each meal. In fact, I created an entire menu around the principle. And if I was at a guest's house and they didn't serve enough liquids, I would down three or four glasses of water in the bathroom before "Tupping." [27]

With practice and a greater awareness of the time factor (it's not necessary to rush but generally you shouldn't wait longer than three-quarters of an hour after eating), the entire regimen became as easy and normal as a diet pill, only without any side effects. I would gorge on my favorite foods, consuming the equivalent of three meals. Then, without resorting to any form of bothersome dieting or exercise, I would unburden myself of the "would-be" mass and body weight within no more than 60 seconds! Once I really got my act together, I could discharge 90 to 95 percent of the repast in under 30 seconds—then return to the table for dessert!

---

[27] "Tupping" is a palatable (pun intended) term I have made up to replace all the negative ones commonly used to describe the process of regurgitating.

As I progressed, I began to use my stomach and throat muscles to greater advantage, making the process that much easier and with gravity doing much of the work.

Gradually, I developed other techniques that combined into a process that has become a mainstay in my existence and all but precludes—if 30 years is enough of a test—the possibility of ever being fat again.

The only problem was the fear of being caught in the act. Remember, this was 1976 and nobody had come out of the bulimia closet. (In fact, the word "bulimia" had not come into common usage.) How could I have explained such a curious, even disagreeable act? And the bigger dilemma—do I tell my family and close friends? You may not believe it, but I never said a word to anyone.

Almost three decades have glided by since that fateful Thanksgiving Day when I chanced upon my "Fountain of Youth." I have never felt younger or healthier. As for my actual weight, it has remained level throughout all these years. And if three decades of diet-free living is any kind of measuring stick—then I am undeniably cured of my problem with obesity.

But this doesn't make sense to you, does it? It might have made sense 25 or 30 years ago—before all those people (including the famous ones) came out of the woodwork to reveal their bulimia tales. Yet here I am, the one and only exception to all that negative bulimia history, telling you what great shape my life is in—when on the face of things you'll sooner think I should be certified as some kind of nut.

Well, I admit the subject will spark controversy, which I could avoid by telling readers that tupping is just another example of my extremism, but then I would have to live with that big lie. And in failing to shed proper light on the subject on which I am the world's greatest expert, I would deny millions of people the benefit of potentially lifesaving insights.

So I'm not going to dodge the issue; I'm going to explain it in detail and let you be the judge. Only, please be objective. Put aside all the negative impressions that are probably rooted in your mind, and pay attention to facts and details. In other words, read what I have to say instead of prejudging it. Not for my sake, but for the sake of millions of people who might be saved from a lifetime of obesity problems and disabilities.

❋ ❋ ❋

Author's note: As this section will trigger controversy and perhaps revulsion among many people, I would like to relate a bit of history before entering this arena. First, the term "bulimia" did not even come into popular existence until the early 1980s. Second, the media has been responsible not only for misrepre-

320 MONUMENT FAILURE

senting eating disorders but also for attaching shame and guilt to the problem. Third, when it comes to issues of oral gratification (which plays a large part in the compelling urge to overeat), I encourage you to be both understanding and objective before making a snap judgment about these issues.

Otherwise you will immediately condemn what I am about to outline, instead of considering its role as a relatively healthy procedure in the overall context of last-resort weight reduction strategies.

To anticipate and respond to inquiries and challenges that will be raised by people concerning the subject, I have chosen a question-and-answer format as the most legitimate way of presenting my case in support of tupping.

> ### *Is there a basic difference between tupping and bulimia?*

Most definitely. Whereas bulimia is essentially an eating disorder, tupping is a modifying tool employed to protect people who suffer from the disorder and want to solve it, as well as other associated problems such as lifetime dieting, being overweight, and obesity.

> ### *Do you recommend tupping as an all-purpose solution to obesity?*

No. I'm not at this juncture advocating any particular solution to the problem (except to keep away from drugs and cosmetic surgery). I'm merely telling my story. However, I will say that tupping should be considered a viable option if you fit into any of the following categories:

1. ***On the road to oblivion:*** Individuals who will otherwise kill themselves from overeating, dieting, exercise, or a combination thereof.

2. ***Can't fit through the door:*** People who are so morbidly obese that they've given up hope of ever being able to deal with the problem, much less live a normal life.

3. ***Prepared to go under the knife:*** Anyone considering surgical means such as intestinal bypass, stapling of the stomach or mouth, or liposuction.

4. ***Druggies:*** Drug-dependent personalities who have been placed on a chemically-oriented weight-reducing program.

5. *Obsessive eaters:* Overweight or obese people who "live to eat"—who cannot control their appetites and will not exercise or practice any other form of weight control, and as a result are under constant and severe physical, emotional, and psychological strain.

6. *Confirmed bulimics:* People reluctant or unable to stop themselves from constantly gorging and purging. For these individuals, it is essential that they at least learn the right way.

> *When you say "the right way," do you mean that there are actually techniques involved?*

Yes. But before I elaborate, let me first describe the "preconditioning" stage. If you're not in fairly good physical condition, you should at least do a bit of basic toning. I'm not talking about anything more difficult than simple deep-breathing exercises and some sit-ups to limber your stomach muscles.

Next, it's important to get your mind off everything else so that you can concentrate on what you'll be doing. I suggest you work on some form of mind relaxation like meditation, yoga, self-hypnosis, or anything that will help you clear your mind of thoughts that will otherwise distract or impede the process at hand.

When you feel ready, we can move on to the practice stage—which should, for obvious reasons, take place in the bathroom.

1. While standing up straight, swallow a small amount of air. Then expel it. No—I'm not kidding. I'm asking you to belch! (Lots of people in different parts of the world are quite proud of their ability to belch.) Practice belching for a few minutes.

2. Once you have your belching act together, bend over at about a 45-degree angle, and rehearse your belches in that position. Adjust your position accordingly.

3. When you feel relatively at ease with the practice of eructing, drink a glass of water, bend over the bowl, and repeat the same procedure again. If your mind is undistracted and you're concentrating on your stomach, what should happen is that the escaping air, along with the pressure of your abdominal muscles (which can be exerted as they are needed), plus the natural force of gravity, will bring up the water and anything else for that matter. **Note:** Until you get the hang of it, you may need to bend (or squat) lower.

That's all there is to it. **Now tell me that slicing, dicing, and stapling your stomach is a better solution!**

One word of caution: Even when practicing with water, be certain to keep your head at a proper angle, so that the water (and later the food) won't run up your nose, which can be quite uncomfortable. With a little bit of practice, it's easily avoidable.

Drill yourself in this simple process over a period of days, before advancing to tupping a meal. During this preconditioning stage, practice your relaxation and stomach exercises faithfully. And when you practice tupping water, try to develop a feel for the technique. By this I mean that you should sense just how much air (if any[28]) you need to swallow, the amount of pulling pressure your stomach muscles have to exert, the position that is most comfortable for you, exactly how to hold your head, etc. Paying attention to all of this will make tupping that much easier when you start doing it with food.

When you have mastered the elements of tupping water, then you have completed your preconditioning program and are ready to move on to the next level. However, you must first commit yourself to following certain Do's and Don'ts. These rules will enable you to proceed without fear of the medical complications that can occur with bulimia.

> *Hold on!*
> *What are the possible medical complications?*

Any number of potential problems can occur, including sore throats, dental decay, esophageal irritation, swollen glands, vitamin and mineral deficiencies, dehydration, disruption of the body's electrolyte and fluid balance, muscle fatigue, stomach rupture, erratic heartbeat, kidney failure, and the ever-present possibility of choking to death.

> *In this case, wouldn't it be wise*
> *for people to consult with professionals*
> *before going on a tupping program?*

A waste of time! Odds are better than dollars to donuts that the people who fall

---

[28] Once you are used to tupping, depending on the type and amount of food ingested, you may or may not find it necessary to swallow air to help you dispose of the meal.

into the six categories I previously mentioned have already been through the maze of doctors, psychologists, psychiatrists, social workers, clinics, known experts in all related fields, etc. They have probably tried every form of therapy, drug, theory, scheme, and diet program on the marketplace—and what good has it done them? Besides, what do all of these so-called experts know about tupping? *Not a damn thing!* I'm the only expert.

To be more precise, 29 years ago I spent an entire day searching through reference files at one of the largest libraries in the world, trying to find anything about induced vomiting. What I found didn't fill one three-by-five-inch index card—most of it was anecdotal stuff about Roman emperors. (During the Roman period of conspicuous consumption and self-congratulation [around 65 B.C.], Roman vomitoriums were relatively common.)

Less than three years later—out of nowhere—a slew of experts, clinics, and associations sprang up to deal with bulimia and anorexia. Hell, bulimia wasn't even widely heard of until the 1980s! And I'd like to know the following: Where did all these newfound experts suddenly come from? Where did they study? When and where did they do their research? I mean, no schools, no curricula, and no body of knowledge were present to draw from.

You want the answer? It's simple: **Once the medical fraternity and insurance companies read the feature stories about famous people coming out of the eating disorder closet, they realized a new cash cow was on the horizon.** Necessity being the mother of invention, they introduced eating disorder clinics, new therapies, drugs, medical coverage, and publicity to harvest the new crop of suffering bulimia and anorexia patients.

If you put these overnight experts together, their combined knowledge of the disorders that they treat amounts to little more than what they gleamed from articles written by bulimics, anorexics, and freelance writers who spent all of three days compiling their facts.

To demonstrate how little they still know, none of these professionals has come up with *simple safeguards* for their bulimia patients. That is why people are still suffering from medical complications to the point of fatality. That is why these people are not being cured of their eating disorders. And that is why they are turning to dangerous surgical procedures. **It need not be!**

> *Are you suggesting that bulimia*
> *was manufactured?*

Out of whole cloth! Bulimia was cultivated just as drug clinics for the rich and famous were created by the insurance industry and the medical fraternity. In both cases, none of the money changers had ever shown a genuine interest in any of the problems related to drug abuse, alcohol abuse, or eating disorders. As soon as they realized that big money could be made, greedy experts emerged from the woodwork and the "spin" was applied to accommodate the carpetbaggers. The ignorant public accepted these artificial new industries without batting an eyelash.

Why? Because they had the unintentional support of famous personalities like Jane Fonda and Princess Diana, whose dramatic testimonies to the horror of bulimia galvanized public opinion. And after 25 years of the eating disorder industry's existence, who's to question their knowledge? Only yours truly. **That's because I'm the only person with the facts as well as the desire to expose the myth and the fraud.**

> *Getting back to tupping, will people*
> *be willing to accept the risks?*

Generally speaking, the people in those six categories will be quite willing to risk just about anything to lose weight. In fact, the greater they weigh, the more risk they'll be willing to take. Being fat is penalized in this society. In fact, the perils of obesity also affect how well (or not) that you are treated by others and even how much you are paid. As a result, when you're overweight, your whole life can become just one big diet. That's why people keep trying over and over again, why they resort to drugs and grotesque surgeries, why they cannot accept their obesity. And unlike loss of a limb or blindness, they can be cured.

> *Okay—what are the Do's and Don'ts?*

First the Don'ts:

1. ***Don't eat "heavy" foods unless you're not going to tup them.*** Chunks of solid meat, green spaghetti, french fries, cauliflower, rice, and the like are quick to go down and slow to come up. Mashed potatoes in place of french fries is a good bet, as are most sandwiches, soups, and light appetizers.

2. ***Don't swallow big pieces whole.*** Chew your food well. You don't want to choke on intake or outtake.

3. ***Don't add salt to your food.*** If you're overweight or obese, salt only adds to the problem because it can cause high blood pressure, which is the main cause of strokes and a major cause of heart attack. Salt also leads to increased anxiety, arthritis, cardiovascular disease, and edema; it can also bring on insomnia and exacerbate water retention. It's a huge no-no for people with weight problems. Instead of reaching for the salt shaker, try tamarind, cumin, pepper, cilantro, basil, thyme, bay leaves, oregano, lemon juice, or fresh garlic.

4. ***Don't wait too long before tupping.*** But this doesn't mean you have to rush your meal. Quite the contrary—enjoy it.

5. ***Don't tup small meals or snacks*** unless it's absolutely necessary because, believe it or not, small amounts are more difficult to bring up. Another important reason for not tupping small meals is that you'll defeat the long-range potential of eventually regulating your weight without having to tup your food.

6. ***Don't try to tup 100 percent of your food.*** You don't have to. Just eliminate the excess, enough to help you inch along to your proper weight.

7. ***Don't "think" while tupping.*** It will break your concentration.

8. ***Don't force it.*** If for some reason you're unable to bring it up, which is more than likely because of the type of food or not enough liquid, don't strain yourself by trying harder. Just relax for a few moments and then drink one or two glasses of water before trying again. That should do the trick.

Now for the Do's:

1. ***Do drink a lot with each meal*** (remember the solution is dilution). *At least* 24 to 36 ounces. The specific ratio of liquid to solid needed to flush out your meal will of course depend on the amount and type of food ingested. Over time you will learn to accurately gauge just how much you should drink with a particular meal, especially if you stick to a tried-and-true menu. For instance, a soup meal will generally require less additional liquid than a sandwich meal. But remember: The more liquids you have with a meal, the easier and safer it will be to tup.

2. ***Do eat as much as you desire.*** You're not on a diet now. (That hasn't worked for you.) So if your objective is to satiate yourself—then do it. But also remember that your eyes can be bigger than your stomach—so be aware of your actual capacity. The balloon can be blown up only so much before its elasticity is strained to the bursting point.

3. *Do tell yourself as you walk to the bathroom that tupping* is *necessary for your well-being and your long-range health.* The truth is that once you have the emotional and psychological assurance that what you're doing is right for you, not only will the process be carried out without strain, fear, or guilt, but you will realize that you are finally on the road leading to full recovery. And that's more than half the battle.

> ***What's to prevent someone from tupping a meal and then going right back to eating again?***

What you're talking about should be addressed for those bulimics who do not tup their meals because, after spending so much time with their fingers down their throats, by the time they're finished they're so damn exhausted and depleted that they need to go back for more food just to regain some strength.

But with tupping, it's quick and relatively easy. You end up so satisfied with yourself that you don't need to stuff yourself with more food. Taking it a step further, a good tup is orgiastic because you're both emptied and satisfied. It's like having your cake and eating it too.

> ***But don't you feel lousy—just having to do it?***

No. I'm eternally grateful. And your question shows just how lacking in objectivity you are. You're not in the shoes of those people who fall into those six deadly categories, so you really can't speak for them. Nor can you begin to imagine how happy they would be to finally be through with all the diets, pills, bills, failed attempts, and the misery they experience throughout their overweight lives. It's all accomplished with a simple *water cure.*

> ***But what about the time it takes?***
> ***And day after day, week after week.***

Truth is, it takes me all of six minutes a day. Tell me—how long does the average diet take? If you could tell millions of dieters that a safe, easy, painless, drugless diet existed that took less than 10 minutes a day—what would they say? My diet is done in less time than it takes you to drive to your pharmacy for your pills! So much pleasure—so little pain.

> ### Is the process of tupping food different than doing it with water?

The procedure is basically the same except that you're bringing up a meal with the water. As much as it will be weightier, it will take that much more effort, especially when you first begin. So it's important to stay aware of the essential process, keep the mind clear of outside influences, relax your body and feel good about yourself and what you're doing. Other than that, unloosen your clothing, find a comfortable position, bend over the bowl[29] at the proper angle, open your mouth wide, then put into practice what you've already learned. With help from dilution, air pressure, stomach power, and gravity, nature will undoubtedly take its course.

But remember—*don't force it.* By all means, start with soft foods like soups or mashed potatoes. Almost anything with a mashed or creamy consistency will work for you. They're great for beginners and help bring everything else up that much easier.

> ### How many times must you do it?

The process of tupping should be repeated three or four times each time you decide not to assimilate a meal. The exact number of reps[30] depends on the type and volume of food and drink ingested, as well as your weight stage. If you still endeavor to lose weight, you will probably want to rid yourself of most of the meal. But if you have already reached your ideal weight, then you only need to follow a maintenance program.

Of course, all these decisions along the road to eventual good health will be made according to your individual need. In any case, whatever your specific requirements are, the sequence of tupping will normally be something like this:

1. The first rep will loosen up your stomach muscles, bringing up a moderate

---

[29] You may prefer to use a plastic tub. Even better—use Tupperware. Ha! As the great Durante used to say, "I'm on a roll now!"

[30] "Reps" is a term used by bodybuilders and weightlifters. Indeed, when used in reference to tupping—it certainly is a weight-lifter.

to fairly large portion of your meal. It will also give you the general feel of things, letting you know if you're going to have an easy time or whether you need to drink more liquid to further dilute and disengage the food.

2. Your second rep, following any necessary intake of fluid, is usually the gusher, the real mother lode, and you will find it infinitely rewarding. Not only will it relieve you of the bulk of your unwanted repast, but it will also alleviate most of the mind and body pressures that go hand-in-hand with stuffing yourself with food and drink. An instant diet!

3. The third, fourth, and subsequent reps will normally produce lighter, although not insignificant yields. These are the ones that actually control your weight and subsequently the way you look and feel. These last labors not only unburden you of the excess food and drink that would otherwise have turned into added body weight, but they also bring the state of buoyancy and euphoria usually felt after completing a diet. In a true sense, that is exactly what you've managed to accomplish, although it's taken you only a few minutes.

And most importantly, even though you now look (and to a certain extent feel) as if you hadn't eaten because you've bottomed out, you *will not* experience the physical and psychological cravings for food that you usually undergo when you haven't eaten.

This is not to say that you will be completely satisfied. **God only knows what it will ultimately take to gratify your deeper hunger, the real source of your pain.** But at least you'll be on the road (or one of the possible roads) to sanity.

> *How can you possibly equate the process*
> *of tupping with being on the road to sanity?*

That's easy. I believe in it. Since I'm as pragmatic as they get, I concern myself with what upholds existence, not merely what appeals to the uneducated masses. I know more acceptable ways to control weight exist—drugs are cleaner, can be purchased over the counter or prescribed, and are widely used and recommended. But they create a growing dependency, can cause extremely harmful side effects (even death), and contribute to all the ills of a drug-oriented society.

Eating disorder clinics and weight-loss programs are famous for their dogmatic opinions and attitudes, but they are miserable failures when it comes to offering people in the six endangered categories a feasible, practical, and affordable remedy to their problems. That's because their solutions are for the most part not viable and often induce people to resort to dangerous surgical means. In a word, they're in business purely for the money.

As for typical moderate methods such as dieting and exercise, they would be fine if they worked for everyone—but they don't. The millions of obese people whom I'm addressing in those six categories cannot or will not avail themselves of normal methods of weight control and appetite satisfaction. So what are they to do? Go to hell on a rocket ship? Continue to suffer through life? Waste their lives? Why? Tupping is a method that can work for the majority of these people. And it does offer the potential of success, sanity, and eventual cure.

> ### Are you cured?

As they say in the military, "Fucking-A I am!" I fall back on tupping only on those occasions when I absolutely must. Then I do it happily because I'm thankful to have a foolproof way of staying at the right weight and remaining healthy.

Although it's not an appropriate comparison (because I *am* cured of obesity), just like a person suffering from hemophilia needs a blood transfusion or a diabetic needs insulin, I'd rather live the way that I do—with its attending problems—than not at all. *Having to continuously diet or fast to extreme at any age, or to remain fat and miserable, unhappy with myself and the world, is not my idea of living.*

Another way of looking at the question is, "What do you mean by 'cured'?" Do you mean feeling good? Remedying the circumstances? Eliminating the illness? Well, I know that in this present life I cannot "eliminate the illness" any more than I can regrow an amputated limb. But as I've managed to alleviate the symptoms, to go about my life looking and feeling good, to devote my energies to living, loving, and creating, instead of being miserable and making others feel bad—then as far as I'm concerned—*I'm cured forevermore!*

> ### What about health and nutrition?
> ### If you're ridding yourself of everything you eat—
> ### how can you be healthy?

You don't rid yourself of everything you eat—only the excess, depending on your specific objectives. Your body retains enough nutritional food to maintain its essential functions. You can safeguard your nutritional needs by snacking on small amounts of healthy foods like chicken, fish, cheese, fruit, vegetables, nuts, a glass of wine, etc., which you do not tup. And if you need vitamin supplements, by all means take them. Remember, the objective is to become a human being of normal weight, something you haven't been able to do using other methods.

> *How long will it take for someone*
> *with a serious weight problem*
> *to become a "normal human being"?*

If the goal is to lead a relatively healthy and balanced life, my general rule of thumb is that you must maintain an appropriate weight for at least one year before you can confidently be on the road to normalcy. I call this one-year-period "gap time," during which that person experiences all the days and important occasions of the year, coming full circle, so to speak, as a new person.

The most common problem with diets is that most dieters quickly regain their weight. They're rarely off the treadmill of diets, pills, programs, etc., for more than a few weeks or months at a time. But once you as a tupper reach your proper weight and complete a one-year cycle, chances are in your favor that you will have adjusted, accepted your new self, and be well on your way to becoming normal.

And it's a thousand times easier to maintain the weight loss over a long time as I have, rather than through shorter cycles of dieting (or whatever the alternative is). Actually, it gets easier as time goes by because you've grown accustomed to the luxury of looking and feeling good; you're not wasting time, energy, and money on dieting; and the tupping regimen, used when needed, has become second nature.

What it adds up to is that you graduate to feeling, thinking, and acting like a person no longer in danger of being fat. And wouldn't you love this!

> *Is there some hitherto unknown and*
> *abstract reason for our hang-ups*
> *and obsessions with food?*

I have a theory on that; I call it the "missing link." It's based on my lifelong awareness that we are missing something because we're never satisfied. That's why we're always yearning for something else and comfort ourselves with things, both material and sensual. For most of us, a common form of comfort is food, which is one of the main reasons contributing to our national problem of being overweight and obese.

Besides food, we drown our sorrows in alcohol, drugs, sex, work, cars, causes, even hope ... seeking salvation or escape from whatever ails our souls.

As to what that missing link is ... picture a perfect universe ... where we live off life, love, and creativity—with or without oxygen—and there is no food chain and therefore no need to stockpile reserves. We sustain ourselves on our creative abilities and the strength of our love for life. That's a planet to strive for!

There's also the possibility that our obesity is caused by a craving for something we can't find on this planet Earth, but previously existed.

Does that sound too abstract for your tastes? Well, maybe we were originally designed that way and then mutated into food eaters, and have spent eons desperately seeking the next meal.

Whatever the answer is, we are now stuck with the results of our food hangups, which have now reached epic proportions in America, so much so that they constitute a national health crisis all their own. And there's no relief in sight from its encroachment because it is fueled by the insatiable conglomerate's cravings as well as our own.

> ### *Do you support websites that dispute that anorexia and bulimia are diseases?*

Before answering the specific question, I must make a clear distinction between bulimia and anorexia. Just as I believe that male and female homosexuality are not one and the same things, I believe that bulimia and anorexia should not be lumped together.

From my point of view, the bulimic wants to eat, while the anorexic wants to starve. That's quite a departure. And while anorexia might be considered a sickness because it is potentially life-threatening, bulimia is basically a disorder that often leads to medical complications of a different origin from anorexia.

In any case, the origins, treatment, and prognosis vary considerably—and it is best that we do not refer to them in the same breath.

Regarding the websites in question, while I dispute that eating disorders are a disease, I do not support these websites because, first, they portray the disorders as philosophies of life; second, they aid and abet the serious potential for a wide range of medical complications associated with the disorders; and third, they are counterproductive in an overall sense because they offer no insights into the root causes of the problems, and they don't suggest other options.

I support my system of tupping because it provides an effective alternative to eating disorders, and offers those people in the six endangered categories (as

stated on pages 320 to 321) protection against the medical complications connected to the disorders. It worked for me for 30 years—and I'm as healthy as
anyone could hope to be. Not a single medical problem.

Prosit!

> ### *If "tupping" is so*
> ### *safe and relatively easy, then why isn't*
> ### *it taken more seriously?*

Tupping has no money in it for the big profit-makers, and it could seriously cut
into the earnings of the eating-disorder industry and the diet-pill companies that
create the likes of Fen-Phen.

The other reality is that the general public may not be ready for it because the
image of tupping causes too much distress for most people. Can you imagine
this: A public that loves to watch (and engage in) violence; goes along with unnecessary (often deadly) extreme surgery; ignores 43,000 road deaths; hundreds
of thousands of drug-related deaths; and 195,000 preventable hospital deaths
a year; supports the killing and maiming of hundreds of thousands of innocent
men, women, and children for political and economic purposes; and ignores many
acts of torture and genocide throughout the world—but they cannot stomach the
thought of individuals using a last-resort water cure to rid themselves of the problem of obesity! What strange values.

In fact, even my close friends and family members are turned off to the idea
and will sooner accept complicated and dangerous surgical procedures over my
plan. That's because the image of regurgitating prevents people from being objective, as does the multitude of lies and distortions associated with bulimia.

The overwhelming fact also remains that all the media people reporting on
the subject are biased and misinformed because they bought into the inaccurate,
misleading information presented by the eating-disorder industry, and thus they
refuse to budge from that impenetrable, the-world-is-flat position.

Because the obesity problem has now swelled into a huge cash cow that gen-
erates billions in revenue, more drugs, surgical procedures, and devices will be
introduced in coming years, including an ultrasound wand that will supposedly
break down fat cells to be consumed by the body's natural mechanisms, as well as
implantable stimulation devices that target the central nervous system.

As long as these companies generate the venture capital to fund these products
and procedures (including high-level marketing strategies), there's little reason
to believe that the obese public (especially people in the highest-risk categories),
will be interested in "tupping."

There's also the fact that the government will soon throw open the door for millions of overweight Americans to make medical claims for treatments such as stomach surgery and diet programs, which will heap another $150 billion into the conglomerate's coffers.

Even on the most practical level, bulimics worldwide will continue to be deprived of the essential tool (tupping) that will at least protect them from various potential medical hazards associated with bulimia. Why? Because the eating-disorder clinics need to pay their rents and big salaries, that's why.

And don't forget that the media can't make any advertising dollars from "tupping" and won't be permitted to give it a fair hearing—and you have a clear perspective on why my method isn't taken more seriously.

My long-range hope is that people who read this book will use common sense and be more objective.

Would you be against the use of an experimental drug or medical procedure on a terminally ill patient who has no hope of survival? Tupping, hardly experimental, is simply a water cure, and could offer hope to countless numbers of obese people in the highest-risk categories—who would otherwise be hopeless. Should they be denied this hope? I think not.

Note: Following my colonoscopy in 2005, I visited my primary care physician to review the surgery, as well as my blood work (which was perfect). In the course of our conversation, I mentioned my work on this book, specifically the bulimia issue. To make a long story short (she questioned me for almost an hour), at the conclusion of our talk she said, (in reference to tupping), "I wish I had known about this four years ago; a close friend of mine, who was also my patient, died of morbid obesity. ... "

By the way, here's some revealing information about tupping: Unless I'm way off-base, I'll wager dollars to donuts that many of the world's champion eaters (the people who stuff dozens of hot dogs down their gullets in record time) have known and utilized some form of tupping for a long time. How else could they do what they do and still remain thin and healthy?

For instance, Takeru Kobayashi won his sixth straight title in Nathan's Famous hot dog eating contest on July 4, 2006, scarfing down 53¾ frankfurters in 12 minutes. How does he do it? Well, I have no insider information, so I'm not about to go on record and say that he uses some form of tupping—while at the same time I have to wonder. I also wonder if those thousands of people who watch him do his thing and cheer him on to greater heights would be as appreciative of his talents if he were to display a disgorging of all those hot dogs?

And what about jockeys? How do you think they make weight for races? Have you ever seen their bathrooms? They're equipped with special toilets designed for "heaving." (Really!) They've also been onto it for a long while. And I never heard of either eating contestants or jockeys going to eating-disorder clinics!

On a final note, you must remember that **the conglomerate wants people to be fat and obese** (all of America if possible!) because you are their gold mine, oil well, and treasure trove. Your fatness leads to diabetes, heart problems, strokes, and a host of other serious, if not fatal, ailments that will reward them with hundreds of billions in added profit each year.

> *Do you see yourself getting*
> *rich and famous with this?*

Here's my fantasy:

1. The definitive book on tupping sells 1.5 million copies in its first printing, and another 7.5 million in 20 different languages worldwide.

2. The American Medical Association recognizes tupping.

3. Fourteen million formerly obese people attain normal weight and remain healthy for the rest of their lives.

4. Obesity declines by 82 percent.

5. Ninety-seven percent of all eating disorder clinics go out of business.

6. Four of the biggest drug companies in the world declare bankruptcy.

7. I win the Nobel Prize for medicine.

> *Seriously, are you trying*
> *to merchandise this?*

No, I'm not out to sell anything. I'm only telling my story. And if it helps anyone, great! Besides, there's nothing to sell! It's a water cure. And you can use ordinary tap water, not the pricey stuff.

> *That sounds well and good, but aren't you afraid that some people who follow your extreme advice regarding dieting may injure themselves or worse?*

That's a crock and I'll tell you why. From the moment we are conceived until we take our last breath of life, there are risks involved with everything we do. That's why there has never been any advancement without trial, injury, or even death. Throughout its span, history has taught us this lesson. We wouldn't have any medicine today, or cars, railroads, airplanes, canals, dams, or reservoirs. Most of the things we take for granted would never have been produced or even invented without someone being willing to stick out his neck and take the risk of trying to push us forward to reduce our pain, suffering, and ignorance. That's life! And I don't for a moment believe it can be any different unless we want to keep on killing ourselves and destroying the planet the way that we're doing now.

As for the true perspective on my "extreme" ideas—as strange as they may seem to the unenlightened mind, the measures I speak of and deeply believe in are truly effective in preventing illness or death and supporting the upholding of existence as I know it. So I'm talking about **saving lives**—not taking them.

From my earliest mention of the six categories of endangered obese people (on pages 320 to 321), I've pointed out that these millions of individuals are dying[31] (many in the very near future from complications of their weight) and that they deserve a fair shot at living. That's what I'm trying to give them.

But despite my intentions, you can bet your bottom dollar that if this book receives national attention, the powers that be will use my beliefs for target practice, labeling me a menace to society. They will attempt to use me as a scapegoat for their neglect, insanity, and outright murder in an effort to shield themselves from the horrendous actions they have been guilty of for so many decades.

They will falsely accuse me of endangering lives or causing someone's death while they ignore their own ignoble deeds, which include the 195,000 preventable and inexcusable deaths in American hospitals every year; the suffering of millions of obese people who deserve a chance to live normal lives; and hundreds

---

[31] A recent study of more than a half-million retired persons suggests that about 19 percent of premature deaths can be blamed on excess weight.

of thousands of drug-induced deaths caused by the cartel of lunatics who head the conglomerate's boardrooms.

Yes, the conglomerate will take ready aim at me, as it does with anyone who dares to enlighten the public and introduce countermeasures to the deadly drugs and medical procedures endorsed by its butchers of man, child, and beast. Chances are better than ever that the public—**YOU**—will believe the conglomerate's representatives because you choose to play it safe, remaining a slave to the will of your masters—rather than take up the good fight. That's history, not my hope. In any case, I have no choice but to stick to my guns.

As for the inherent dangers of my advice, even ordinary aspirin, if taken in large enough quantity, can kill. And in case you haven't heard, Tylenol is abused on a massive scale; more than 56,000 emergency-room visits a year are due to Tylenol overdoses and 100 people die annually as a result. Likewise, if you fail to follow written directions on drug labels, you can develop cancer or even die. If you don't drive safely, well, you know what happens.

What I'm saying is that a certain level of danger exists in almost everything we do. If we ignore rules and common sense, we get hurt. And following my extreme ideas and theories are no different: Obey my instructions, and you'll be fine. In fact, you'll be healthier than ever.

> *While we're on the subject of extremes,*
> *what about fasting? Do you recommend it?*

Fasting is a huge topic in itself and I certainly endorse its use, both for losing weight and cleansing purposes. I particularly favor Thakur's four-day fast (which I did for the first time just prior to getting married in 1970), losing anywhere from 7 to 17 pounds, depending on the level of activity during the course of the fast.

Thakur's Four-Day Fast

Day 1: At 10:00 A.M.: One full glass of water and a bowl of brown rice with a green banana[32] mixed in. Nothing else.

Day 2: At noon: One full glass of water and a bowl of brown rice with a green banana mixed in. Nothing else.

---

[32] These are edible green bananas, found in most Latino grocery stores. String beans or another green vegetable can be substituted for the green banana, but these are not quite as effective.

Day 3: At 2:00 P.M.: One full glass of water and a bowl of rice with a green banana mixed in. Nothing else.

Day 4: Nothing.

Two important rules are key for Thakur's Four-Day Fast. One, I had to rest and meditate as much as possible. Two, the daily meal was to be prepared by someone else and served as an "offering." This offering was something that I didn't know how to relate to, and it would be several years before I fully understood the meaning of this gesture.

However, the rest and meditation were difficult to follow because I don't like to be at a standstill for any length of time, especially when dieting. It's too much of a reminder of what I'm missing. I end up dreaming about banquets or food orgies, smelling bacon, eggs, and toast in closets, hallways, even under beds! I decided to forsake as much of the rest and meditation as I thought acceptable, and with time growing short, I plunged ahead on my first legitimate fast.

Ever since the day that a supply officer at Sampson AFB told me I had to lose 50 pounds or be cashiered out of the service, I have experimented with a variety of homespun diet methods and programs, many of which were extreme, such as 89 days on Metrical (losing 109 pounds!). I wasn't uptight about a mere four-day fast, presuming that it would be easy to handle.

Just shows ta go ya! I was irritable every minute of the first three days, my temper flared at the slightest innocent provocation, I was cold to almost everyone, and for the first time in 16 years of dieting, I begrudged anything that anyone had to eat, even if it was only a lousy cup of tea or a piece of lettuce.

Even worse, I felt hate for anyone who had the right to eat while I could not, a total persecution complex if there ever was one. I figured out that this was exactly what the sly Thakur had in mind. It was just some of the "poison" leaving my system.

The fourth day, however, was a piece of cake. "No sweat" was the sentiment of the day. That last day also taught me a very fundamental lesson about my diet temperament. I will sooner go with total abstinence of food and drink than have a small portion of something that doesn't satisfy me.

That last night of the fast, I went to sleep dreaming not about food, but about how much fun it was going to be to buy a new suit of clothes for my wedding day. When I awoke at 11 the next morning and weighed myself, I had shed over 17 pounds.

Thanks Thak!

> *And what about your 31-day total fast?*

I am part camel and part bear, by which I mean that I can go without water for incredible, record-breaking lengths of time. I can also go into my own form of hibernation, where I reject the need to eat, and my body shuts down entirely. Having started six years earlier with Thakur's four-day fast, I had worked up to seven days of total abstinence at a time. Now I was going to put my professional weight-losing career to the ultimate test. I was going to completely stop eating and drinking for an indefinite period of time. I was going for broke.

(For those of you who are utterly skeptical about one's ability to abstain from eating or drinking anything for more than a few days, this is not surprising because Western society has long accepted this premise. However, people in other parts of the world [certainly India] have consistently practiced total fasting without even water for weeks and months at a time. There is much documented evidence to this effect.)

I knew that this complete fast would put me through exhaustive changes, so I decided to record my thoughts and feelings throughout the experience. Here is an abbreviated account:

18 hours: Feeling very hungry and angry. Also dizzy and headachy. I wish I could be strapped into a seat at a movie theater for a couple of weeks.

24 hours: I want to quit. The urge is so great. Just give me a good reason and I will. But I know it won't happen. I can't accept defeat.

36 hours: Physically worn out. Don't feel like doing a damn thing. Don't even want to talk. I wish I couldn't smell or feel.

48 hours: Today I tried to sleep through the worst of it. But I couldn't. Instead of lessening the agony and thirst, it heightened it. Even a short nap was painful. Tossed and turned like a baby with a rash. And I kept daydreaming about food. What a horrible feeling clawing at my insides.

60 hours: I'm staring at the ceiling and walls of my bedroom, watching (hallucinating) everything change shape and form. The light fixture has become a potato pancake, the painting over the bed mashed potatoes, and the phone is a roast chicken. Everything else in the room is a juicy hamburger. No shit.

72 hours: It's Sunday morning and someone is cruel enough to be cooking ham and eggs and toast and coffee. I could kill them! They have no right to make me suffer. Yes, I'm paranoid. Wouldn't you be?

84 hours: Angry with the world. With God and karma. And with people. And the angrier I get, the more I try to deny it. Thank God Nan isn't taking the brunt of it. (At least I hope not). I play-act for her. I was always a good actor.

96 hours: *Toughest part seems over. And I've lost 14 pounds. Great. But I feel disoriented and confused; why am I doing this? Am I going to keep on going? Why not stop now? Can't. It would have been a wasted effort.*

Day 6: *Headachy feeling and drowsiness gone. Feel very weak—but I sense I'm not getting any weaker. Even slept a few hours at a time, between reading, thinking, wondering about life. No "food" dreams—thank God!*

Day 9: *No feelings of hunger or thirst. Everything has shut down. I'm in hibernation. But fully awake.*

Day 10: *A great feeling—no persecution complex! People can do what they want—and they can't bother me. I'm out of danger. In a state of grace.*

Day 11: *Moving about more. Not quite floating. I've lost 20 pounds thus far. Look great at the waist. I can get into my best pants. Very comforting.*

Day 12: *My strength is returning. Amazing! How much of it is in my mind? How much is real? I think it's real.*

Day 14: *I should be reading, listening to music, sleeping more. (I would think Gandhi did that.) But my body craves activity. Is my body going crazy?*

Day 17: *I've been 16 days without food or water. Feeling light, refreshed, normal. More like a healthy young man than a deprived person.*

Day 18: *No poisons left. Feel clean, airy. If only I could begin a fast at this point!*

Day 19: *It's a romp! Feel like working. Running.*

Day 20: *I've gone back to work! Resumed administrative responsibilities. Also writing. Most people assume I'm off the fast. All the better. Fewer questions to answer.*

Day 21: *Creative urge is titanic. For the first time in my life I've tried my hand at poetry. Wasn't too bad. Made Nan laugh. Here's an example: "Two tulips kissed and became four lips."*

Day 22: *Today I played football for two hours—and I perspired! The doctors and experts and Western record books obviously don't know what they're talking about. Or am I an isolated case? Or a freak? Or both?*

Day 23: *A great feeling of lightness today. Not "weight" lightness—but "brain" lightness. All my thoughts are extremely clear, sharp, defined. And I can actually feel the different parts of my brain (and brain cells) in operation, as if they were separate gears working independently of one another.*

Day 24: *Extremely sensitive to everyone around me. Very aware of their thoughts and problems. Perception keener than ever.*

Day 25: *Ran a group today. An impromptu affair. Everyone thought it was the best group they had ever been in. I felt akin to mystical power. There's nothing to interfere with thoughts being relayed to me. On target with absolute ease. Today*

I'm a guru!

Day 27: *Everything normal. No complaints. Played a great game of football. Invented a submarine style of throwing the ball. It traveled 50 yards! Did it any number of times. This is great!*

Day 31: *I feel I could go on this way for at least two more months. But I've decided to stop at my favorite number. There's nothing more to gain, no weight to lose, nothing to prove by continuing. I think I will open a bottle of champagne.*

And I did!

*Author's note: I **do not** go on record in support of this extreme starvation diet because most people attempting such a total abstinence of food and drink would be unable to handle its effects and consequences.*

You must remember that I am an endurance freak; hiking long distances, staying underwater for almost two minutes, conducting more groups and 40- to 60-hour marathon sessions than anyone in history, and dieting to excess for many years. So fasting was a ready-made strategy for me. But even then, I had expert guidance from Indian masters like Thakur, and only graduated to the 31-day fast after many years of practicing fasting.

> ### Isn't it dangerous to lose a lot of weight so quickly?

Here we're dealing with mythology again. I've never seen an ounce of evidence that proves the contention that it's dangerous to lose lots of weight quickly, except in situations where someone's weight loss is attributed to disease, in which case death is caused by overall physical deterioration.

The medical guidelines that instruct obese people that they shouldn't lose more than half of a pound a week flies in the face of all but anecdotal evidence. Point of fact: It's a hell of a lot more dangerous for you to carry around all that excess weight than to rid yourself of that bulk in a relatively short time. Every day that you remain obese brings you a step closer to any number of diseases and life-threatening conditions. (If you're not overweight, try carrying 60 to 100 extra pounds of weight around for a day or even a few hours. See what it does to you).

As for the effectiveness of the quack medical directives against quick weight loss, get this: You're telling people who are anywhere from 60 to 150 pounds overweight to lose no more than two pounds a month. Translated into reality, it will take someone who is 60 pounds overweight two-and-a-half years to reach his proper weight, and someone with an extra 120 pounds can look forward to attaining her objective in five years. Guess what? That successful result rarely happens.

This explains why most obese people are yo-yo dieters, ending up using diet drugs or opting for extreme surgery—both of which benefit the conglomerate and feed into the quick-fix mentality of our misguided society.

Needless to say, everything is relative. Someone who's already suffering from diabetes or an aggravated heart condition probably can't handle the physical and emotional strain of shedding pounds quickly. It's highly unlikely that they would even try. But most people would be able to handle the quick weight loss—and be better off for it.

One example: Arkansas Governor Mike Huckabee lost 110 pounds in less than two years and in 2005 ran a marathon in just over four hours. I think I'm on safe ground when I tell you that the governor and his family and friends all supported the relatively quick weight loss.

The clincher is that the conglomerate supports extreme surgery that either triggers a high rate of weight loss over a relatively short time or a sudden loss of many pounds of fat, **and the medical profession doesn't say a word against it!** Likewise, dozens of magazines feature stories about quick weight-loss programs every month, and the powers that be never object to them.

····   ····

In all my years of dieting and fasting, I have never suffered any ill effects from sudden weight loss. I have actually found it health-giving, exhilarating, and profoundly gratifying in every sense. So don't pay attention to the conglomerate nonsense. It only wants you to stay fat so it can continue to deliver its deadly goods to you.

Going back to tupping, you're basically talking about vomiting. Isn't it disgusting?

For the sake of argument, let's say that vomiting is disgusting. But ask yourself where that impression comes from. You have to recall your initial introduction to throwing up as a child. What I remember (after eating a hotdog at the circus) was a bad stomachache, extreme discomfort and pain, lying in bed sick, retching over and over again, and terrible smells and a horrible aftertaste in my mouth.

Yes, you might characterize that as disgusting. But that disgorging of something festering in your stomach and bowels has *nothing to do with tupping*—which involves fresh food, no bad smells, no pain, no audience, and no bad memories.

So there's nothing disgusting about it, except the predisposed attitude that tells us it is quite revolting.

To take it to another level, what, pray tell, isn't disgusting? How about urinating and defecating? And giving birth? And bleeding? Not to mention old age and death? Aren't they all disgusting? Or is it all in your mind? In any case, you should learn to live with such things.

Also, don't write off tupping because of your revulsion to the act of regurgitating. That would discriminate against millions of people in those six categories who desperately need help. Think about them. **Please.**

Author's note: **In the largest study of its kind (over a half-million retired Americans), conducted by the National Cancer Institute and published by the** New England Journal of Medicine **in August 2006, it was reported that obesity can triple the risk of death.** *That probably doubles for people in the six endangered categories.*

> ### Don't you feel guilty when you tup?

I think you're confusing "guilt" with "shame." From an early age in our society, we are taught that the act of vomiting is a shameful thing rather than a potentially cleansing act, which it certainly can be. In fact, many aboriginal tribes practice it for that very reason. And there's nothing wrong with that. What's inherently wrong is the idea of guilt or shame being attached to natural acts. Our society would be better off if it stopped to consider the acts we really should be ashamed of... and have reason to feel guilty about. Tupping is not one of these truly shameful acts. It upholds existence.

> ### But don't you think there will be some sort of stigma attached to it?

Let's look at some history. Jane Fonda was probably the first celebrity to reveal her bulimic past, and it didn't do her any harm. In fact, she sold more health-related books and videos than anyone else. And what about Princess Diana? She gained the affection of the world. So who's to say that someone engaged in tupping is going to be negatively labeled?

I hope the opposite happens; people close to those who finally succeed in controlling their weight problems should cheer them on, instead of pulling attitudes and forming negative impressions. And they should also realize that the cure is certainly no worse than the disorder. So take away the stigma and guilt, and half the battle is won.

> ***If you feel this way, why haven't you***
> ***told anyone about your tupping?***

I have lots of reasons. For one thing, why bring attention to it? What purpose does it serve? Can you imagine how you would feel every time you get up from the table? The looks, hidden or otherwise, might not be as reassuring as you would like, so you're better off simply going about your business.

On the other hand, let's assume your friends are ultra-liberal, capable of treating it lightly. Can you picture the scene when you get up from their dinner table, and your wife turns to the host as you depart for the bathroom and says, "Excuse my husband for a few minutes, he's just going to throw up your lovely quiche!"

All joking and seriousness aside, you have little to gain by informing on yourself, unless you're looking for sympathy. However, if you find it difficult to maintain your tupping program without the support and understanding of family and friends, I urge you not to tell them until after it's a proven success. They'll have a much easier time swallowing it (I couldn't resist that one!) when they see tangible results. At least one should hope as much.

Of course, all this is really a moot point because chances are they'll find out anyway, in which case you can follow your instinct and either discuss it openly or pass it off as nothing to be concerned about. And if people close to you cannot accept your way of dealing with obesity—it's their problem.

> ***What about the waste? All that food and drink***
> ***going down the bowl?***

Your perspective is way off. The real waste, material or otherwise, comes when a person is unhealthy, unhappy, and not functioning creatively. This state of misery is not only wasteful, it can be deadly—not only to the individual, but to his family and friends as well. I'd rather see it all going down the bowl—where it can't do any widespread damage—than save it at the expense of remaining unhappy and unhealthy.

> *All right, waste aside, isn't this pretty costly?*

Well, there are ways of cutting down on costs. For instance, with some meals—like chili con carne—it's possible to tup into a bowl, then reheat and serve again!

> *Now that's gross!*

No doubt. But infinitely practical—if you're thinking of cost.

> *Do you have any other practical ideas?*

A Tups restaurant (I've already created the menu); a Tups picnic grounds, with specially designed bathrooms equipped with a pulley and hoist that enable you to hang upside-down while tupping (talk about gravity!); and a Tups compost pile for all the environmentalists. And a Tups recipe book. I'll mail you one.

> *What will you think of next!*

Contests! An annual Tups-Out! World-class stuff. In fact, we'll hold the event in conjunction with an eating contest!

> *Oh, God, have you no shame?*

If you really want the truth, I'll tell you a story that illustrates the absolute reaches of my lack of shame.

> *Go right ahead. I just can't wait to hear it.*

One evening I was sitting at a small table in my room at the Acropolis House

Hotel in Athens, Greece, reading the sports pages of the *International Herald Tribune* and finishing off the last of four *souvlakies* and two bottles of Coke. Just as I reached for the glass and raised it to my lips, my hand began to shake. Now I've always been an intense person, but never so nervous that my hands would shake, so I became quite worried.

Suddenly my hand became even more agitated, shaking quite violently. In a moment my whole body began to tremble. You can't imagine how frightened I felt.

A split-second later I was relieved to realize that nothing was wrong with me because my table was also shaking. So was the room! In fact, the whole damn hotel was shaking and rattling—along with the entire city of Athens!

In less time than it took me to grab for my shoes, I was visualizing scenes from the movie *San Francisco*, when the 1906 earthquake hits. I had seen the movie numerous times, had read many accounts of major earthquakes over the years, and now I was in one—in the flesh!

I couldn't quite believe it and didn't feel frightened (because it was still striking me as a movie scenario). But in fact, people were screaming all around me, the hotel was rumbling as if a cataclysmic explosion were about to go off—and then the lights went out.

In another moment, a strange and terrifying sound began emanating from the very depths of the earth's bowels. That sound is locked within my memory forever, yet I cannot describe it adequately. It was like a sound wave or a sonic reverberation, as unnerving as anything I can ever remember.

At that moment I knew it was for real. Instantly my mind switched from the theatrical aspect of the experience to the reality of surviving.

I managed to lift myself into a standing, albeit tottering, position, and began to head for where I hoped the door would be. But when I got there, I couldn't open the door because it was locked, with the key on a side table near the bed.

Now I really felt scared. I was in the middle of an earthquake with the lights out, and I couldn't find the key to open the door!

Somehow I made my way to the bed, and after grappling blindly and frantically for a few moments, located the key. Thank God it hadn't fallen on the floor!

Then I crawled on all fours to the door, unlocked it, and stumbled into the hallway, which was on the second floor of the hotel.

There I was, 15 feet from the staircase with access to escape from what could momentarily become a pile of concrete and destroyed furniture—with me under it!—and what do I do? Instead of heading for the staircase and safety, I felt my way along the hallway until I fell against the door to the bathroom. And in the midst of an ongoing 6.8 earthquake, I took the time to *do my thing!* And you want to know if I have any shame?!

> *After hearing that story, I have only*
> *one other question to ask.*
> *Is there no other alternative for you?*

You still don't get it, do you? Look, the chemistry was wrong from the beginning. I never had a chance to be normal. It took 40 years for me to finally solve the problem. So now what should I do? Look for trouble? I'm too old for that. And my family is better off this way. Believe me. Besides, when you come right down to it, if I had been eating these 30 years without tupping, by conservative estimates, *today I would weigh 8,176 pounds!*

Part IV.
The Best Damn Workout Ever

Before beginning my workout plan, I want to pay tribute to my two workout mentors, both sports champions in their own right, without whose guidance and genuine support I would never have learned the do's and don'ts of working out.

Chris Tolos was part of the wrestling Heavyweight Champion Tag Team of Chris and John Tolos. Chris first brought me to the Mid-City Health Club in New York City in 1965, and it was there where he introduced me to Kimon Voyages, who placed second in the 1945 Mr. America Contest in the Most Muscular category.

Between these two true experts in their field, I discovered the secrets of what I would need to carry me through a lifetime of physical conditioning and longevity. I have never forgotten what they taught me, and I hereby pass it on to you, in the hope that it will add significantly to your physical well-being.

The Best Damn Workout Ever

Judging from the fact that seven out of 10 American adults don't exercise regularly despite the proven health benefits, and that many of those who do merely follow a course of leisure-time physical activity, rather than *really working out,* is a clear indication of just how bad a shape most Americans are in. Alongside our tens of millions of overweight or obese people and America's deplorable healthcare system, this is a deadly one-two-three punch that is seriously incapacitating our nation. In fact, it is directly related to the deaths of at least a million people a year.

Why are so many people unwilling to commit to an effective workout program? Are they dense, dumb, lazy, or is it that they don't give a damn? Or perhaps—as I've explained in dozens of ways in "Monument To Failure"—we are so addicted to drugs, doctors, hospitals, and the entire conglomerate way of life that we have lost our sense of reality and personal responsibility to ourselves, families, country, and civilization.

Whatever the causes may be, when it comes to working out regularly, the general attitude of the American public is one of malaise, indifference, and sloppy thinking. Better believe it! And it grows worse day by day.

What it comes down to is a simple choice: Do you want a quality existence throughout your life or do you want to steadily move toward the inner lane of physical weakness, disease, and the death-dealing devices that are waiting for you at the hands of the conglomerate? There are no other choices. You will live or die with these two options.

If you want to get in the fast track toward a quality existence, then you must work out regularly. Mind you, I say *work out,* not just exercise, because too many Americans choose the leisure-time exercise program, which will not provide enough in the way of the physical activity you need to get in good shape and maintain your health. Note: The only exceptions to this health equation are generally limited to long-lifers in other parts of the world who are regularly occupied with farming, fishing, or other arduous physical activity that provide the same benefits derived from working out.

With this in mind, if you decide in favor of working out, then it's time you drop all of your defenses about this heavy-duty physical program. That includes such questions as "Why should I work out? Is it really worth it? Can't I just work out 30 minutes a day three times a week?" You must also rid yourself of attitudes like, "I don't like exercising. I find it boring and not fun. I always hurt after I work out. Why should I continue?"

Now that I've made this point clear, if you're ready to move on—LISTEN UP!

❋ ❋ ❋

Putting it frankly, **most people who work out don't know what they're doing.** It's no surprise that they suffer from overall health problems—even if they work out regularly. So let's get to the fundamentals.

For starters, if you want to avoid the commonplace physical problems usually attributed to age, such as back problems, sore knees, tired legs, weak joints, lack of flexibility, poor circulation, slowed reflexes, tight muscles, and various injuries, **you must learn the proper way to prepare for any physical workout.** In fact, the very first thing that Chris Tolos and Kimon Voyages told me was, "We have to teach you the right way to stretch and warm up—before you work out."

And teach me they did! The results have been fantastic. At the age of 70, I'm as limber as I was when I was 26; I never suffer from any strains or pains in any part of my body; I maintain tone, strength, and stamina; and I feel that I can go on this way for another 40 years!

Conversely, the major problem with almost every young person who works out is that because they're still young and generally haven't begun to experience the physical decline and breakdown attributed to older age, they fall into bad habits, the first and foremost of which is *they don't stretch or warm up properly.*

Most people, including trainers, hardly pay attention to their workout preparations. They simply take their bodies for granted, and therein lies the great danger. *And it will catch up with you.*

Even professional athletes fail to consider the importance of proper preconditioning before actively engaging in a particular sport. The worst offenders appear to be baseball players. This not only accounts for the frequency of injuries suffered by both pitchers and position players, but also for their shortened careers and serious physical deterioration and impairment of retired players in their 40s and 50s.

These setbacks and illnesses are usually attributed to accidents, grueling schedules, the wear-and-tear of long years of competition, and so on. But I don't buy it because there are sports figures who rarely, if ever, suffer serious or long-term injuries (look at Cal Ripken, who broke Lou Gehrig's endurance record) because their entire bodies are properly conditioned and toned without the use of steroids or other drugs.

One prominent negative example among many baseball players is Ken Griffey, Jr., who is known by teammates to shun stretching exercises. It's no surprise that in the last six seasons, after being traded from the Seattle Mariners to the Cincinnati Reds, he has suffered one injury after another, seriously limiting his playing time and altering the course of what was once a classic Hall of Fame career.

On the other hand, if you're looking for the perfect example of excellent preconditioning *(perhaps the only such example in all of major league baseball),* just watch Ichiro Suzuki, arguably the best all-around baseball player in America. He's out on the field hours before other players, going through a highly disciplined routine of stretching, warming up, and preparing his body and mind for the game ahead.

And the results are profound. In his first six seasons in the major leagues, Ichiro has broken hitting records that have stood for many decades, establishing himself as one of the most durable players to ever step on the field. It's no wonder. No other major league player is willing to do the preconditioning that Ichiro does. They're just too lazy and spoiled by the excesses connected to fame and fortune, and in numerous cases dependent on drugs instead of conditioning.

Similar to Ichiro, I put myself through a grueling preparation routine that other people are unwilling to do. And they're foolish enough to think that they can get away with it—without paying the piper somewhere down the road.

To be redundant: If you want to be able to maintain great physical health into your 50s, 60s, and right on through your 90s and beyond—you absolutely must be willing to put in the time and effort necessary to prepare you for strong physical activity such as working out. **There is no other way.**

Furthermore, even if you don't use drugs, eat nutritional food, and stay in good shape—it still doesn't make up for a proper preconditioning regimen. Get it?

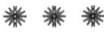

So let's get started!

When I speak of stretching, I am referring to the physical activity associated with extending, stretching, holding out, even straining muscles and muscle groups beyond normal or reasonable limits for an extended period of time (30 seconds or more).

Warming up refers to the general act of stimulating (and warming up) your entire body by putting it through a range of physical actions that will prepare it for a strenuous workout.

To a certain degree, stretching and warming up are interchangeable in that the act of stretching will aid in warming up the body, while warming up will also stretch muscles.

Stretching and warming up are both necessary; one without the other constrains the body and prevents it from attaining full physical energy and stamina, and can result in any number of injuries or disabilities.

Depending on the type of workout you're doing, you might begin by either stretching, warming up, or doing a combination therein. For instance, if I'm doing a leg workout, or preparing to run, skip rope, or box, I find it best to warm up prior to stretching. If I'm doing a heavy upper body workout, it's best to start with my stretching routine, followed by the warmup.

I should also mention that stretching is not necessarily a static process; you can be in motion as you stretch, and you can also vary the nature and intensity of each stretch, according to your particular need. For instance, if a specific part of your body is tight or sore, begin lightly and build the stretch gradually. If necessary, repeat the stretch several times before going on to another part of the body.

I also like to incorporate some form of dynamic tension (also referred to as "isometrics," or by The Arnold as "Iso-Tension"), which was pioneered by the world-famous Charles Atlas over 75 years ago. There are numerous, although similar, definitions of the technique, which can be used as a full-scale workout routine as well as a preconditioning technique.

Isometrics can involve either contracting (by flexing, pulling, or pushing) the muscles and holding them in the same place for a period of time, or pushing on an immovable object for a given time (try standing in a doorframe and pressing against its sides). I find that these tension-based exercises reach areas normally missed in training, and give the body a more chiseled look.

As for the actual stretching and warmup techniques:

1. **Each stretch should be held for a minimum of 30 seconds.** This is absolutely necessary. I constantly see people doing a basic hamstring stretch for about four to 10 seconds, followed by one or two other stretches such as an arm-chest stretch, one side at a time, again for about four to 10 seconds—and that's it!

    Wrong, WRONG, WRONG! Stretches that are too brief are very detrimental because you're led to believe that your body is actually ready to work out—when it's not. That's why there are so many pulled muscles and strains, even among young people, and professional athletes.

2. **You must stretch your entire body, not just your legs and chest.** People don't even bother stretching their back, shoulders, biceps, triceps, forearms, wrists, neck, abdomen, etc. Note: Younger people are especially prone to foregoing a full body stretch because they think that they can get *away with it.*

But like all other weaknesses in life, not doing so eventually catches up with them. By the time they're 40, they're hospital cases!

Scan your body and focus on those areas that feel tight, sore, and weak, or need special attention. Use your instincts here: Move each part of your body around a bit; sway, roll, and get in touch with how everything feels; pinpoint where weaknesses exist; and then use laserlike focus to *stretch them out.* Your stretching routine should take a minimum of 15 to 20 minutes.

Note: As fitness instructors limit the stretching and warmup phases of their classes because they would take too much time from the overall sessions, you should do your own stretches and warmup before any exercise class.

3. **Warm-ups can consist of any type of movement or dancelike exercises that engage the body in an entire range of possible motions.** Don't worry about your form (I'll get to that): just "act-as-if." (The "act-as-if" is an effective therapeutic tool, an intellectual, emotional, and physical device that takes you from the point of pretending [acting] that you are capable of carrying out a specific objective to gradually feeling as if you are actually achieving your goal, then to successfully fulfilling it. By acting-as-if, you become capable of realizing ambitions that would normally be out of reach.)

    This will help loosen up your body from head to toe. Use your full torso here; twist and turn it from left to right, up to down, in as many directions as possible. (Twists are great!) As with stretches, use your instinct to listen to what your body is telling you, and then warm up this part of your body. As a further warmup, I like to do a few minutes of shadow boxing (pretend you're in a boxing ring and dance about and throw punches at an imaginary opponent), followed by two to three minutes on the heavy punching bag. This warmup phase should take you eight to 12 minutes.

4. **Cap off your preconditioning with a three-minute jog** (the Boy Scout pace will do) to get your heart rate up a bit. If you have no space to actually run, do it in place. If you prefer to do jumping jacks or skip rope, that will do just as well.

Now you're ready to work out! (Although the regimen that I've outlined may already seem like enough of a workout!)

Following any workout, cool down by doing some stretches and deep breathing. This is necessary because your muscles will need to start recovering, so ease your body back into a calm and restful state.

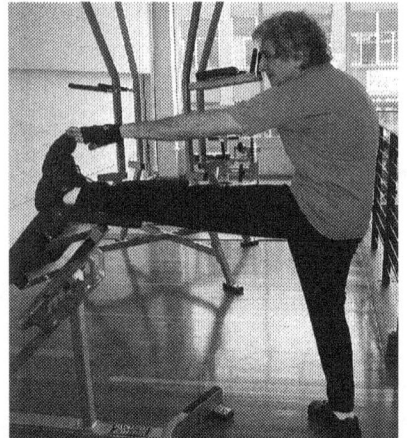

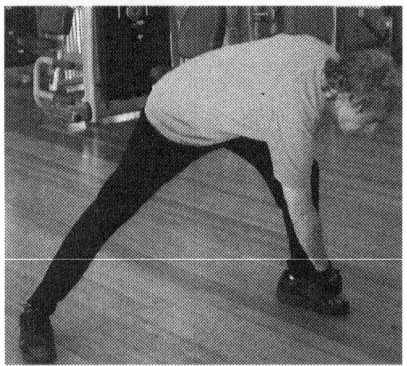

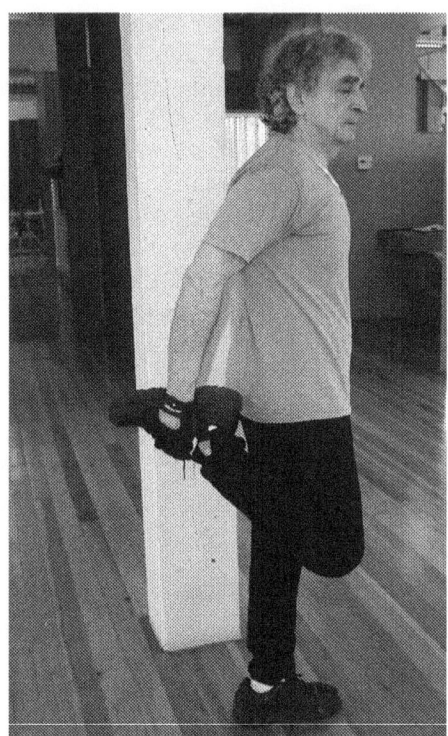

Preconditioning, with various motion and static stretching exercises, while working out at Rain Fitness in Seattle, Washington. *From top left, clockwise: leg and back; hamstring; gluts and legs; quadriceps and warmup; and back, chest, and hip flexors.*

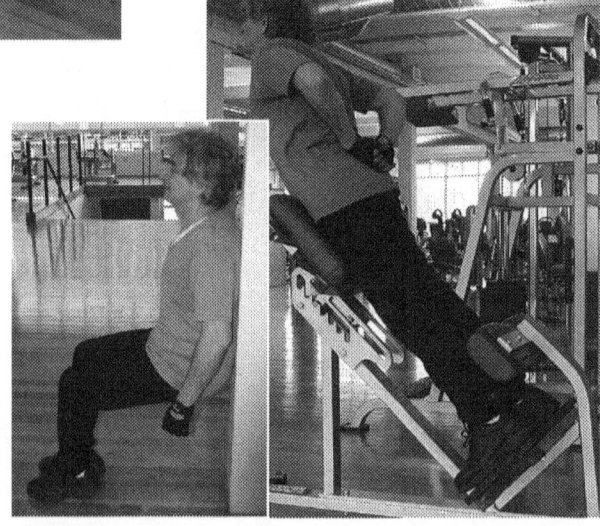

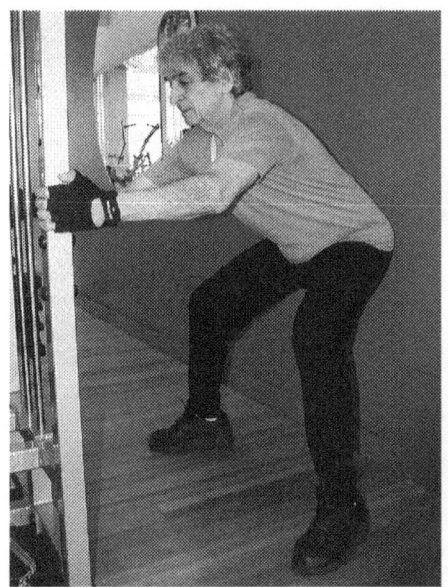

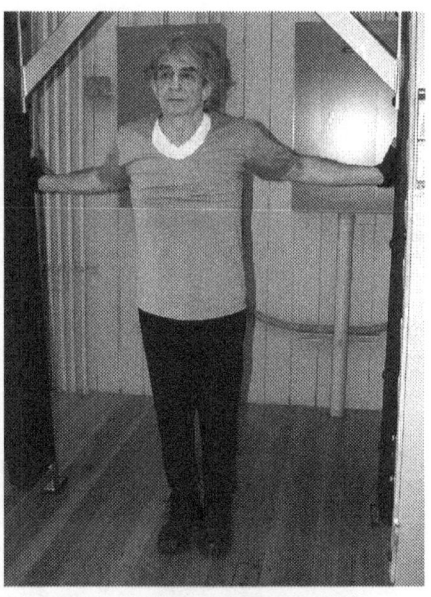

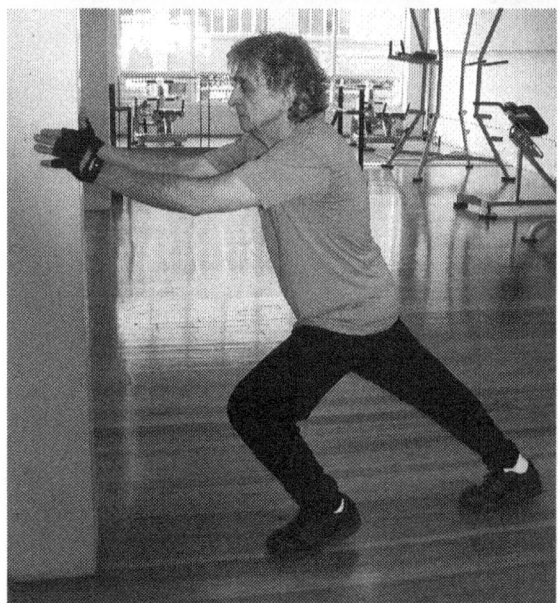

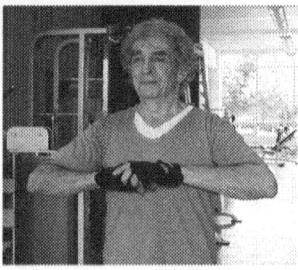

***Isometrics or dynamic
tension exercises.*** *These
contract muscles by flexing,
pulling, or pushing on
an immovable object for
30 seconds or more.*

*Clockwise, from top
left: upper back; lats,
shoulders, and arms;
arms and shoulders;
and back and legs.*

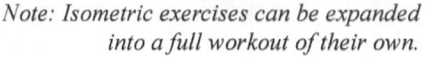

*Note: Isometric exercises can be expanded
into a full workout of their own.*

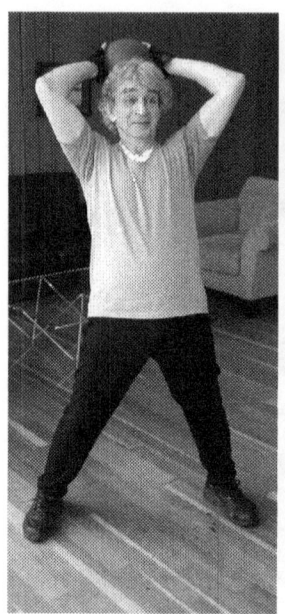 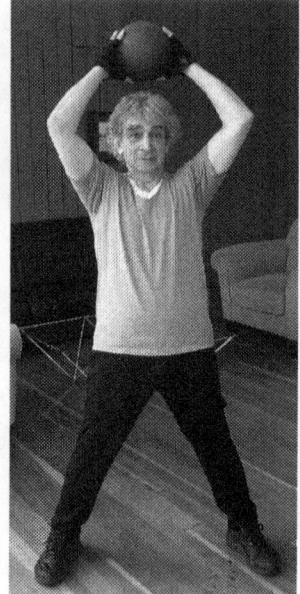 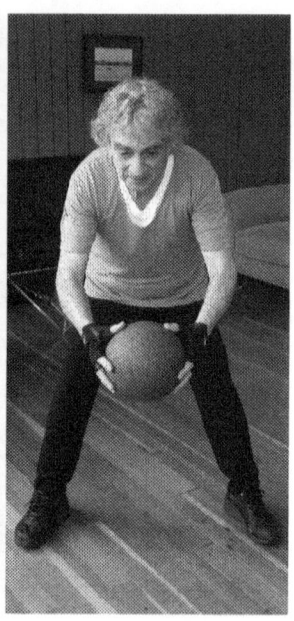

Stretching and warming up, continued.
Twisting and turning (with weighted medicine ball) and full-body torques.

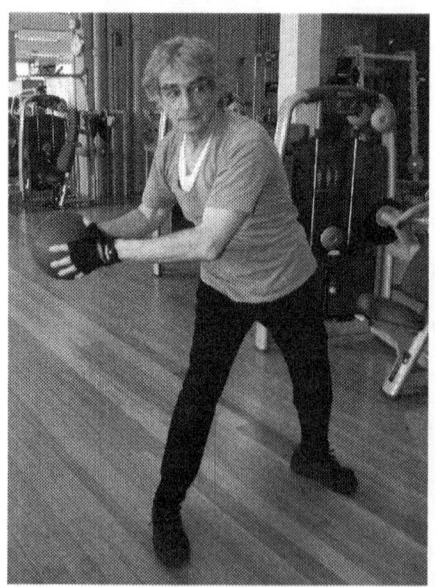 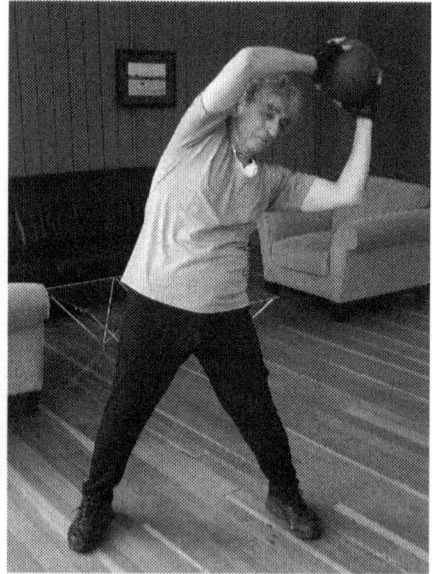

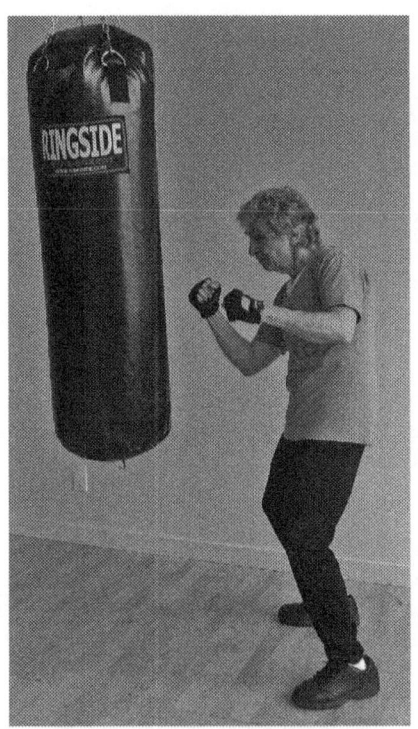
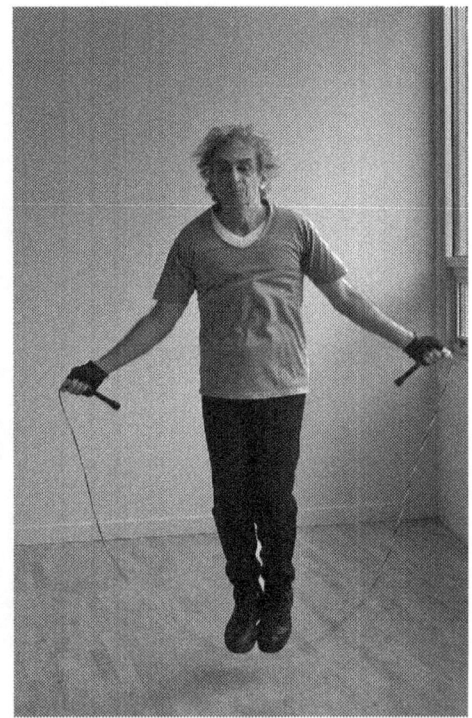
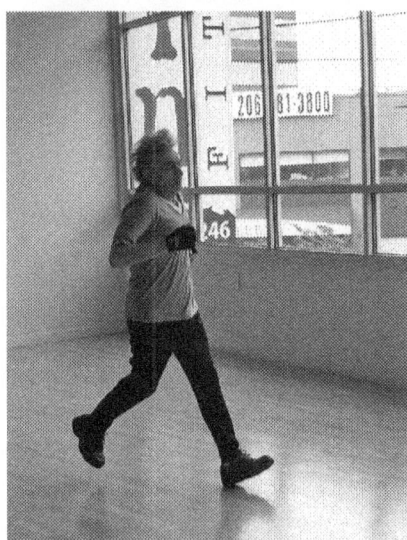
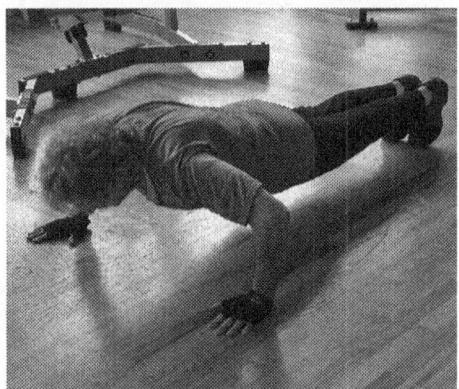

Warming up and getting the heart rate up.
Clockwise, from top left: punching heavy bag; skipping rope; pushups, and jogging.

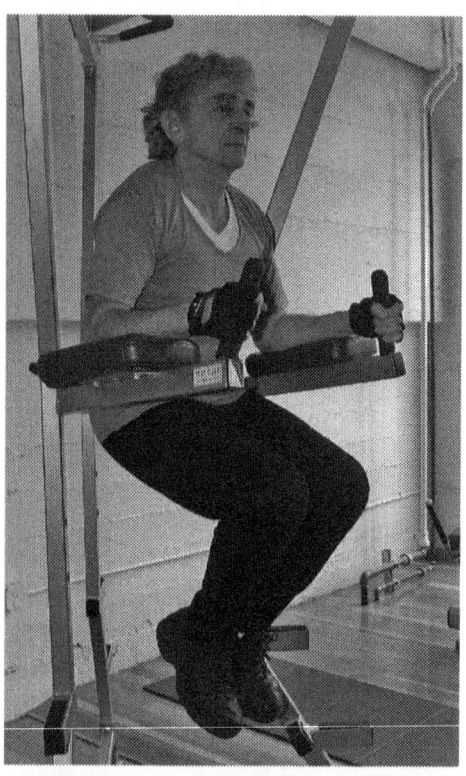

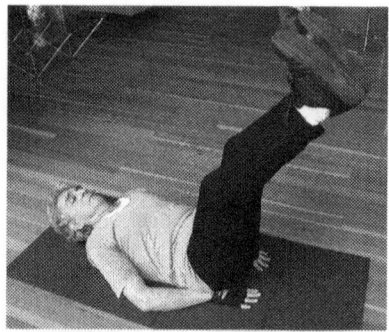

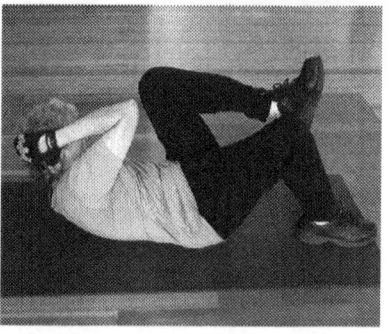

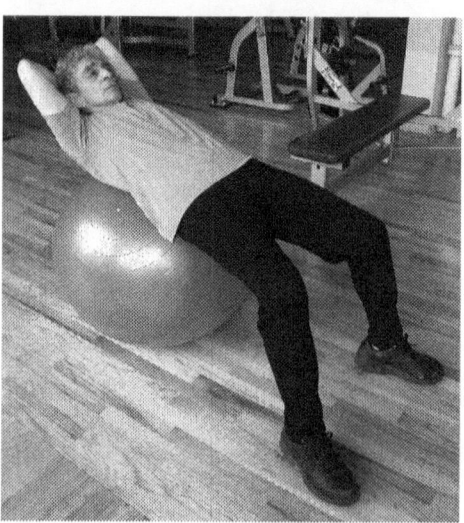

Stomach work and abdominals.

From top left, clockwise: Captain's chair for abs; leg raises for lower abs; bicycle for obliques; and on the Swiss ball for upper abs.

Don't be foolish enough to think that you can use vibrating machines or various massage devices in place of working your abs. No way.

All those easy fixes are worthless—pure ripoffs.

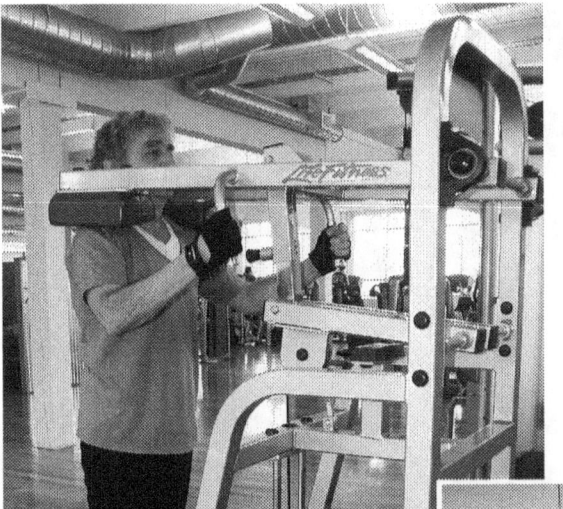

Leg workout.
From top left, clockwise:
standing calf (for the
gastrocnemius and soleus);
leg press (for quadriceps,
hamstrings, gastrocnemius,
soleus, and glutes); abductor
(for tensor fasciae latae,
and gluteus maximus); and
leg curl (for quadriceps).

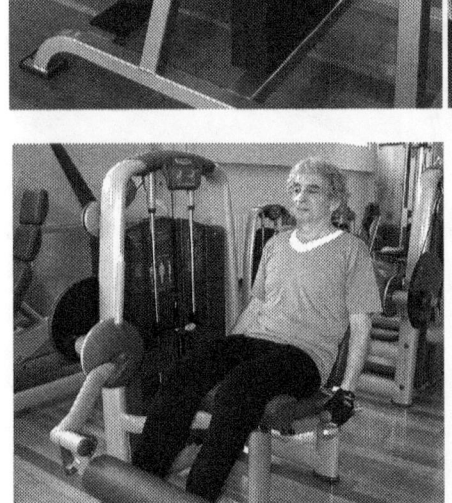

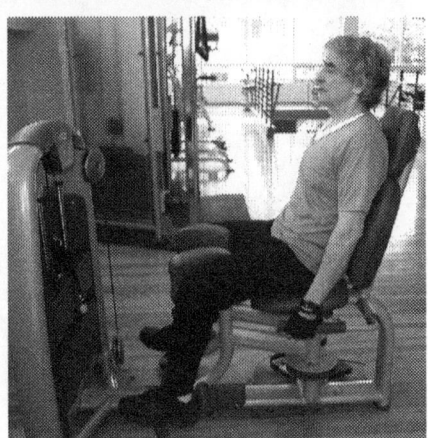

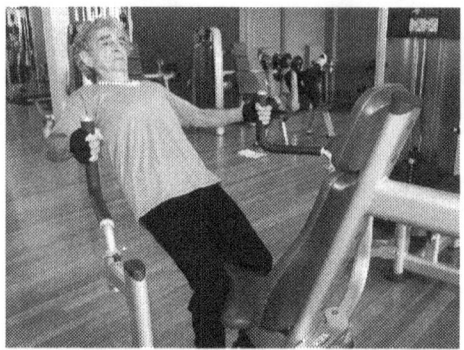

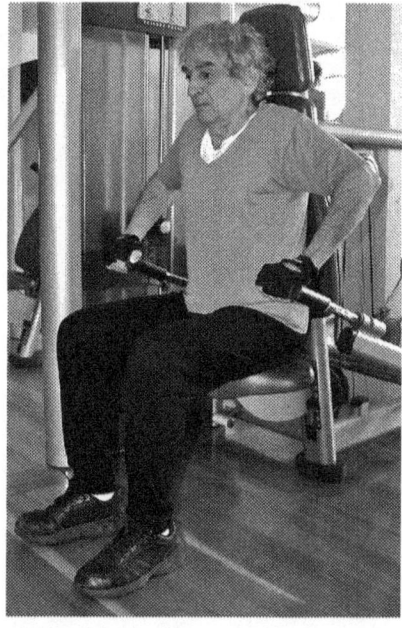

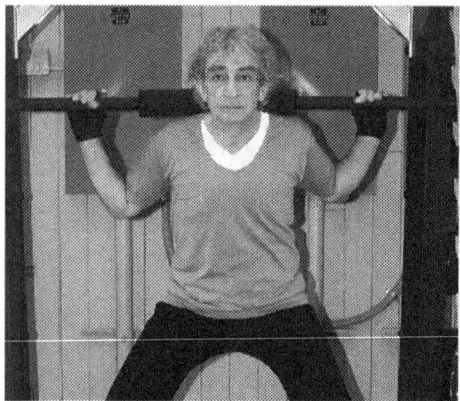

Weightlifting session. *From top left, clockwise: Fly work for upper back, lats, biceps, forearms, and wrists; triceps press; biceps curl; chest press; and squats for glutes.*

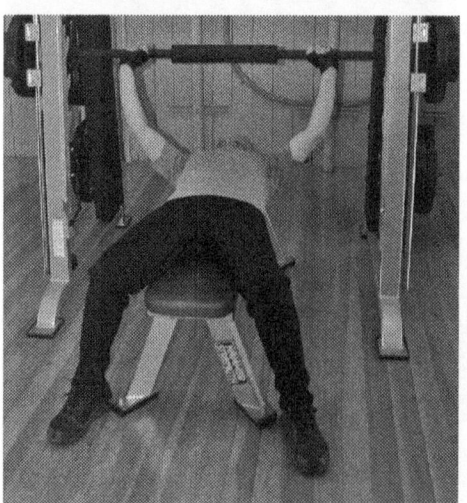

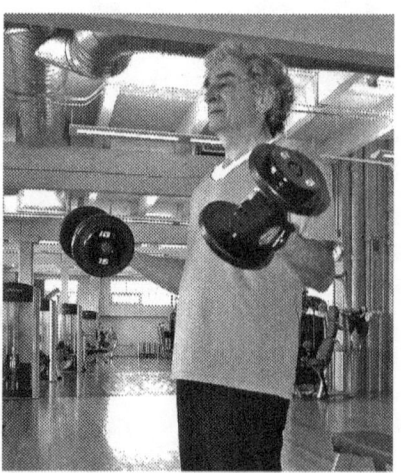

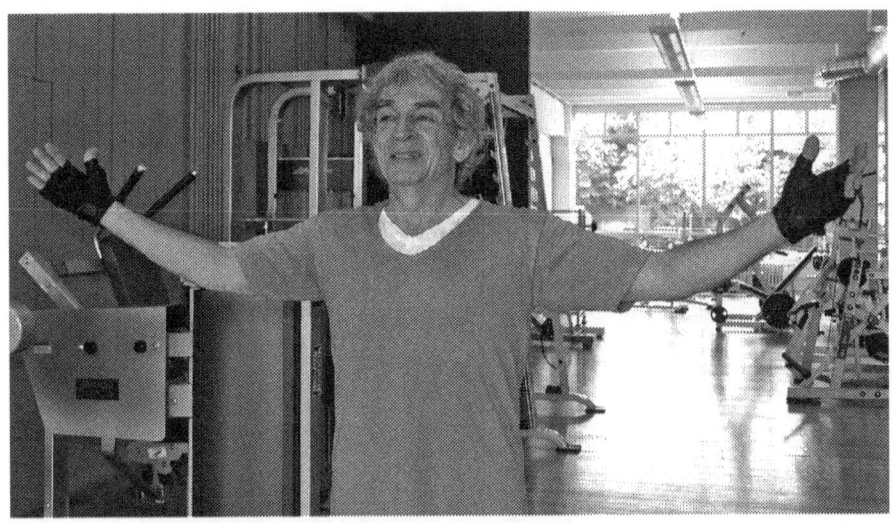

Before and after working out.
Above: Facing a long, grueling workout with a sense of joy and determination.
Below: The exhilaration and charge that you feel when
you've done it again is unimaginable!

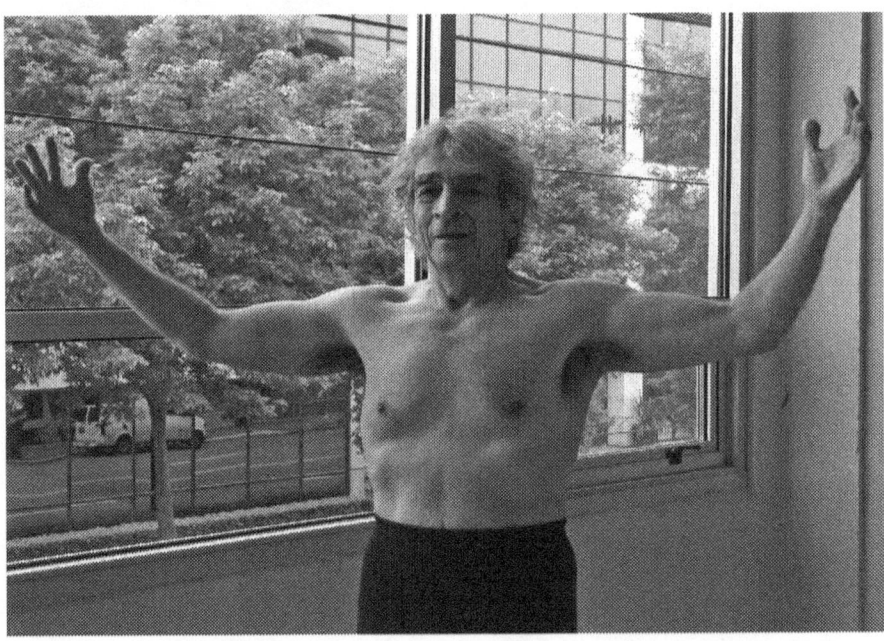

> *Any important tips related to cooling down*
> *after a heavy workout?*

One thing that will help you immediately after a workout, especially an aerobic one, is to inhale deeply but gently through your nose, then exhale slowly through pursed lips (as if you were whistling). This reduces your recovery time and also helps maintain the correct balance of oxygen and carbon dioxide in your blood.

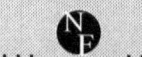

· · · ·   · · · ·

The preconditioning routine will take about 30 minutes, which may seem like a lot of time BUT—putting in that extra time before each workout may eventually save you *years of wear and tear and visits to your doctor and hospitals,* not to mention all the pain and fatigue you'll save your body. That's a hell of a good tradeoff!

Continuing with fundamentals, it's vital for you to know some basic underlying concepts of bodybuilding and weightlifting. Here are the ones that you must understand and adhere to:

1. **Do what works for you, and don't do what doesn't work for you.** There are thousands of exercises and hundreds of training programs. Your objective is to discover those that will help you attain the physical condition you want to be in. It's a selection process from beginning to end.

> *How do you learn which exercise to select?*

There are several ways:
- Watch those people who are in good shape and who seem to know what they're doing, and learn from them. Between my early sessions with Chris Tolos and Kimon Voyages, I would watch other pros and pick up tips from them. It was a steady

process of observing and asking questions. Very basic stuff. And gradually I adopted a training routine from what I saw other people doing.

By the way, in seeking out role models, don't just look for individuals with big builds (especially upper body) because that's not the only indication of good body development and workout techniques. Some of these top-heavy weightlifters don't pay enough attention to core development and, as such, could lead you to following an unbalanced training program.

- Speak to a trainer. S/he will usually be happy to get you started on a basic program that you can build on from one workout to another.

- Don't be afraid to experiment. You'll be surprised at how many techniques you'll come up with if you listen to your body's signals and messages.

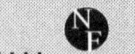

Of the many exercises you try, chances are that you will find that some are more suitable to your needs and physicality than others. Also, you may find that some exercises are—for whatever reason— causing you either strain or pain. If that's the case, then don't do them. For instance, I discovered that chin-ups, as much as I liked doing them, caused some sensitivity in my elbows. As I could find no effective way of strengthening my elbows, I stopped doing them. No problem; there are hundreds of other exercises to take the place of chin-ups.

2. **Make certain you're working out your entire body, not just specific areas.** Of the many thousands of people I've seen working out over the years, only a small fraction of them work their entire body. In the process, they often overwork certain muscle groups and neglect other vital areas of the body, setting themselves up for all sorts of physical problems in the future.

3. **Pay strict attention to your "core."** In training circles, the core consists of

the muscles in your lower back and abdominal areas, the muscles associated with the spine, and the hip flexors. These muscle groups work in harmony to stabilize the body and provide the normal transfer of power from one part of the body to another. Neglecting the core will result in serious long-range health problems, while strengthening the core will result in untold physical benefits.

Along those same lines, we all know that wrestling is an "act." Nonetheless, wrestlers suffer fewer injuries because their training routines place strong emphasis on training their glutes, backs, and abdomens—the "core." These core components—and their fitness level—are disproportionately more vital to wrestlers' athleticism than any other parts of their bodies.

So whether you're a pro, semipro, or just working out for fun and good health, establish a training routine that is holistic and a bit top-heavy with abdominal as well as back work.

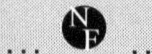

· · · ·   · · · ·

There are as many abdominal exercises as Carter has little liver pills. Here's the trick: You don't have to do all of them, just as long as you do lower, upper, and obliques. You must also realize that there are various attitudes about what constitutes the best abdominal workout—and as I've already said, do what works for you. Whether that means crunches, situps, or work on an exercise ball (sometimes referred to as a "Swiss" ball) depends on your level of training and how good you want your abs to look. I personally stick to three or four basic exercises that suit my temperament and needs. See page 358 for examples.

Note: Some people believe that you should work your abs as often as possible, while others think they need just as much recovery time as other parts of your body. I fall somewhere in between, working my abs three to five times a week, with some workouts more extensive than others.

4.   **Be certain to include squats in your program, as they are extremely important to overall physical well-being.** Why? Your legs carry the brunt of your physical activity, whether it's walking, running, cycling, or any other active sport or recreation. By doing squats you add a vital power compo-

nent, strengthening the glutes (the buttock muscles) and taking some of the pressure and strain off your legs. It really works! I also recommend that you include pushups in every workout, as it is a great overall exercise (which can also be done at home or while on vacation, etc.) and the old-fashioned "clean and jerk," in which the barbell is first lifted from the floor to the shoulders (the clean) and then from the shoulders to a position overhead (the jerk). With or without weights, it is a staple exercise that gives your body a well-rounded stretch and warmup.

5. **Besides doing squats, work your legs accordingly.** In my case, I walk-jog at least five times a week, skip rope, box, and work my legs strenuously. So I don't have to add much in the way of additional leg work. But I still do calf raises, leg presses, and hamstring exercises (see page 359). It's a matter of striking the proper balance, so that it's neither too much or too little.

> *If I do loads of crunches,*
> *will I trim fat from my midsection?*

I hate to tell you, but even if you do 2,000 crunches a day, you won't lose body fat. Only diet and lowering your weight will cut the gut. However, with all those crunches, your muscle tone (below the fat) will greatly improve.

6. **No training program is complete without the use of weights.** As you get older, you become susceptible to osteoporosis and related bone diseases. Weight training helps build new bone and speed the recovery process, even when you're older. That's why you can lift progressively more weight—it's not just muscle you're building.
    Regarding weights, these are the terms most often used:

    •   **Reps (repetitions)** are the number of consecutive times you do a particular exercise.

    •   **Sets** are the number of times you repeat reps of the same exercise, with a short break (30 to 45 seconds) in between.

    •   **Super-sets** are usually two different exercises for the same muscle group, done back to back, with no break in between. You can also super-set two different forms of exercise. An example is an isometric exercise followed by push-ups.

> *Any special training tips for weightlifting?*

When you are counting your repetitions silently or otherwise (for instance, 1 through 12), don't count them in one long succession (1–2–3–4–5–6–7–8–9–10–11–12). Instead, count them out in threes: 1–2–3, 1–2–3, 1–2–3, 1–2–3. Why? It's a big psychological advantage; the mind treats 1 through 12 as a much bigger obstacle than 1–2–3 four times. In fact, I find that I usually add a few reps this way. It really works! Remember—75 percent of your workout is mental.

Weightlifting general rule of thumb: If you are overweight or obese, use lighter weights and do more reps (20 to 30); if you are on the thin side, use heavier weights and do fewer reps (8 to 12). The reason is simple—if you are already bulky, you don't want to add more bulk—you want to tone and firm up. If you are thin, you do want to bulk up.

Depending on your training program, you may do anywhere from one to four sets of a particular exercise. You may also vary each set by either increasing or decreasing the amount of weight and number of reps per set.

Weightlifting involves three dynamics: pushing, pulling, and resisting. At one time, weight training was called *resistance training*, which focused much of the dynamic on lowering the weight slowly, all the while resisting the tendency to simply drop the weight down. However, as it now stands, I see lots of pushing and pulling, but very little resisting. Don't neglect it! Whenever you lower a weight, do it slowly and resist (control) the force of gravity. In doing so, you will gain more strength and endurance. Resistance training can be accomplished by using either free weights or stationary machines. In both cases, the principle is the same.

> *How do I reduce my chances of injury?*

Adjust physical weaknesses by strengthening specific muscle groups. For instance, I know many cases where people suffered from shoulder problems—even though they worked their shoulders strenuously. These folks need to strengthen their upper backs and lats—the muscles that *support* the shoulders. Likewise, as I mentioned earlier, your legs may be quick to tire because your glutes are weak; and your back may be vulnerable to injury because you don't work your abdominal muscles enough. So whenever you have a particular weakness or debilitation, you should analyze the physical situation that contributes or plays a direct part in the problem, then figure out how to adjust it by reinforcing another muscle group. It's all a matter of knowing how to strengthen and balance all your muscle groups and develop full body symmetry.

Form is enormously important to your training program, and for that matter, to all physical activity. Without proper form, you not only look awkward at what you're doing, but the results of your movement and activity are limited by physical ineffectiveness and inconsistency. With proper form, you have the style, manner, and design that shapes and structures your every movement. In other words, **your form should be your own work of art.**

Form also distinguishes people at various levels, from the ordinary, to good, great, exceptional, extraordinary, one-in-a-million. Joe DiMaggio had form, then more form, and even more form. Even when he struck out, it was a thing of beauty. And when he ran to catch a fly ball, he glided like a gazelle. Similarly, Arnold Schwarzenegger's posing form put him in a class by himself. As muscular and cut as he was for competition, when he went into his varied poses, he made the other bodybuilders look ordinary in comparison.

Are you born with form? Can it be acquired? The answer to both questions is yes. Some people are born with natural form, while most others have to develop it over a period of time.

When I started dancing at Arthur Murray's back in 1959, I had no form. Consequently, I not only didn't look like a good dancer, I couldn't do things a good dancer had to do. Likewise, without good form, you can't carry out your objectives when you work out. Without knowing it, you have built-in handicaps that will prevent you from progressing at a normal pace, and you will look and feel inept and ponderous in the process.

So how do you attain proper form? You start by creating a model in your mind, a vision of who you want to be, how you want to look, move, run, dance, lift weights, and carry yourself. Mind you, **your vision must not be an unattainable one;** you can't add another five inches to your height or restructure your bones and muscles to be a Greek god any more than you can walk on water. That doesn't mean that you must be realistic to a fault, and only see yourself as a slightly altered person. It means that, given what your physical and creative attributes are, **you're capable of becoming a very advanced version of yourself.**

Once you've created the mental model of the *new* you, you must apply the time-honored principle of **"act-as-if"**—until you gradually develop your form and become that person you envision.

And you know what?—it works! You can go from being a klutz on the dance floor to a medal winner. Maybe it won't be an Olympic gold medal, but a medal winner nonetheless!

Here's a good opening "act-as-if": The simple act of improving your posture—

by holding yourself up high but relaxed (like a dancer).

The key to any successful act-as-if is patience; you've got to give it time to work. It won't happen overnight. But if you stay with it, you'll transition from the physical to the mental and then the emotional (just as you do when you learn to ride a bike or drive a car), and actually become the person you envisioned. And it will feel natural. One way to help it along is to see yourself as being a healthy, young, spirited person—with no handicaps or physical weaknesses. Walk down the street that way, acting as if you are that person. And remember, **75 percent of all physical activity is mental**—and leads to the proper form.

You must combine proper form with *technique* (the correct way to do a particular exercise), follow the act-as-if principle, apply your intelligence, artistic temperament, and *be and become* the physical personality that's in you. The rest is old-fashioned hard work and desire. That triangle will reshape your life.

> *Are there any other primary*
> *workout elements besides form?*

Focus is certainly one of them. As weightlifting and bodybuilding are meditative exercises (just like hypnosis), they require the highest possible level of concentration on the varied objectives such as lifting, pulling, pushing, stretching, and resisting.

In simple, practical terms, this means that you must be completely focused on your objective, almost as if it were a matter of life or death. Nothing else can matter. There must be no interference in what you're training your mind and body on doing. And unlike the method actor, whose attention is focused on the character being played but must still maintain at least 5 to 10 percent of his vigilance on external objects that might affect his portrayal, the person working out cannot afford to withhold any measure of focus or energy. It's as if **nothing else exists!** Even the slightest distraction can make a big difference between a good workout and a great one.

So *focus*—and go for it!

※ ※ ※

Before rounding things out with my canon of do's and don'ts, I want to indoctrinate the uninitiated into Nick's personal list of extreme training attitudes:

- **Wearing earphones and listening to music during a workout is a no-no** because it's a perfect concentration breaker. Music is fine for walking, running, swimming, and classes (where it helps keep everyone working in unison), but not for general workouts. Focus on your workout—not distractions.

- **Wearing one of those monitoring devices that give your heart rate, blood pressure, etc., is a lot of nonsense!** Unless you're under strict doctor's care (which is not the case with these folks because most of them are young), you're just indulging in some medical tomfoolery that won't truly help you get in better shape. These devices are just another distraction, a crutch (as if you were sick) and part of an image game of showing off. They're pathetic, counterproductive, and don't serve any meaningful purpose.

- **Leave your cell phone in your locker.** It's bad enough having to put up with them in so many public places, where they are a genuine nuisance of the first order, but in an athletic club they are even worse. They interfere with your concentration, literally force others to listen in on your life, and make me want to grab them out of their users' hands and fling the rotten contraptions out of the nearest window. You're there to work out—not to conduct business or be social.

- **If you can afford a private trainer, be very selective** and choose an individual who is both aware of your background and your needs, an individual who will not coddle you. Trainers are generally careful not to push you beyond your ability, which is fine providing they don't err on the side of being too sparing and delicate with you. (From over 40 years of training experience at 30 different athletic clubs in a number of countries, I have never seen a single trainer push someone beyond their capabilities. That's especially true of people who are not in good shape, have come off an injury or illness, or suffered from a serious infirmity. In fact, trainers usually are also very aware of the dangers of being sued.)

I strongly suggest that you also establish some basic ground rules for yourself and the trainer, such as **focusing on your workout and keeping the incidental talk to a minimum.** Perhaps that sounds callous, but I witness too much gabbing during training sessions, along with strolling around and drinking lots of water, which takes away from concentration and hard work. (It's also quite costly; at typical private training rates, this talk isn't cheap!) Save the talk for a time when you feel that you have accomplished something. Remember, you're there to get in shape, not to socialize.

While we're on the subject of working with a trainer, here are some other pointers: There are trainers—and there are *trainers*. The novice trainer (like the novice dance teacher) will stick to basics and be more apt to follow a workout program that is limited in scope and effectiveness. For instance, I constantly see trainers introduce older clients, who have been sedentary for many years, are overweight, and are in very poor shape, to a combination of balance exercises on a bosu (a curved, rubber balance device) and lunge exercises carrying very light weights. Oy vey! That's not what's needed!

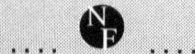

Lunges are rock-bottom great. However, I can tell you from many years of witnessing out-of-shape people start out on training programs that focus on balance and lunge exercises that they rarely, if ever, keep up their training. That's because **it's the wrong exercise for startup programs.** These people look all around at the people doing the free weights, machines, and classes, and then feel frustrated, intimidated, and that they're not "getting with it." And then they get bored by the balancing and lunging act! Save it for a time when the individual can look back on progress and be more committed to a long-range program.

You need to get into action. Get into motion! Lots of motion! And that means your entire body.

Otherwise, you'll get no place fast, and after not seeing quick results, you'll be discouraged and want to quit. I've seen it a thousand times.

What's more, after these older and out-of-shape people finish their initial training course—usually in two to three months—I rarely see them return to the club to work out on their own or participate in classes. So tell the trainer to save the balance stuff (which is fine once you have gained some tone and strength) and get your body activated.

Look in the mirror and analyze what you see, then imagine what you *want* to see—and go for it! Tell your trainer to customize a program that will get you rocking!

- **Don't drink a lot of water during workouts.** The "experts" (the water police) are sure to gang up on me about this one! But the story they run on everyone about dehydration is another myth that's gained wide acceptance in spite of the fact that it's **nonsense.** (It's been around so long that everyone accepts it without question.)

As for studies that recommend you drink six to eight glasses a day, that's sound advice for those of you with normal metabolisms who do not retain excessive fluids and maintain normal weight. But if you are among the weight casualties of America—it's a sure way of adding even more weight to your already overburdened body because you don't just pee it away. Like it or not, your body retains too much fluid. That's why overweight people use and abuse laxatives.

I've watched people who haven't even begun to work out go to the water bottle for a big drink—and these same people wonder why they're overweight and can't lose the pounds! (You can just imagine how many javas and sugar-laced drinks these people put away each week.) These "drenchers" spend more time drinking water than working out, never build up a sweat, and act as if they are moving mountains.

Because of this overblown myth about water needs and supposed dehydration, hundreds of thousands of overweight and obese people guzzle water and other fluids, acting as if they will otherwise become dehydrated and quickly die. They never stop to realize that 60 percent of their body weight is already water and they will be okay if they cut back a bit on the guzzling.

Remember, there's a huge difference between feeling dryness of the mouth and actual dehydration. Like day and night, salami from cream cheese.

When I work out—and I really work out—I have an occasional sip of water when I need it. Otherwise, I trust my body's signals, which are very clear and direct, so I don't need to overdo it out of some ridiculous fear of becoming dehydrated.

On another "water-dehydration" level, I have earlier in this book outlined the 31-day fast that I completed. No doubt the "experts" scoff at the notion than anyone can live more than a few days without water. Well, in October 2004, a 17-year-old girl who had been reported missing was rescued from the car in which she had been trapped for eight days in Redmond, Washington, during which time she had not had a single drop of water or food. She survived the experience and is alive and kicking in Seattle.

To beat a dead horse (because I think this point is important), tens of thousands of cases exist of people surviving without water for extraordinary lengths of time, but the experts—many of whom are the conglomerate's charter members– would rather you believe that you will quickly die if you go without water for more than a day or so. As always, ***they want you to feel weak and inadequate in the face of what should be relatively ordinary life situations.*** Why? Because it makes you all the more dependent upon their doctors and pill-pushers—that's why!

And in case you don't know it, being bloated from drinking too much fluid makes breathing properly more difficult, and breathing plays a huge role in maintaining proper form and training habits.

So drink moderately, only when you really need to. Remember, you need to drink only enough fluid to replenish what your body needs. Nothing more, nothing less. Just **use common sense.** Don't dehydrate yourself, and don't bloat yourself.

A final thought on fluid intake during workouts: If you ever watch a boxing match, you'll see that after each round the boxers go to their corners, sit on a stool, and are attended to by their respective managers, trainers, cutmen, and seconds. And almost immediately the water bottle appears and they are given a drink. However, you will also see that they usually spit most of it back into a bucket. The reason? If they didn't—the first time their opponent hit them in the labonza—you would witness a big splash all over the ring! So they know better than to get bloated.

- **Earlier I spoke of general lifestyle changes and one area that is most neglected is *speaking your piece.*** No one seems to realize that *this sucking up to people's ignorance and arrogance also affects your overall health and lifestyle.* This attitude also supports the disregard and weakness of our society, so don't think of this cowardice as an insignificant thing that I'm running my mouth about. Apropos of this:

- **When you're working out, cover your mouth when you cough,** even if you haven't got a cold or the flu, because it's a good habit, common courtesy, and respectful to all those around you. This practice is something that we see less and less in our health clubs. I'll take this a step further and ask you to tell others to do the same thing. You might suggest to the management of your club that they put up a large sign reading: *"Observe proper club etiquette and cover your mouth when you cough or sneeze. Please wipe down the equipment after using it."*

You would think that health clubs (or their clientele) wouldn't need to be reminded about such basic essentials, but the reality is that I've suggested this simple health-giving idea to at least 20 clubs over the years. Guess what? Not one of them was willing to do it because of a fear that it might offend someone.

It's no wonder that I appreciate the Singapore model for things such as outlawing spitting in public (which is a national disgrace in this country), urinating in elevators, etc. I'm old-fashioned that way. So by all means, uphold everyone's existence by taking it upon yourself to be a model and an agent of change.

Furthermore, if a health club official is afraid to offend someone, tell them that three-year-old children should know enough to cover their mouths when they cough or sneeze—so why shouldn't an adult be as accountable? In other words, don't be afraid to offend someone who's behaving like a jerk—including the health club. **Just tell them that the word "health" encompasses more than just working out.**

It's amazing and unconscionable that health clubs totally ignore their members' offensive behavior and refuse to do a damn thing about their clients inadvertently infecting countless people with colds and flu. So protect yourselves and others. Yes—**offend the offenders!** Give it a shot.

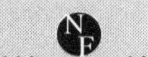

Nan and I went to grocery store recently, and when we got in line to pay for our goods we noticed that the grocery clerk was coughing steadily while at the same time handling customers' groceries. Later, we figured that within the course of just one day, this person probably potentially infected 200 people with his cough. And when you figure out how many people those 200 individuals subsequently infected, you get the picture.

Imagine what might happen in the case of a flu pandemic!

For those of you who still, after all this time, take exception to my extreme attitudes, please understand that I'm not advising against these things because of some strange cranky fixation. Hardly. What I'm trying to do is to instill proper exercise and general health habits in people, so they will see better results more quickly. Anything that interferes with this goal is counterproductive and often leads to disappointment, futility, and eventual failure. So stick to the basics! Forget the unnecessary trappings and self-indulgence.

Furthermore, when I take these ideas to the extreme, I am trying to get you to break the habit of following doctors' advice at every turn; exercising in moderation, drinking loads of water, and unnecessarily checking blood pressure are part of the conglomerate's scheme to make you obey their instructions or else pay the consequences.

As a result, you follow blindly; you also accept myths and distortions along with any constructive treatment. In the process, *you become enslaved to the madness of accepting sickness and eventual breakdown as the norm*, relying on the slave master to provide cures in the form of drugs, hospitalization, and lifelong observance of the rules set down by this unholy conspiracy. Wake up! Be sharp!

✳ ✳ ✳

Whether you do it at home or in a private club, these are the do's and don'ts of working out. **These do's and don'ts are geared toward people of all ages, not just senior citizens.**

THE DON'TS:

1. **Don't ask your physician for advice (or permission) about working out unless he truly knows what he's talking about.** I caution you to remember that most doctors aren't interested in healthy patients because they don't want to lose their sick patients. Unless you have damn good reason to believe that your doctor has the prerequisite expertise to advise you about a training program AND is also really concerned about your health—not just his bank account—don't waste your time talking to him about working out (or nutrition, for that matter).

    If your physician is in poor physical condition (which well may be the case), that's another sure tip-off not to involve him in any discussion about physical activity, since he obviously lacks any personal understanding of the subject. And don't let him run the "Do as I say—but not as I do" number on you. (You might even ask him why he looks paunchy and why his teeth are in such poor shape.)

    Instead, do some research, read up on the subject, talk with a sports therapist, and visit a health club and discuss the matter with a trainer. Depending on your overall physical condition, this on-the-job approach should get you started on an effective training program.

2. **Don't be so quick to pamper yourself.** That's not to say that, after years of more or less sedentary behavior and very little (if any) strenuous physical exertion, you should act like you're a dormant Arnold Schwarzenegger or Jack La Lanne and go hog-wild to prove it's still in you. BUT, by all means, do not

allow yourself to fall into the trap of treating yourself as if you've already got one foot in the grave.

3. **Don't ignore the importance of supplementary training in the form of daily walks (at as good a clip as you can manage) or even some light jogging to get that heart pumping again.** I wholeheartedly suggest the old Boy Scout run, which consists of 100 paces jogging and 50 walking at a quick pace, repeated two to three times, three times a week for the first few weeks, then increased incrementally until you're doing about six to eight of them three times a week, or about 15 minutes of combined walking-jogging per run.

> *How important is walking as part*
> *of an exercise program?*

While I don't wish to create yet another controversy and as much as I don't want to burst anyone's bubble, walking as exercise is highly overrated. Why? Because most people walk at a relatively leisurely pace, which doesn't amount to much in the way of genuine exercise.

An unhurried stroll through the park can be a lovely experience. It feels good, sounds good ("let's go for a walk"), and soothes the soul. But that's pretty much as far as it goes. And no matter what the doctors tell you, it hardly contributes to an effective exercise program. Worse, if you're over 50 and dumb enough to think that you're getting adequate exercise because you walk every day, you are actually weakening yourself—because your walks will not be enough to compensate for the years of inactivity, sedentary work, and lack of dedication to fitness. And you'll be fooling yourself all the while—thinking that you're getting sufficient exercise.

The only way walking adds up to measurable and effective exercise is if you do it at a fast pace and over a distance of at least three-quarters of a mile. In other words, get your heart pumping! Otherwise, go for a stroll, sing a song, have a great day—but don't expect to regain and maintain optimum health and fitness.

4. **Don't lapse into thinking that you need to follow a training program for only a few months and that then you can return to sedentary ways.** This is especially true if you're past 50. If you want to avoid the ills of old age that are mostly due to poor physical conditioning—and which can be avoided—then you must keep at it year-in and year-out. Take this into account: **The older**

you get, the more you must compensate; exercise that might have been easy in your earlier years will take that much more willpower and energy in later years. In other words, you must work harder to catch up and stay in good shape.

I hate to let you in on this reality BUT—when you get past the age of 50, every time you slack off on workouts—even if it's only for a few weeks— you're going to lose ground. Better believe it! You will not maintain good condition unless you stay the distance—which really means **the rest of your life.**

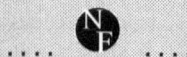

If you should ask how it feels—at the age of 70—knowing that I can't let up from working out, not even for a few weeks, and that I will be dragged into my grave still pumping iron, the answer is ... fantastic! Does that mean I love working out? Hell, no! I would rather be planting tomatoes, and be sitting before a roaring fire, champagne in hand. But it's still as good as it gets because **I love being healthy** and looking great. I wouldn't want to spend my remaining years (decades!) taking drugs, going to hospitals, and generally falling apart because I was too weak and ignorant to accept that working out was the way to go. So don't feel sorry for yourself. Feel privileged to be among the smart ones.

5. **Don't use lack of time as an excuse to skip workouts.** Even if time commitments are heavier than usual, you can still do a basic maintenance program (at home, the office, in an airport lounge, etc.) consisting of stretches and warmups, pushups (one of the greatest all-around exercises and conditioners), situps, clean and jerks, and squats. It takes only 10 to 15 minutes a day.

6. **Don't think that because you're elderly and in poor physical condition that you cannot regain body tone, muscularity, and energy.** *Nothing could be further from the truth.*[33] I'm not saying that you will look like a million

---

[33] William J. Evans is a physiologist with the Veterans Administration Medical Center in Little Rock and director of the Nutrition, Metabolism, and Exercise Laboratory at the Donald W. Reynolds Department of Geriatrics. He pioneered aging and exercise research and wrote breakthrough studies more than a decade ago to show that elderly subjects well into their 80s and 90s could gain strength by lifting dumbbells and other light weights. Of course the majority of doctors didn't collectively buy into this proposition for years.

in short order. I AM saying that if you start training with a vision of how you want to look and feel in 12 to 18 months, go at it in a committed way, eat properly, stay active throughout the day, and keep off "junk" (unless you cannot function, stay the course without drugs)—you will regain a measure of tone, energy, and strength. You will also look and feel much younger.

7.   **Don't ignore the rest of your "activity potential,"** such as walking up stairs instead of riding the elevator, using your feet instead of driving, and striding at a brisk pace instead of strolling leisurely. Use everything to your advantage. I try to get in mini-runs as often as possible while crossing a street or doing the Boy Scout run for a couple of blocks.

8.   **Don't listen to outside advice (or agitation) from old friends or family members** who tell you things like, "Stop exerting yourself so much—it's bad for the heart." These people don't know what they're talking about and for the most part are envious or jealous of anyone's physical improvement. Remember that "misery loves company," and unless you really do have a heart condition or suffer from an illness or disease that would preempt an exercise program, stay true to your workout commitments.

THE DO'S:

1.   **Do join classes that are provided by health clubs.** Try to select a class that offers you an opportunity to try a wider range of activities than those to which you are normally accustomed. Most clubs will permit you to observe classes, and if you feel up to it, participate on whatever level you can. Don't hesitate out of fear that you can't handle the class. You will generally find that you don't need to attempt certain exercises in a class that you presently find too difficult, while a majority of them are quite within your range. Don't be concerned with your image in front of others. You're not there to prove anything to anyone but yourself, and no one expects you to do otherwise.

Classes can be enormously beneficial because they literally shame you into working harder than you would if left to your own devices. As such, they pound you into submission and give you a sense of what could be—if you get with it. Conversely, I have seen more home-gym equipment end up in yard sales, in thrift shops, and in advertisements than almost any other product. As good as these contraptions can be (and some of them are highly rated), most people— especially those in poor shape—fail to use this equipment because of their lack of motivation and commitment. In other words, it's hard to do it on your own.

So take advantage of the classes. Submit yourself to the will of the instructor. You'll build confidence, improve your reflexes, look and feel better, and become disciplined. And whereas private trainers can be costly, most classes are free with club membership.

2. **Do eat small, healthy meals throughout the day,** especially several hours before working out and an hour or two following your workout. Most importantly, be aware that eating less and exercising more—which is a basic weight-loss strategy for millions of people—doesn't necessarily work to your advantage because the body responds by slowing your metabolism down, making you hungrier and doing a number of things to hormones that cause you to gain your weight back. You're better off having smaller but more frequent meals during the course of the day, and you'll also be providing your body with the fuel and energy it needs to maintain an efficient training program.

    I put together a meal consisting of salmon, broccoli, garbanzo beans, grated cheese, and olive oil, along with fruit and nuts, which I eat three to four times during the day at two-to three-hour intervals. Delicious and nutritional!

3. **It is also essential that you maintain the proper balance between sodium and potassium in your diet.** Numerous studies have shown that a low-potassium, high-sodium diet plays a major role in the development of cancer and cardiovascular disease (heart disease, high blood pressure, strokes, etc.) Conversely, a diet high in potassium and low in sodium is protective against these diseases. Researchers recommend a dietary potassium-to-sodium ration of better than 5:1 to maintain minimum health, which is 10 times higher than the average intake.

    Note: Our bodies require no more salt than is supplied in the food we eat, so we are in no great need of adding more salt to our diet because we're working out. However, potassium lost in sweat can be very significant, so people who regularly exercise have higher potassium needs.

    From personal experience, one of the best sources of potassium is bananas. In fact, when I worked out at the Mid-City Health Club in New York (where numerous professional weightlifters and bodybuilders exercised), the management of the club always provided huge amounts of bananas for the athletes.

4. **Cut down on the caffeine.**[34] If you must have some, let it be of the green tea variety.

---

[34] A study, published in the March 8, 2006 issue of Journal of the American Medical Association, suggests a correlation between coffee consumption and heart-attack risk, depending on how quickly your body breaks down caffeine.

5. **Do go dancing regularly.** Dancing is great exercise in and of itself, as well as a solid confidence-builder at any age. Coupled with a good training program and meditation, it can add flavor and excitement to your life, making you feel and look a lot younger. Try salsa!

6. **Do buy yourself some new clothes to reflect the reshaping and remodeling of your body.**

7. **Do feel proud of your emerging self.** Don't get humble at this point in life. Let it hang out a bit. Talk about how it feels. Share your new wealth and encourage others to get on the same bandwagon.

8. **Do let yourself fantasize about being young again.** No matter what anyone tells you, it's a healthy way to go about life, because it feeds the upholding of existence, energizes your brain cells, and actually revitalizes you.

This is no cornucopia of dreams and would-be philosophies. It's a workable plan that can lift you out of your malaise, spreading cheer throughout your whole body and mind in such large doses that you will go from "*acting*-as-if" to "*thinking*-as-if" and then "*feeling*-as-if."

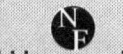

The "act-as-if" mindset is a great therapeutic tool BUT it doesn't work when you're on drugs. Brain cells work naturally.

Again, this is not some pie-in-the-sky daydream. **In my 70th year, I've reversed the aging process!** That doesn't mean that the lines on my face have disappeared or that my gray hairs have reverted to their original color. It does mean that I now feel, think, and behave like a very healthy young man—which is why I'm boxing again, doing 50 pushups at a stretch (even after a long workout), able to do hundreds of situps at a sitting, and finishing my biweekly, one-hour body-sculpting and boxing classes feeling stronger than all the young men participating (who then sit in the locker room and moan and groan about how tough the classes were). All of which leads me to sprint down the street like a happy-go-lucky teenager.

I don't give a damn what my birth certificate says because I know beyond a shadow of a doubt that I'm barely 30 years old—**and getting younger every day!**

✳ ✳ ✳

If you're wondering how the "No pain—no gain" adage applies to people who start training at a health club, you better believe it when I tell you that it's as real and meaningful to the novice as it is to a world-class bodybuilder.

I'll go even further and say that the sourness and pain in your muscles experienced 24 hours after a hard workout is as good as it gets—providing you're smart enough to capture those moments in your life and **treat them with affection and joy—instead of running to your doctor or medicine cabinet for pain relief.**

Yes, it's marvelous to feel what you should be feeling, that your body is responding, not lying half-dead. Just remember to give your muscles adequate recovery time—two to three days—between heavy workouts. In between, do those stretches, warm-ups, and light runs.

> ### *What about exercising to extreme?*
> ### *Isn't that dangerous?*

Ho, ho, ho, and a bottle of rum! Another big fat myth to contend with! To begin with, the only people I've ever known who exercised to the extreme were professionals who knew what they were doing, or people who exercised like jerks because they didn't know what they were doing. In between, I've known runners who ran themselves into the ground training for marathons without the prerequisite skills, and that can be very dangerous.

Otherwise, moderation is not necessarily the way to go. Not that it can't work. For the average person, it's probably okay: just what they're looking for and enough to get by on. Its major drawback is that for most people the very meaning of the word *moderation* can be somewhat confining because it often places the wrong kind of restraints on people—and for the wrong reasons. Some examples:

- If you want to set a higher standard for yourself, moderate exercise won't work.

- If you're looking to be among the elite (which is A-OK) then moderation and $2.75 buys you a moderate cup of coffee.

- If you're extremely overweight or obese, in terrible shape to begin with, or suffering from a physical weakness that calls out for a big stretch of the imagination as well as the body, then moderation is sure to kill you. Only dumb doctors will try to keep you on this moderate track—of Mickey Mouse exercise combined with drug therapy.

- If you follow such typical moderate thinking, you're good for another five years—along with some diabetes, extreme medical bills, and nothing in the way of a healthy and exciting future. So you're better off going to extremes. At least that gives you a crack at more than just bare survival.

- I watch all those who exercise moderately, and you know what? They stay the same year after year, going nowhere, and not getting the level of physical or mental satisfaction they need in the process. They're also continuing to get sick. *They're the first ones to get the flu, run to the doctors, take unnecessary medications—all of which wears down their immune systems.*

If you are among the legions of people who will undoubtably argue against exercising to extreme for any number of reasons, including not having enough time or energy, not being in good enough shape, or unwillingness to suffer the pain (as in "no pain—no gain"), I can only tell you that, like everything else in life, it's a matter of choices and priorities. I choose to work out to an extreme because my priority is to live a full, active, healthy existence without drugs, doctors, medical procedures, and hospitals—and my extreme workouts are a major part (in many ways the foundation) of maintaining this lifelong goal.

As for extreme exercising:

- All you need to do to protect yourself from any danger of extremism is to do the right kind of exercise and build up your stamina, strength, and capability as you're going along. And when you get to the point where you're in a steady groove, can see the sights ahead, and are ready to go for broke—then take your shot!

- As for any danger of grueling exercise endangering your immune system, that's more hogwash put out by the same experts who tell you that rest and drugs are the correct way to rehab an injury. I use myself as an example: At the age of 70, I exercise to the extreme, and my immune system is overjoyed! It's not only getting some time off, it's getting a boost, a charge, preparing itself for the long haul.

- Don't be afraid of taking something to extreme; if that's your nature and you have the ability to make the big stretch to the highest level—go for it. Otherwise, you're falling in line with everyone else and whether you know it or not, practicing the misery-loves-company routine for the sake of others less inclined to reach for the next rung.

In other words, the word *moderation* is much like the word *interesting;* it's a sure way of keeping yourself in the middle, a boring place to be. I kid you not.

To make this topic more personal, I go back to my first love relationship; Jean used to tell me, "Everything in moderation" (wasn't she the one to talk!). Had I followed her advice, life would have been a lot easier, I would have saved money, not taken risks, and died an early death of boredom and frustration. I'm not the fella for moderation.

Another way to view moderation and extremes: If you're trying to deal with an acute problem, and you treat it with moderation, chances are that you will move about a quarter of the way to the center—and in short order fall right back to where you started.

On the other hand, if you behave as an extremist, and move all the way to the opposite end of things, chances are that you will gradually fall back to a new position—in the center of things. Right where you want to be.

The aforementioned way of looking at moderation and extremism is something I taught in groups for many years. It's a therapeutic tool that works!

❋ ❋ ❋

Along with physical exercise, you should take up other meaningful activities that will contribute to your overall health. You may recall that your immune system grows, so you should exercise it regularly by abstaining from any unnecessary use of medication; by guarding against any intrusion that will weaken it; and by talking to it—yes, talking to it! Give your immune system the same boost of confidence that your personality and character need. Specifically, meditate (focus) on your immune system's vast powers and direct that energy to all areas of your body, especially those that need assistance or adjustment.

Most importantly: **Exercise your immune system by trusting it.**

Another vital part of your exercise program (and one that is almost always ignored) is emotional exercise. As I've mentioned in many different ways in this book, our emotional health is as important as anything else, so it requires an ongoing exercise program that will reinvent its original purposes, adding a key ingredient to your overall health plan.

Before going into specifics, I'm going to go to the extreme of trying to force you to understand this underlying but least accepted fact about overall health. In other words, I'm about to trip out!

In a broad sense, we've done to our emotional health what we've done to our immune system: betrayed it, rendering it next to useless and obsolete. Even worse, **we've created monsters out of our natural emotions,** turning them into something they were never meant to be—freaks! A perfect example: **Anger management is to our emotions what drugs are to our immune system—a systematic reversal of intent and purpose.**

The net result is that we Americans are the most unemotional people in the world. Women can't get angry, men can't cry, we think there's something unnatural about fear, and we become intimidated or anxious at any normal display of emotion. In place of showing natural emotions, we act tough, and either strut around like fools or hang our heads looking for sympathy—all quite unnatural and superficial.

In fact, the only time we really show our emotions is when it's societally considered perfectly safe to do. On June 8, 1969, I attended Mickey Mantle Day at Yankee Stadium. While the Mick was driven around the perimeter of the field in a golf cart, over 50,000 fans showered him with raw emotion. Men of all ages and descriptions shed more tears in those minutes than they had offered up in their entire lives. That's because everyone else was doing it. Finally, they felt it was safe. Those same people go to family funerals and keep a close check on their feelings, their daily lives devoid of true emotion.

On a different level, when we drive, we often show our worst feelings; all our unexpressed rage, all the pain within our souls, and all our impatience and frustrations spill out against people we don't even know. We stick our fingers in the air, curse, threaten, and act like semibarbarians. That's because our emotions are held in check everywhere else: at our jobs, in stores, on the street, when dealing with bill collectors and corporate people. At those times we're meek, frightened, and obedient to our personal and collective restraints.

This collective form of trained emotions is as much a national health problem as obesity, drugs, and violence. You might say it's violence to ourselves, but we're too dumb to know it. **And this bottling up of emotion contributes to our early decline and death.**

In practical terms, you must exercise the following emotions:

- **Anger:** Having worked with over 4,000 therapy groups, I can state categorically that unless you can express anger appropriately, you cannot attain good overall health at any age. So you must exercise anger—**not hostility**—regularly. How? Join a sensitivity group or workshop, or just practice with a friend or loved one. All you need to do is repeat the words *"I'm angry."* While you're doing it, truly let yourself feel the anger.

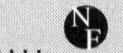

Having trained hundreds of people (both in acting classes and therapeutic groups) to express feelings, I know full well that dealing with anger is not as simple as it should be—had we been raised in an atmosphere that welcomed the display of normal emotions.

You might begin by using the act-as-if technique (mentioned on page 353) to gradually become an emotional human being, which is healthy and desirable. That includes the ability to express appropriate anger, pain, and fear.

Living in today's world—the here and now—one is subjected to a constant flow of personal and collective experiences that are provoking and angrifying. As such, it is not that difficult to get in touch with anger. All you need to do is be truthful to yourself, then examine, reflect upon, and express that anger.

You can also use "I'm angry at you," "I'm angry at life," "I'm angry at the world," "I'm angry at being hurt," or "I'm angry at being frightened." Whatever it is that makes you feel anger.

The important thing is to dig down into your gut and get in touch with your anger (it's there), express it without hostility, and clean it out of your system—so it can no longer fester inside you and weaken your entire emotional health.

Women especially must exercise their anger because they normally keep far away from this normal emotion, just as men keep away from pain.

It is equally important that you exercise your ability to take in anger. Have your friend, partner, or loved one work on that with you. It's a sure way to improve the health of any relationship and to prevent typical hostility.

If you're still confused by the distinction between anger and hostility, here's a further clue to its workings. When I tell someone "I'm angry" at them, I'm expressing something I feel inside me, a pure emotion. And by expressing it, I clear away my resentment, maintaining my good feelings for that person.

But if I take that anger and express it venomously with "You're a rotten son-of-a-bitch and I'd like to kick your teeth in," I'm turning it into hostility, masking the underlying emotion of anger, building resentment, creating a sense of guilt within myself, and fostering negative feelings in both parties. All of this works against your emotional health.

I go so as far as to say that this same dynamic (or lack thereof) plays the major role in relationships between countries in conflict—if only they could learn. *So manage your hostility—and exercise your anger.*

- **Pain and hurt:** Exercise this emotion the same way you exercise your anger. Use simple words like "I feel hurt," "You hurt me," or "I feel so much pain and hurt." Just as you have to cleanse your gut of the anger, the same goes for this emotion. Dig it up, express it cleanly, and then rid yourself of it. **The best thing that a man can do for himself is to cry.** Yeah, that's what most men hide from and it takes a huge toll on their emotional health. And remember this: *You can collapse from unexpressed pain just as much as you can from a purely physical ailment. So bring those tears to the surface and let them flow.*

- **Fear:** Follow the same process as with anger and hurt. Dig it up, get it out in front, then get rid of it. There are dozens of exercises you can do with fear: Challenge it by diving off a board into a pool repeatedly until you're no longer afraid of the height; have someone stand behind you and fall backward into their arms; search your mind for the things that really frighten you—then treat them as worthy adversaries to be denounced and put in place. **Turn that fear into excitement!**

- **Love:** Surprisingly enough, we don't exercise this emotion as much as we think we do. Hardly. We throw out the words as if real emotion were involved, but usually we miss the mark because we don't really dig down and get in close touch with it. Thakur said it perfectly: "Just love before you speak of love."

  Along with giving and taking anger, giving and taking love are the most difficult and vital emotions to express. (I recommend that you use the words *Balo Bashi* [Hindu words that translate into "I live in your good"] instead of "love." It expresses so much more.)

- **Joy:** This is a misunderstood emotion because we have been schooled in the false art of pretending to feel joy through the use of joking, fooling around, drinking, smoking marijuana, etc. These quick fixes and image games get us away from the true joy that is in all of us. Try feeling the real McCoy: Practice being light-hearted and free of worry. Go out of your way to express joyous thoughts about people you love—even yourself. Remember what it's like to play with your children and get out of yourself—be and become that giver and taker of glad tidings and fun-loving mirth. And try to laugh as often as possible. That's great medicine! Go a step further and laugh at yourself!

On that note, here's an email I received from my friend Neil Selden:

You trying to smile, dear Nicko, is a powerful psychospiritual strategy—I began a sort of yogic smile practice 10 years or so ago when Lee's sister Dawn was dying and I had been diagnosed with prostate cancer, walking up from Tribeca to St. Vincent's Hospital to spend some hours with her every day. I do it as a breathing meditation as I walk or whenever. Breathing in and breathing out, I smile the radiant compassionate radha-soami smile of perfect loving, healing emptiness and pure joyful, healing awareness, calming, cleansing, healing, and blessing all those I see, hear, speak to, touch, hold, or think of.

And you are often one of those I think of in my smiling, and it's quite delightful how people passing my smile on foot or in their cars respond, probably thinking they know me, or wish they did.

By exercising our emotions we add the vital component that goes along with good physical health, eliminating many of the causes of cancer, other diseases, and premature death. In fact, it's a spiritual as well as an emotional and mental exercise. And it actually alters the body's chemistry, which in turn boosts its immune system.

So exercise these emotions as if your life depended on it. Failure to do so will deplete your health reserves.

* * *

Yet another form of exercise that is sorely missed in our everyday lives (although most of you will deny as much) is mental exercise. We are, most unfortunately, ignorant and backward. Because we refuse to accept this reality, we get dumber by the day. So if you really want to clean up your act and become a healthy person—give your mind and brain cells a daily workout. How? Here's a short list:

- Read a newspaper every day and select three articles (topics or stories—whatever interests you) and pick them apart. Question, dissect, obliterate, rearrange, or rewrite them all—as if you were teaching someone about that particular subject matter. It doesn't so much matter how you view these topics but that you push your mind to go in different directions than usual. If you vote Republican—go Democrat in your thinking; if you have an opinion about such topical things as abortion, gun control, legalizing marijuana, or capital punishment, reverse your opinion and build a case for the other side. Again, it doesn't matter what your opinion presently is; the idea is to stretch your mind and initiate new processes of thought.

- Start asking others what they think and really take in what they have to say as if you knew nothing at all. By doing this, you deal with your mind and your ego at the same time. (Questioning is like letter writing and conversation; it is a lost art. If you're wise enough to revive it in your life, it will add significantly to your mental vigor and thus your overall health.)

- Take up some new creative venture, one that's difficult for you, and tax your mind and those brain cells to grow creatively and intellectually. Try dancing, singing, painting, acting, writing, mechanics, sky-diving, learning another (or new) language— whatever will test your abilities and reinvigorate your life.

- Write letters! And keep journals! Express hidden thoughts, fears, and whatever else has been lying dormant in your mind all these years. And, while you're at it, broaden your vocabulary (another form of exercise) and force yourself to construct sentences in altogether new ways. Try learning three new words every day. And use them when you speak or write.

SO WORK OUT IN A DOZEN NEW AND EXCITING WAYS!

❋ ❋ ❋

Along with your workouts, I recommend that you take up some form of meditation, which will strengthen your willpower and determination to stay the course of your overall training objectives. I have used self-hypnosis for many years and it fits in perfectly with my overall training program.

"Hypnosis" comes from the Greek word *hypnos*, which means "sleep." With a rich history that dates back to the ancient Egyptians and Greeks to scientific discovery by the famous Franz Mesmer (mesmerism), Sigmund Freud, Ivan Pavlov, and Milton Erickson, hypnosis has gone from being a remarkable cure-all to an utter fake and back to respectability again. It is now accepted as a legitimate medical treatment by the American Medical Association (AMA).

Hypnosis involves open and active thought with the subconscious mind by guiding the hypnotized person through different states of awareness, memory, and creativity. The process relies on meaningful questioning, self-examination, and feedback (called "posthypnotic suggestion") to help the hypnotized person adopt new behaviors and relinquish old ones.

So powerful is the mind's focus when under hypnosis that one can create an imagined sensation, feeling and believing just as though it were real. Thus, hypnotized people can actually change their own physiology, such as decreasing blood pressure and heart rate, even blocking out the pain associated with fear.

Hypnosis is a marvelous tool that can also be used to help you deal with migraine attacks, smoking, obesity, road rage, and various other forms of compulsive behavior. You may recall that I suffered through many years of the worst type of migraine attacks before being cured through one hypnotic session. It actually works! The documented evidence is overwhelming, which is one reason why the AMA finally placed its seal of approval on it.

In a way, nothing is really surprising about the power of the many forms of hypnosis. Haven't we all practiced, at one time or another, different types of intense mental focus such as concentration, visualization, imaging, getting psyched up, "getting in the zone"? It's all one and the same.

Hypnotic techniques and approaches vary. One can be "put under" by a professional (and you don't need someone with the title of "doctor") or you can simply practice self-hypnosis. There is also the matter of degree. Most hypnotists, working with clients who are trying to overcome basic problems like smoking and obesity, take them to a subconscious level just below the normal level of consciousness. This is where many of the basic ingredients of human behavior, such as common sense, reside.

For more traumatic problems, the hypnotist takes the patient deeper, perhaps into a trance-like state, to uncover experiences long buried and forgotten. But this is advanced hypnosis, and under most normal circumstances it's wholly unnecessary, even ill-advised, especially for the beginner.

The important thing for the newcomer to know is that the Hollywood notion of hypnosis has little to do with its practical application and contributes mightily to the lack of clear understanding about its basic workings. There's nothing magical or mystical about hypnosis, and the hypnotist need not be a Svengali- or Dracula-type personality, whose penetrating stare makes you fall into a deep trance.

Another thing I must debunk is the idea that a hypnotist can make you do something against your will. That's sheer nonsense. S/he can only suggest and encourage you to do things you want to do. ***The hypnotist can't force you to lose weight or stop smoking or acting out in whatever way you do unless you want to.***

So it comes down to this: You must first want to change something before you enter any form of hypnosis, or you will be completely wasting your time. As an example, many years ago I went to a hypnotist in an effort to cure my road rage, which was advancing to a dangerous point. After listening to me describe my behavior and attitude toward other drivers, she told me that she wouldn't even attempt to put me under because it was obvious that I wanted to hold on to my rage toward these drivers. And she was perfectly right. She told me to come back when I was ready to give up that venom (hostility). That's the only way it works.

Unless you have a need to go into something much deeper (like past-lives therapy, which you shouldn't attempt unless you've been in hypnosis for quite a while), the basic act of focusing your mind and expanding your thought process can be a relatively simple task. It can also help you change the way you perceive your world and your place in it.

To get back to my suggestion about using self-hypnosis to strengthen your will-power and determination to stay the course of your overall training objectives, the way to begin is to think of it as a method of tweaking your subconscious mind to do what you really want. All this requires is your conviction that you actually do want to work out and improve your health. If that's what you want, then read on.

Self-hypnosis is one of the easiest and most relaxing exercises you can do. However, people who try it tend to fall into an enormous "trap": They expect something to happen quickly—just like with a pill—and most of these people also expect to feel something different or unusual. When this doesn't happen, they tell themselves that hypnosis is a lot of nonsense and a waste of time. Those of you who have read my autobiography will remember my story about the hypnotist in Cleveland. I was so damn sure that nothing had happened, when lo and behold, my migraine headaches were cured for life!

So don't go into hypnosis thinking that you're supposed to reach some altered state or suddenly feel like a new person. It doesn't work that way.

❋ ❋ ❋

How does hypnosis work?

Except for those cases where the hypnotist knows something you don't (like my wanting to suffer headaches because of hidden feelings of guilt) and is able to quickly connect you to it and thus rid you of the block, hypnotism works **cumulatively.** These effects take place in imperceptible increments but are nonetheless happening, although you are not immediately aware of them. As you continue layering these effects, the total result is strengthened (you might call this synergy), and you gradually begin to feel the change.

The key to success is consistency. That's the only way it will work. If you just "try" it—forget it! (And that's true of almost anything.) You'll quickly feel disappointed and quit before anything can happen. Likewise, if you don't do it regularly—**every day**—you'll give up on it.

So first and foremost, for the sake of your decision to make your health the top priority in life, commit yourself to a daily minimum 10- to 15-minute session of meditation and self-hypnosis, preferably in the morning, before you delve into your active day. Better yet, commit to both a morning and evening meditation. I do my evening meditation just before going to sleep.

Who plays the part of hypnotist?

Here are several options:

- Ask someone whom you really respect, like a close friend, family member, teacher, or even a stranger with a clear and soothing voice, to do a simple tape recording of your meditation, which you can play each day. The important thing is that the voice must command your respect and attention.

- Instead of using an actual recording of the voice you chose, just hear it in your mind, saying the same words of the voice you chose that would otherwise be heard on a tape or CD. For many years I have used the voice of my dear departed friend Edmund Spencer for my meditation and self-hypnosis sessions.

- If you prefer, you can contact a professional hypnotist or hypnotherapist and ask them to record the meditation.

As for the actual script of the meditation, here's what I use (and you can certainly alter it accordingly for your own purposes):

Spencer: "Good morning, Nickolas ... Let's focus on my voice ... and we'll count down from 100 as we do and reach that subconscious, meditative, hypnotic level where you can go over the important things of the day and make decisions that will carry over posthypnotically to your conscious life today. ...

... Okay ... Let's begin ... Close your eyes, relax every part of your body, starting with your toes, then work your way up to your ankles and shins, then your knees, thighs, groin area, abdominal muscles, your lower back, chest, upper back, hands, forearms, biceps, triceps, shoulders, neck, jaw, cheeks, eyes, forehead, entire head. ...

Now take a deep breath and slowly let out the air ... 100 ... Drift down, down, down to that well of souls, that wonderful place in the universe where all creatures reside in complete harmony ... peace ... contentment ... and calmness ... another deep breath. ...

... 99 ... Drift further and further down ... to that place in the universe where there are no pills, bills, or therapies ... where there's only harmony, peace, contentment, and calmness ... Take another deep breath. ...

... 98 ... Drift further down ... toward that place where there are no problems or conflicts, no cash to raise, no banks to go to, no accounting ... no worries ... where there is only harmony, contentment, peace, and calmness ... Another deep breath. ...

... 97 ... Drift further down ... free-falling now ... toward that sea of tranquility and bliss and calmness ... Take another deep breath ...

... 96 ... Drift down and down ... toward ground zero of all that calmness ... Now take a final deep breath. ...

... 95 ... and drift all the way down ... to the center of all the calmness in the universe ... that island of calmness ... where you are enveloped by calmness ... and you become one with the calmness ... You become calmness itself ... calmness of soul and spirit ... body and mind ... being and personality ... and emotion and memory ... complete calmness ... You are calmness. ...

... Now, Nickolas, how does your day shape up?"

At this point in the meditation and self-hypnosis routine, I (you) take over and talk (in my mind or softly out loud) about the plans for the day: shaving, showering, dressing, work, tasks, special problems or highlights, hopes, expectations, and of course—my workout.

I conclude by saying, "And with everything else, I will stay calm throughout the day … not ruminate about anything … not let anyone or anything get to me … be productive … creative … positive … and 'believe.'…"

Spencer: "That sounds like a great day, Nickolas … Now let's take a deep breath and slowly count back up to 100 … then awaken and begin the day … 96 … 97 … 98 … 99 … 100 … 'Joy guru'…. "

❋ ❋ ❋

I must again stress the word "cumulative" and advise you that the exact choice of words you use in your meditation will play an important part in the cumulative effect, which is why I use the word "calm" repeatedly. As a way of illustrating this, three years ago I experienced a personal storm in my life that was deeply painful and terrifying. It rocked the very foundation of my life, leaving me in the worst emotional and mental state of my adult life (and if you've read my autobiography, you know that I've been through severe times).

All I had to fall back on besides my excellent physical health was my meditation, which would have to carry me through the early stages of the healing process. I knew from many years of experience that I could depend on it, as long as I was consistent and believed in it. And the word "calm" was the key word—because what I needed most during this crisis was calmness—to face its problems, pressures, and emotions, and ground myself in order to come out of it in good shape.

I did come out of it … feeling calmer than I ever have in life. And the cumulative effects have been extraordinary; I walk down the street every day feeling so calm that it's ridiculous! That's the power of meditation and self-hypnosis. And it can come from a single word.

Once you have created your meditation routine, whether it be a recording or someone's voice that you will hear, the process is as follows: While lying either in bed or on a comfortable couch, and in a quiet place where you will not be disturbed, close your eyes and begin. It's that simple.

❋ ❋ ❋

Besides what I have outlined under this section on working out, feel free to engage in any type of physical activity or therapy, including yoga, isometrics, reflexology, acupuncture, acupressure, herbal therapy, primal therapy, cleansing, or anything else you know of or want to try. The objective is to mount a coordinated attack against whatever ails you, be it physical, mental, or emotional.

Don't be afraid to be inventive. Use your imagination and try out different things, even if you're totally unsure of what you're doing. For instance, without any prior thought or intention, one evening six years ago I stared at myself in the bathroom mirror and began to seek out the tension points in my body and to attack them with a vengeance. I stretched, massaged, probed, pressured, even growled at each and every spot that needed attention, trying to release its tension and set my body free of any anxiety. In the process, I released energy, pain, anger, fear, and frustration, all for the good of my body and mind.

I tried this same type of exercise many times over the course of the last six years and was grateful for the results. But I never realized that I was only scratching the surface of what was to come. On Thursday night, December 29, 2005, I hit the mother lode.

Three nights earlier, Nan and I, having heard a glowing review of the new movie *King Kong* from our daughter Jenny, went to see this latest version of the classic Merian C. Cooper tale. True to Jenny's enthusiasm for the film, Nan and I loved it. The next three days found me still reenacting many of the thrilling movie scenes in my mind.

That's what was taking place that Thursday evening as I finished flossing and brushing my teeth. I stared in the bathroom mirror and began to envision Kong pounding his chest and bellowing at his enemies. It was both fun and therapeutic in that I was also adding to the Kong fantasy by using the stretching, massaging, probing, pressuring, and vocal techniques I had experimented with for the past six years.

During the following minutes, as I continued to stretch and pound, I also recalled a group therapy marathon I ran at Hofstra University back in the 1970s, when I experienced an adrenaline rush so powerful that I was able to drag 10 people across a room. I had never approached such a feeling of raw energy again. But now as I began to mentally enter into a primal state—that of a beast with enormous physical power—I began to drift toward that convergence of superhuman strength. Combining the radical stretch with the primal urge (like King Kong), and not only pounding the chest but opening it and my entire body, was the desired effect.

And then it happened: Like an animal suddenly unchained, bursting out of its bonds, I let loose all physical and emotional restraints and unleashed forces never before dreamed of.

As I stretched from head to toe, I moaned, groaned, bellowed, confronted the world, the universe, God and man. I awoke everything!

At that moment, I felt as strong and invincible as Kong, Godzilla, Superman, and Spiderman combined, letting go on all 24 cylinders, as if I could tear down walls, destroy everything in my path, conquer cities. It became a chain reaction, like atomic energy, and it was real, not just a thought or emotion! **It was the primal force that exists within all of us.** We are all Supermen. And we can control this force and use it to our great advantage as a basis for both physical exercise and emotional growth.

I call this new therapy "The Monster Stretch." (It sounds like a 1950s song or dance craze!) It's the ultimate workout. Within minutes, you can experience a phenomenal sensation that leaves you tingling with earthly vigor and wholeness. I especially enjoy doing a number of short monster stretches, which I call *outbursts*, which focus on a specific area of the body and then EXPLODE like an atomic cannon! They're orgiastic! It's like the universal Big Bang theory!

The monster stretch also has cleansing implications; the very act of unleashing inner forces physically, mentally, and spiritually purifies the whole body.

I should mention that you will need a few days to recover from this monster stretch. Since this initial experiment lasted only about 20 minutes, I took it for granted that it was not a full workout and went to my club the next day for my regular workout. Was I in for a surprise. I was burnt out. I had nothing. I had given it all up the night before.

Here's a warning about this all-out monster stretch: **DON'T** attempt it until you're ready for it—which will take some weeks of steady full-body stretching (as outlined previously). Otherwise, you'll tear yourself up and you might even disintegrate. After all, you're not King Kong—yet. But just wait!

Note: For those who would chide me for having reinvented yoga, I will tell you that although certain elements of meditation, breathing technique, and certainly stretching are involved, the monster stretch is not yoga as known or defined. Whereas yoga uses very defined postures and controlled techniques, my program is entirely spontaneous and geared toward moment-to-moment discovery and action. It avoids subtlety, depending on explosiveness and extreme ranges of raw power surges.

So reach for the sky, let loose, and rejuvenate your physical being!

※ ※ ※

This same inventiveness can hold true for different forms of dieting and fasting. Either try something you've never done (like Thakur's four-day fast [on pages 336 to 337] or an Isagenix cleansing [see pages 304 to 305]) or create your own model with the intention of releasing your body's toxins, cleansing and purging all the crapola you've taken in over the decades.

Remember, unlike cuts, bruises, and injuries caused by accidents, your cancers, acne, weight, asthma, and diabetes didn't happen overnight. They're an accumulation of life's problems, traumas, and poisons, and it will take a concentrated, concerted effort to set your body straight. So go for it!

❋ ❋ ❋

Continuing on the general theme of taking back your life, once again I ask you to realize that good health isn't just a matter of proper diet and exercise or staying away from drugs, hospitals, and the claws of the conglomerate—although that's a hell of a good start! Good health involves every aspect of living, and that includes the condition of your soul. On that note, our deficiencies may well exceed all our physical and emotional problems tenfold.

No, I'm not about to run some religious thinking on you. I'm talking about something a lot simpler and more basic than any form of holy-rolling. I'm talking about what you do during the course of your days, especially how you earn your money. Does that uphold your existence?

For instance, if your work requires you to hurt other people or put fear in their hearts—say a job involving calling people who are late on their payments for their house, car, or TV, and threatening them with foreclosure, serving papers, repossession, or legal action—you might just as well let your obesity or illness take you to hell on a rocket ship for all it matters. This is because you are aiding and abetting all the conglomerates in America and upholding no one's existence—certainly not your own. You are damaging your soul.

I must take this a step further: We think of torture as a brutal form of physical punishment and humiliation, but it's only one way of carrying out immoral and sadistic acts to achieve a specific purpose. The corporate world has established a form of torture that brutalizes our minds and emotions. It has trained tens of thousands of young men and women to use vile and immoral methods to extract payment of debts. As an example, they leave messages telling you that a close relative or friend has died, to get you to contact them.

These collectors often work in teams, ganging up on debtors as if they were criminals, sharing their ugly tales of success and pretending to be honest and honorable people merely trying to collect a debt. To make their behavior more loathsome, these people think of themselves as being *cool*. And whenever they are called into question for their tactics and cruelty, they all hide behind the same rationale of "I'm just doing my job."

Yes, these Americans torture fellow Americans, having become so adept at *forcing payment* that they act as if the debtor *cum* victim owes them personally.

I call them by their rightful name: sick vermin—who sneak around like thieves in the night and invade people's sanctity, serving them court papers or driving off with their cars. For the sake of money, they would do anything, even become executioners. The only ones worse than them are the lawyers they work for. These repo artists are uncivilized and soulless.

✳ ✳ ✳

Then we have the actors and athletes who do the pill commercials on TV. They're as guilty of peddling death and destruction as the rest of the conglomerate clan. And their souls will suffer for it. This also holds true for the advertising agencies that create the bullshit spins about the conglomerate's deadly products. These Madison Avenue whiz kids are no better than Joseph Goebbels, the Nazi propaganda minister. **Their lies and pitch tactics about drugs kill more Americans than the Nazis ever did!**

Again we witness their rationale of "It's just a job—not my way of life. I'm a good person." I have news for you. They're as deluded as the good people who run the slaughterhouses, export jobs to countries that exploit child workers, support police brutality, ignore someone's screams for help, or legislate laws that deprive people of their civil liberties.

Furthermore, if their rationale for your involvement with a destructive occupation is, "I only follow orders," that's what Hitler's henchmen also used as their excuse for war crimes against humanity.

Remember, we humans are pretty impressionable, and a negative job can shape our character down the line without our even realizing that it's happening. We are easily trained to obey and then rationalize all the sick things we do.

I recall the story of a young Greek farm boy who was enlisted to guard Greek communist prisoners during the Greek Civil War in the mid-1940s. Within only weeks of orientation, this innocent boy of 17 was torturing fellow Greeks. The same thing happened in 2005 at Guantanamo Bay and Iraq, where young American men and women soldiers tortured and killed Iraq prisoners.

So don't take your negative jobs that lightly, any more than you should take your road rage or poor health lightly. They affect your character, community, country, and the world, contributing to the eventual downfall of society. If you doubt that, just take out any book on world history and read up on what's gone down through the centuries.

In today's world, with its nuclear arms, biotechnical capabilities beyond description, an environment endangered from all sides, inferior leaders who are both illiterate and psychotic, and multinational conglomerates that don't give a damn for human life—your life and the way you support or fail to support existence play a much more important part in what will eventually happen to this misguided world than you realize.

Better you should go homeless and impoverished before you add to humanity's suffering. Be sharp—you can't play both ends. You're either on the side of humanity or in cahoots with the sick conglomerates throughout the world. So cut your losses and find another job.

On that note, to facilitate the objective of helping people cut loose from negative and destructive forms of employment, I recommend that we pressure Congress to create a new holiday: National Quit Your Lousy Job Day. Just think about it: Every year hundreds of thousands of people could cleanse their souls and start living like loving human beings again. What a celebration!

※ ※ ※

On another level, you can never attain good health if you disregard your basic obligations to the elderly, whether they are family or strangers. *Nowhere on the face of this earth is there such disrespect shown to the aged as in the U.S.* It's so bad that younger people don't even want to bother talking to anyone from an older generation.

In places like Hollywood, younger people ignore anyone over 40, unless they happen to be famous. It's as though 60 percent of our population isn't worth knowing. And that extends to not hiring people over the age of 60, a deplorable reality.

I have to get rather personal here: When I reached the age of 70, I had to go through the five stages of death and finally accept the reality that most people under the age of 40 would no longer relate to me. Although I look much younger than I am, feel like I'm 30, and behave like a young, healthy, energetic, and highly creative individual, it doesn't matter to young people because the American social mentality dictates that I'm no longer worth knowing.

These age barriers extend into all areas of life to the point where it is almost unheard of for younger people to engage in any social interaction with older folk. I mean, not even as much as sitting down and having a cup of coffee with them. That's how bad it is.

This age discrimination is part of our caste system. It divides people in much the same way that one's economic and social position determines where our place in society is. Those of age are outcasts.

The pitiful truth of this ugly and dismissive social doctrine is that it perpetuates itself and its current practitioners will eventually suffer the same consequences, isolated from the general population because they have lived to a certain unenviable number.

Not that older people don't play their part in the problem; if they stopped *acting* old and useless, they might get more respect and attention, too. At least they would have a fighting chance. So I would hope.

※ ※ ※

These matters of the soul play as much a part in your poor health as anything else that you're having trouble with, and all the more so if you're a young person. So you would do well for yourself to check out every corner of your life, see what you can do to regain your higher being before it's too late, and aid others to do the same.

※ ※ ※

In closing my story, if you're one of the tens of millions of people who are overweight, obese, overmedicated, overhospitalized, going nowhere but to early graves, and putting up with a poor quality of life because that's the rut you've been in for many years, then you've really got nothing to lose by trying a radical departure from so-called normal living.

You may get hung up wondering if it's worth going through all the bother and hard work necessary to rebuild your life from the bottom up in order to regain your health. Well, I remember a young person at Encounter back in 1967 who, after coming out of a very intense group session, walked up to my friend Neil Selden and said, "I really don't know if this is for me—going through all this pain and conflict. What's the point of it?"

Neil looked at him, smiled, and then said, "I don't know if it's worth it for you, but I'm doing it because I want to 'groove' in life when I'm 70 years old."

For the record, Neil is past 70—and he's still grooving. So just remember, as Thakur said, "Life is for living and for love—not for death."

※ ※ ※

Every story deserves a kick-ass ending, and here's mine.

Over the years of practicing my fountain-of-youth obesity cure, I've completed some 20,440 mini-diets (if you want to call them that), and indeed I'm healthier than ever, looking and acting like a man 30 years younger. In fact, women are now telling me that I look "hot," which goes to prove that **the joy is in the eating—not the digesting!**

Be safe....

Part V.
J'accuse!

In Tribute to All
Who Have Needlessly Died

This may seem like overkill—especially after the previous chapters—but I feel a strong need to conclude this book in a spirit of compassion for the tens of millions of people who have died premature deaths as a result of the conglomerate's deadly actions.

*On a personal level, my father, my best friend, a former wife, and numerous other dear friends and associates are among the **missing in action.** Their lives were disfigured and cut short by the sick deeds of those who were supposed to "First, do no harm."*

As a tribute to those who have passed away, I must once again confront the archvillains responsible for this horrendous betrayal of their trust.

What separates this confrontation from all the others contained in this book is a hitherto unexposed reality that I wish to make public, in the hope that all reasonably minded people—including those who would otherwise disclaim my contentions—will see the glaring truth of my accusation.

J'accuse!

Iaccuse the American Medical Association (AMA) of knowingly conspiring to cover up the deadly effects of smoking for more than 100 years.

Just as the American Dental Association (ADA) has concealed the deadly effects of dental amalgams (mercury-metal fillings), the AMA consistently looked the other way, all but ignoring **what every doctor knew to be true,** namely that smoking caused lung cancer, heart disease, emphysema, and many other serious diseases and health complications. In fact, this cover-up was systematic and involved the unflinching support of the entire chain of conglomerate conspirators. It caused the premature death of more people than those who died from all of the world wars combined.

Let's first look at the systematic process of minimal clinical interventions (much of this information is listed on the National Center for Disease Control's Tobacco Information and Prevention Source website):

1. Until the first Surgeon General's report on smoking and health in the United States in 1964, the subject was kept in the closet by the medical fraternity.

2. The Federal Cigarette Labeling and Advertising Act of 1965 (Public Law 89-92) required that the warning "Caution: Cigarette Smoking May Be Hazardous to Your Health" be placed in small print on one of the side panels of each cigarette package. The act also prohibited additional labeling requirements at the federal, state, or local levels.

3. In June 1967, the Federal Trade Commission (FTC) issued its first report to Congress recommending that the warning label be changed to "Warning: Cigarette Smoking is Dangerous to Health and May Cause Death from Cancer and Other Diseases."

4. In 1969 Congress passed the Public Health Cigarette Smoking Act. Officially known as the Federal Cigarette Labeling and Advertising Act Amendments, Congress passed the law (Public Law 91-222) in 1970. It prohibited cigarette advertising on television and radio, requiring that each cigarette package contain the label, "Warning: The Surgeon General Has Determined That Cigarette Smoking Is Dangerous to Your Health."

5. By the mid-1980s, scientific evidence revealed that smokeless tobacco use causes oral cancer, nicotine addiction, and other health problems. The Com-

prehensive Smokeless Tobacco Health Education Act of 1986 (Public Law 99-252) required three rotating warning labels on smokeless tobacco packaging and advertisements: (1) WARNING: This product may cause mouth cancer. (2) WARNING: This product may cause gum disease and tooth loss. (3) WARNING: This product is not a safe alternative to cigarettes.

6.   On June 26, 2000, the FTC announced a settlement with seven of the largest U.S. cigar companies, requiring health warnings on cigar products. Health warnings must appear on the principal display panel to ensure that warnings are easily seen. The agreement also calls for warnings to be placed on various types of advertising, such as magazines and other periodicals, point-of-purchase displays, and catalogs, with every cigar package and advertisement requiring warnings that cigar smoking *can* cause cancers of the mouth and throat, even if you do not inhale; *can* cause lung cancer and heart disease; increases the risk of infertility, stillbirth, and low birth weight; are not a safe alternative to cigarettes; and increases the risk of lung cancer and heart disease, even in nonsmokers.

Needless to say, all the Surgeon General's reports and public laws passed by Congress had little effect on the smoking (and chewing) habits of Americans. In fact, in 1981 the FTC issued a report to Congress concluding that health warning labels had little effect on public knowledge and attitudes about smoking. The reasons for this lack of public attention are easy to evaluate. To be more precise:

- The Surgeon General's position in the hierarchy of the medical world is dubious at best. From the public's point of view, it's no more than a fancy title that holds no real weight and moves no one to action. Note: Former U.S. Surgeon General C. Everett Koop (Surgeon General from 1982 to 1989), who waged the most determined campaign against smoking, the leading cause of preventable death and disability in the United States, than any other federal official before or since, can now be seen on television advertisements selling emergency alarms.

- The overall planning and direction of the Surgeon General's office and Congress left little doubt that they constituted barely a half-hearted minimalist effort to alert the public to the dangers of smoking and the use of smokeless tobacco.

- The wording on the labels was conceived to dilute the seriousness of the danger. Words like "may be hazardous" and "can cause cancer" fall on deaf ears, all the more so because the labels appear in small print on only one side of the panels of each cigarette packet.

- Congressional leaders were lobbied by the tobacco industry and had no intention of going against the wishes of the people whose donations kept them in office. In case you're not aware, lobbying is a form of direct bribery. In the case of smoking, the tobacco industry bribed our Congress to allow the continued genocide of millions of Americans and to ignore the perjury of tobacco industry officials. This was obviously done in collusion with the conglomerate, **and the medical fraternity did not intervene.**

  Furthermore, the entire series of Surgeon General reports and public laws regarding warning labels was a fraud from beginning to end. These minor actions were meant to mislead the public and maintain the status quo for the smoking empire—and even when the CEOs of various tobacco companies perjured themselves repeatedly before senate committees, Congress took no action to finally force the issue and safeguard the public.

  Although Congress (finally) passed the Public Health Cigarette Smoking Act, which prohibited cigarette advertising on television and radio, the death-dealing Marlboro Man's advertisements were soon replaced by the conglomerate's pharmaceutical advertisements, so the public went from the fire into the frying pan!

As a child, I remember listening to the Jack Benny radio show and hearing these words every week: "A recent survey shows that more doctors smoke Camels than any other cigarette." Bravo doctors! You were aiding and abetting both the conglomerate and the tobacco industry even back then.

* * *

But all the above pales in comparison to the hitherto unrevealed reality of the AMA's direct involvement and complacency in the deaths of hundreds of millions of people. As I've never been known to pull my punches, I will now outline the tragic and gruesome details involved in this genocide that has gone unchecked for at least 100 years.

Let's use common sense:

- From the time when autopsies were first performed and death certificates were issued, what were the medical findings and conclusions regarding deaths of smokers caused by lung cancer and emphysema (to name the more obvious smoking-related diseases)? Is there anyone in his right mind who can say that until as late as 1965 (when the first warnings were placed on cigarette packages—and that only indicated *may be hazardous to your health)*—doctors had not identified smoking as the cause of death?

- Cadavers are examined in all medical schools, are they not? Did our good ol' buddy Doctor Warpick absent himself from these examinations? Was he blind to the fact that smoking caused cancer? Is that why he never told my father that smoking was dangerous? Or are you fool enough to believe that millions of men and women have gone through medical school without studying lung tissue, without being trained to identify the causes of lung cancer and emphysema? Or were they all told that each and every dead body that bore the signs of smoking-related disease had in fact worked in coal mines?!

    Sure, that's taking it to the ridiculous, but this demonstrates how far you have to go to believe that the doctors and the AMA did not know for absolute certainty—**for more than 100 years**—that smoking caused these deaths. **HOW COULD THEY NOT HAVE KNOWN?!**

An added note: In a 1950 study, Sir Richard Doll, a British scientist, established a clear link between smoking and lung cancer. The epidemiologist was credited with preventing millions of premature deaths in England. However, his American counterparts all but ignored his research. *Consequently, the first Surgeon General's report on health and smoking wasn't made until 14 years later.* How many millions of premature deaths in America might otherwise have been prevented?

All of which begs these questions:

- Why didn't the AMA petition Congress to take strong action against the tobacco companies to prevent the premature deaths of millions of people?

- Why did the AMA continue to ignore its responsibility while the evidence piled up higher and higher?

- Why did doctors pussyfoot with their patients about smoking-related health issues?

Let's go a step further:

- What reason would any doctor give for not telling—ordering—their patients to stop smoking? They would not hesitate to tell them if they needed surgery or to lose excess weight, so why did they shy away from confronting the issue of smoking?

- What prevented the AMA—before and after the first Surgeon General report on smoking—from turning to the American public and informing it of the full truth regarding smoking and tobacco use? **Why didn't the AMA make it a major issue?**

- Why didn't the AMA and all its affiliated organizations and agencies march on Washington, D.C. and demand full-scale action to prevent the ongoing genocide? Are you telling me that a million doctors, dentists, and care providers all rising to the occasion wouldn't have an effect on the public?

- You can bet on this: If the issue was tort reform, the nation's doctors would go to no ends to see that their grievances were heard. They would march, picket, demonstrate, create voter initiatives, and do everything in their power on behalf of themselves. But for their patients and the public in general—hell no!!!

The bottom line should be obvious to everyone: **The AMA, in consort with the tobacco industry and the conglomerate, has for over the better part of a century stood by and allowed hundreds of millions of people to die of smoke-related illnesses.** Of that, there can be no doubt. And whereas the AMA should be the first line of defense against the ravages of tobacco and the conglomerate, it has walked hand-in-hand with these sick-minded people and corporations—all the way to the bank. **And it still continues on this same path!**

Those millions of individuals who died for the sins of these madmen deserve something for their human sacrifice.

✳ ✳ ✳

While I'm on this deathly subject, I must also speak out for those victims of asbestos-related diseases, which have, since the 1930s, taken more than 300,000 lives. Once again, the AMA sat back on its haunches and paid only minor attention to this growing epidemic.

Chalk up another genocide to those sworn to "First, do no harm."

※ ※ ※

On behalf of all who have died as a result of neglect and indifference ... I accuse the AMA and the conglomerate of CRIMES AGAINST HUMANITY ... of which they must be charged and judged accordingly.

Be safe....

Bibliography

All entries here are listed sequentially rather than alphabetically, to help readers locate the author's sources more easily.

I.   MONUMENT TO FAILURE

3   McCaughey, Betsy. "Coming Clean." *The New York Times,* June 6, 2005.

3   Fouad, Dr. Tamer, M.D. "Study Shows Hospital Staph Infections Cause 12,000 deaths, Cost $9.5 billion." The Doctor's Lounge.net, August 11, 2005. http://www.thedoctorslounge.net/ infections/articles/nosocomial/staph_hospital/index.htm (July 10, 2006).

6   Abrams, Jim. "Congress Still Grappling with Pension Bill." The Associated Press, June 30, 2006.

6   Fitzgerald, Jay. "Health-care Expenses Keep Rising for People in Retirement." *Boston Herald,* March 7, 2006.

12   The Associated Press. "Panel Recommends Routine Cervical Cancer Shots for 11-, 12-Year-olds." June 30, 2006.

15   The Associated Press. "UNICEF: Poor Nutrition Kills Millions of Kids Each Year." May 3, 2006.

21   Cook, Gareth. "Scientists Find Regenerating Heart Cells." *The Boston Globe,* February 10, 2005.

21   Wade, Nicholas. "Plant May Have Backup of its Genome." *The New York Times,* March 23, 2005.

23   Cowell, Alan. "Better in Britain? In Matters of Health, Yes." *The New York Times,* May 3, 2006.

24   Cromie, William J. "Suicide High Among Female Doctors." Harvard University *Gazette,* February 3, 2005.

26   PR Web. "Rising Health Care Costs and Drug Complications Lead Americans to Explore Other Options." http://www.prweb.com/releases/2006/5/prweb384692.htm (November 12, 2006).

28   Starfield, Barbara. "Is U.S. Health Really the Best in the World?" *Journal of the American Medical Association* 4: 483–5 (July 26, 2000).

29   Herbert, Bob. "Doctor Recommends Strong Medicine for Nation's Health Care Ills." *The New York Times,* June 28, 2004.

30   The Henry J. Kaiser Foundation. *Kaiser Health Poll Report Survey.* August 2005.

31   O'Connor, Kathleen. "Involve Public in Health Care Reform." *Seattle Post-Intelligencer,* January 18, 2005.

33   Donn, Jeff. "Health Care Is 'Equally Mediocre,' Survey Finds." The Associated Press, March 16, 2006.

32   Hargrove, Thomas. "FBI Issues Statistics on Missing Children." Scripps Howard News Service, March 10, 2006.

33   Svensson, Peter. "U.S. Lagging on Maternity Leave." Seattle Post-Intelligencer, August 1, 2005.

35   Healthfinder.gov. "Hundreds of Thousands of U.S. Veterans Denied VA Health Care." U.S. Department of Health and Human Services, January 25, 2006.

35   Barker, Allison. "Soldier Injured in Iraq To Get Refund for Body Armor." The Associated Press, February 9, 2006.

35   Operation Helmet. 2006. http://www.operation-helmet.org (September 8, 2006).

35   The Associated Press. "Wounded Soldiers Left in Debt." April 28, 2006.

35   Barber, Mike. "Fisher Houses Offer Refuge to Vets' Families." *Seattle Post-Intelligencer,* April 26, 2006.

36   www.eyewitnesstohistory.com. "The Bonus Army." EyeWitness to History, 2000. http://www.eyewitnesstohistory.com/snprelief4.htm (July 9, 2006).

43   Bakalar, Nicholas. "Evidence Can Be Lacking for Drug Effectiveness." *The New York Times,* May 31, 2006.

43   Johnson, Gene. "Genetic Tests May Prevent Drug Reactions." The Associated Press, January 25, 2005.

43   The Associated Press. "Bad drug reactions send 700,000 to ER yearly." October 17, 2006.

44   Bridges, Andrew. "Millions of Pills Recalled over Metal Bits." The Associated Press, November 10, 2006.

44   Saul, Stephanie. "Sleeping Pill Ambien Tied to Traffic Arrests." *The New York Times,* March 8, 2006.

44   Food and Drug Administration. "U.S. Marshals Seize Lots of GlaxoSmithKline's Paxil CR and Avandamet Tablets Because of Continuing Good Manufacturing Practice Violations." Press release, March 4, 2005.

45   Industry Canada. *Clinical Trials in Canada: Quality with Cost Advantage.* Executive Summary of report prepared for Industry Canada, 2003.

45   Tanner, Lindsey. "Cough Syrups Don't Work, Doctors Say." The Associated Press, January 10, 2006.

46   Schmid, Randolph E. "Asians Warned on Cholesterol Drug." The Associated Press, March 3, 2005.

46   Harmon, Amy. "Young Play Doctor with Mood-altering Drugs." *The New York Times,* November 17, 2005.

47   Lyons, Kim. "Guard, Doctor Charged in OxyContin Ring." *Pittsburgh Tribune-Review,* December 22, 2005.

47   Families USA. "New Report Links High Prescription Drug Prices to Marketing Costs, Profits, and Enormous Executive Compensation." July 10, 2001. http://www.familiesusa.org/resources/ newsroom/press-releases/press-release-new-report-links-high-prescription-drug-prices-to-marketing-costs-profits-and-enormous-executive-compensation.html (June 4, 2006).

48   Scout News LLC. "Abbott Labs To Pull Controversial ADHD Drug." 2005. http://www.healthcentral.com/newsdetail/408/1505984.html (June 4, 2006).

49   The Associated Press. "FDA Withdraws Approval for ADD Drug (Pemoline)." October 24, 2005.

49   Bridges, Andrew. "Drug Companies Falling Through on Study Promises." March 4, 2006.

52   Bowman, Lee. "Doctors Order Needless Tests, Say Experts." Scripps Howard News Service, May 20, 2006.

54   Shukovsky, Paul. "Ex-UW Team Doctor Sentenced." *Seattle Post-Intelligencer,* May 10, 2005.

55   The Associated Press. "Kids' Behavior Drugs Use Soars." May 17, 2004.

56   Carey, Benedict. "More Kids Getting Anti-psychotic Drugs, Study Finds." *The New York Times,* June 6, 2006.

57   The Associated Press. "Feds Recommend Warnings on ADHD Drugs." February 9, 2006.

57   The Associated Press. "FDA Orders Antidepressant Warning." October 15, 2004.

57   Johnson, Linda. "Attention-Deficit Drugs Now No. 1." The Associated Press, May 17, 2004.

58   Pyle, Encarnacion. "Even Babies Getting Treated as Mentally Ill." *The Columbus Dispatch,* April 25, 2005.

58   Elias, Marilyn. "Strong Warnings Expected on Antidepressants for Kids." *USA Today,* September 8, 2004.

58   National Alliance Against Mandated Mental Health Screening and Psychiatric Drugging of Children. 2006. "Stephanie Died from Ritalin Used for ADHD at Age 11." www.ritalindeath.com/ ritalin-death.htm (October 14, 2006).

59   Harris, Gardiner. "Sleeping Pill Use by Youths Soars, Study Says." *The New York Times,* October 19, 2005.

60   Bakalar, Nicholas. "When Images Speak Louder Than Doctors." *The New York Times,* May 31, 2006.

61   Gardner, Amanda. "FDA Panel Calls for Strongest Warning on ADHD Drugs." HealthDay News, February 9, 2006.

61   Medical News Today. "New Sleeping Pills Are Effective, But None Stands Out As the Best." January 1, 2006. http://www.medicalnewstoday.com/medicalnews.php?newsid=35586 (June 26, 2006).

62   Forliti, Amy. "Exercise Helps Treat Depression." The Associated Press, March 17, 2005.

63   Columbia University TeenScreen Program. 2006. www.teenscreen.org (June 26, 2006).

66   Davidow, Julie and McGann, Chris. "High Court Deals Blow to Medical Marijuana." *Seattle Post-Intelligencer,* June 7, 2005.

67   Boone, Rebecca. "Judge Blasts Lack of Drug-rehab Centers." The Associated Press, November 22, 2005.

68   ESPN.com News Services. " '96 MVP Admitted Steroid Use, Fought Drug Problem." November 3, 2004. http://espn.go.com/classic/obit/s/2004/1010/1899091.html (July 10, 2006).

68   Hargrove, Thomas. "Heavy NFL Players Twice as Likely to Die Before 50." Scripps Howard News Service, January 31, 2006.

68   The Associated Press. "Steroid Penalties Much Tougher with Agreement." November 15, 2005.

69   Canseco, Jose. *Juiced: Wild Times, Rampant 'Roids, Smash Hits, and How Baseball Got Big.* New York: Regan Books, 2005.

71   Arangura Jr., Jorge. "Palmeiro Suspended for Steroid Violation." *The Washington Post,* August 2, 2005.

72   Baseballlibrary.com. "Gaylord Perry." 2006. http://www.baseballlibrary.com/ballplayers/player. php?name=Gaylord_Perry_1938 (November 8, 2006).

72   Brown, Maury. "BALCO Founder Conte Gets Eight Months." The Associated Press, October 18, 2005.

73   The Associated Press. "Meth Supplier Gets 107 Years in Prison." November 19, 2005.

73   CNN/Sports Illustrated. "Bonds Exposed: Shadows Details Superstar Slugger's Steroid Use." *Sports Illustrated,* March 7, 2006.

74   Miller, Ted. "Bonds Exposed: Saga Begets Outrage, Shrugs." *Seattle Post-Intelligencer,* March 8, 2006.

74   Brown, Sherrod. "U.S. Trade Rep Helps Powerful Drug Industry." *Seattle Post-Intelligencer,* June 28, 2005.

76   Abrams, Jim. "House Oks CAFTA on 217–215 Vote." The Associated Press, July 28, 2005.

76   Stevenson, Mark. "Pot, LSD, Coke—Small Amounts May Soon Be Allowed in Mexico." The Associated Press, April 29, 2006.

77   Harris, Gardiner, and Koli, Eric. "Dozens Died, But Drug Was Still Kept on Market." *The New York Times,* June 10, 2005.

79   Johnson, Linda. "Arthritis Drug Vioxx Recalled." The Associated Press, October 1, 2004.

80   Marchione, Marilynn. "After Vioxx, Safety Doubts Raised on Celebrex, Other Pain Relievers." The Associated Press, October 7, 2004.

80   Wikipedia. "Thalidomide." 2006. http://www.en.wikipedia.org/wiki/Thalidomide (June 28, 2006).

81   CBS Broadcasting, Inc. "Pfizer to Halt Celebrex Ads." December 20, 2004.

82   NewsMax.com. "Painkiller Vioxx Might Return to Sale." 2005. http://www.newsmax.com/archives/articles/2005/2/18/92207.shtml (February 18, 2005).

82   NewsTarget.com. "FDA Scientist Dr. David Graham Forced to Blow the Whistle by FDA Negligence." November 24, 2004. http://www.newstarget.com/002551.html (June 28, 2006).

83   Nesmith, Jeff. "Pain Drugs' Benefits Offset Risks, FDA Panel Decides." Cox News Service, February 19, 2005.

83   Harris, Gardiner and Berenson, Alex. "FDA Panelists Have Ties to Drug Makers." *The New York Times,* February 25, 2005.

84   Agovino, Theresa. "Merck Sought to Alter Vioxx." The Associated Press, June 23, 2005.

85   Berenson, Alex. "Merck Loses Vioxx-related Lawsuit." *The New York Times,* August 20, 2005.

86   McConnaughey, Janet. "Jury Finds Vioxx Is Not to Blame For Man's Death." The Associated Press, February 18, 2006.

87   The Associated Press. "Administration's Praise of FDA Provokes Outcry." December 20, 2004.

87   Henderson, Diedtra. "FDA Orders 'Black Box' Warning on Anti-depressants." The Associated Press, October 15, 2004.

89   Bridges, Andrew. "Unchecked, Tobacco Could Kill 1 Billion in This Century." The Associated Press, July 11, 2006.

89   Roxe, Hilary. "Reduced Penalty in Tobacco Trial Decried." The Associated Press, June 10, 2005.

90   Lichtblau, Eric. "Lawyers Opposed Cut in Tobacco Penalties." *The New York Times,* June 16, 2005.

91   Holland, Gina. "Court Won't Let Bush Push Tobacco Penalty." The Associated Press, October 17, 2005.

91   The Associated Press. "Judge: Big Tobacco Guilty of Decades of Deception." August 17, 2006.

92   Marchione, Marilynn. "Turning Back Heart Disease?" The Associated Press, March 14, 2006.

92   Meier, Barry. "Patients Not Told of Device's Flaw." *The New York Times,* May 24, 2005.

93   The Associated Press. "Guidant Recalls Heart Defibrillators." June 18, 2005.

93   Meier, Barry. "FDA Had Report of Short Circuit in Heart Devices." *The New York Times,* September 12, 2005.

94   Chang, Alicia. "Drug Studies Under the Influence." The Associated Press, May 26, 2005.

95   Donaldson, Jake. "Medical Schools Should Be Immune to Influence." *Seattle Post-Intelligencer,* February 20, 2006.

96   Tanner, Lindsey. "Report Finds Old Health Studies Wrong." The Associated Press, July 13, 2005.

96   Bowman, Lee. "Obese May Be More Sensitive to Pain." Scripps Howard News Service, March 2, 2006.

98   Phinney, Susan. "Study Finds a Clear Link Between Obesity and Mood Disorders." *Seattle Post-Intelligencer,* July 4, 2006.

98   Bowman, Lee. "Life for Older Americans Improving, Report Says." Scripps Howard News Service, March 10, 2006.

101   Bent, Stephen, et. al. "Saw Palmetto for Benign Prostatic Hyperplasia." *The New England Journal of Medicine.* February 9, 2006. http://content.nejm.org/cgi/content/short/354/6/557 (June 29, 2006).

103   Mercola, Dr. Joseph. "Vaccines and Immune Suppression." 2005. http://www.mercola.com/article/vaccines/immune_suppression.htm (August 1, 2006).

104   Johnson, Carla K. "Report: Flu Shots for Elderly Not Saving Lives." The Associated Press, February 15, 2005.

105   Bowman, Lee. "Study Casts More Doubt on Flu Shots." Scripps Howard News Service, February 25, 2005.

107   Lumpkin, John J. "New Flu-shot Supplier Approved as Vaccine Season Nears." The Associated Press, August 31, 2005.

108   The Associated Press. "Flu Preparations Expected To Cost at Least $6.5 Billion." November 1, 2005.

108   The Associated Press. "Nations Not Meeting Bird Flu Commitments." June 4, 2006.

108   *Seattle Post-Intelligencer* staff. "Bush's Plan To Fight Flu Doesn't Thrill States." *Seattle Post-Intelligencer,* November 2, 2005.

109   The Associated Press. "U.S. Not Prepared for Flu Pandemic." November 21, 2005.

109   The Associated Press. "Leavitt: States Will Ration Bird Flu Vaccine." June 7, 2006.

110   Paulson, Tom. "Lots of Vaccine, So Where Is It? Retailers Have Plenty; Health Providers Go Wanting." *Seattle Post-Intelligencer,* November 10, 2006.

112   Gay, Lance. "Clean Hands Fight School Germs, Kids Are Told." Scripps Howard News Service, September 22, 2005.

112   Lumpkin, John J. "FDA Panel Targets Claims of Anti-bacterial Soaps." The Associated Press, October 21, 2003.

113   Franklin, Deborah. "Not All Sanitizers Live Up to Name." *The New York Times,* March 21, 2006.

113   NSF International. "Millions of Germs and Bacteria Await Kids at School." Press release, NSF International. September 15, 2005.

115 Bartley, Nancy. "Woman Who Took Son From Hospital Is Charged with Kidnapping." *The Seattle Times,* June 26, 2006.

118 Tanner, Lindsey. "Study: Estrogen Pills Raise Risk of Dementia." The Associated Press, June 22, 2004.

118 Neergaard, Lauran. "Hot Flashes? Night Sweats? Hormone Therapy Still Rated Best." The Associated Press, September 30, 2004.

118 Phinney, Susan. "Estrogen May Help in Preventing Heart Disease." *Seattle Post-Intelligencer,* February 14, 2006.

119 Kolata, Gina. "Studies Challenge Traditional Breast Cancer Treatments." *The New York Times,* April 12, 2006.

119 The Associated Press. "Birth Control Pills Cut Risk of Heart Disease, Cancer." October 20, 2004.

120 Nozawa, Randall. *Inside Dentistry: Everything You Need To Know.* Bellevue, Wash.: Elfin Cove Press, 2000.

120 Davidow, Julie. "2 Studies Vindicate Mercury Fillings: No Link Found to Impairments." *Seattle Post-Intelligencer,* April 19, 2006.

121 Dreyfuss, Ira. "Limbering Up? It May Be a Stretch To Find Benefits." The Associated Press, August 14, 2004.

122 The Associated Press. "Millions Get Needless Pap Tests, Says Researchers." October 8, 2004.

122 Pollack, Andrew. "Aspirin Isn't Always What Doctor Ordered." *The New York Times,* July 20, 2004.

123 Shane, Scott. "New Thinking on Gulf War Illnesses." *The New York Times,* September 24, 2004.

124 Bridges, Andrew. "No Such Thing as Gulf War Syndrome, Federal Report Says." The Associated Press, September 13, 2006.

124 Tanner, Lindsey. "Obesity Surgery Can Cure Other Problems, Too, Research Finds." The Associated Press, November 5, 2004.

124 Donn, Jeff. "Liposuction May Not Make You Healthier." The Associated Press, June 17, 2004.

125 Smith, Stephen. "Once-touted Vitamin E Fails As a Magic Bullet." *The Boston Globe,* November 26, 2004.

125 Carey, Benedict. "Mom's Anti-depressant Use May Cause Babies To Have Withdrawal." *The New York Times,* February 4, 2005.

125 Bowman, Lee. "Moms Taking Anti-depressants May Put Unborn Babies At Risk." Scripps Howard News Service, May 18, 2005.

126 Grady, Denise. "Childbirth Study Says No Need To Delay Epidurals." *The New York Times,* February 17, 2005.

128 Johnson, Carla K. "More Research Casts Doubts on Benefits of Episiotomies." The Associated Press, May 4, 2005.

129 The Associated Press. "Ovary Loss May Hurt Women, Study Says." August 1, 2000.

129 Neergaard, Lauran. "Breast Implant Ban May Be Lifted." The Associated Press, April 14, 2005.

130 Davidow, Julie. "Teens Taking Depo-Provera Can Recover Lost Bone Density." Seattle Post-Intelligencer, February 8, 2005.

130 Cortez, Michelle Fay. "High-fiber Diet and Cancer: Prevention Claims Disputed." Bloomberg News, December 14, 2005.

131 Kolata, Gina. "Big Study Finds No Clear Benefit of Calcium Pills." The New York Times, February 16, 2006.

131 Johnson, Linda A. "Women with Lupus Can Use Birth Control Pill, Studies Say." The Associated Press, December 15, 2005.

132 Kolata, Gina. "Study Tying Longer Life to Extra Pounds Draws Fire." The New York Times, May 27, 2005.

133 Marchione, Marilynn. "Health and Fat Don't Mix, CDC Chief Says." The Associated Press, June 3, 2005.

133 Bowman, Lee. "Vitamin C Won't Stop a Cold—Unless You Run Miles." Scripps Howard News Service, June 28, 2005.

134 Tanner, Lindsey. "Doctors, U.S. Panel at Odds Over Worth of Yearly Exams." The Associated Press, June 28, 2005.

135 Tanner, Lindsey. "Review Finds Fish Oil Doesn't Cut Cancer Risk." The Associated Press, January 25, 2006.

135 Stengle, Jamie. "Soy Vey! Maybe Tofu Isn't So Great After All." The Associated Press, January 23, 2006.

135 Wein, Harrison. "Different Trials, Different Results: How To Explain Them?" The National Institutes of Health, August 2004. http://www.nih.gov/news/WordonHealth/aug2004/story03.htm (November 12, 2006).

135 Davidow, Julie. "Low-fat Diets Didn't Lower Cancer Risks." Seattle Post-Intelligencer, February 8, 2006.

135 Raloff, Janet. "Do Meat and Dairy Harm Aging Bones?" Science News, January 13, 2001, Vol. 159 (2): 20.

135 The Associated Press. "Research: Third of Study Results Don't Hold Up." July 13, 2005.

135 Cole, Kristen. "Consider the Source When Weighing Contradictory Health Advice." George Street Journal, September 14, 2001.

136 Allen, Scott. "Review: Hospital Errors Are Major Cause of Death." *The Boston Globe,* July 28, 2004.

137 Francis, Raymond. "A Nation At Risk." Beyond Health, 2006. http://www.beyondhealth.com/nation-at-risk.htm (July 10, 2006).

137 CIA. The World Factbook. "Rank Order: Population." June 29, 2006. https://www.cia.gov/cia/publications/factbook/fields/2119.html (November 12, 2006)

138 Bowman, Lee. "Medical Workers Are Often Mum On Mistakes." Scripps Howard News Service, January 27, 2005.

139 McCaughey, Betsy. "Clean Up Hygiene in U.S. Hospitals." *Seattle Post-Intelligencer,* June 7, 2005.

141 The Associated Press. "Surgical Tools Washed in Hydraulic Fluid." June 13, 2005.

141 Bowman, Lee. "Hospital's Bottom Line Tied to Surgical Mistakes." Scripps Howard News Service, June 8, 2005.

142 Heavey, Susan. "U.S. Leads Way in Medical Errors." Reuters, November 3, 2005.

142 Berman, Steve W. "Hospitals Take Advantage of the Uninsured." *Seattle Post-Intelligencer,* June 2, 2005.

144 Asplin, Brent R. M.D., et al. "Insurance Status and Access to Urgent Ambulatory Care Follow-up Appointments." *Journal of the American Medical Association* 294 (10): 1248–1254 (September 14, 2005).

144 The Associated Press. "Report: ER Care in U.S. at 'Breaking Point'." June 14, 2006.

145 Stobbe, Mike. "C-section Rate Sets a Record of 29%." The Associated Press, November 16, 2005.

149 Badam, Ramola Talwar. "Foreign Surgeons Attract U.S. Patients." The Associated Press, September 25, 2005.

152 Tanner, Lindsey. "Obesity Procedures Riskier Than Thought." The Associated Press, October 24, 2005.

154 Klein, Steve L. "Medical Liability Crisis Full of Myths." *Seattle Post-Intelligencer,* November 3, 2004.

155 Tanner, Lindsey. "Fearing Suits, Doctors Practice Alarming Rate of 'Defensive Medicine'."The Associated Press, June 1, 2005.

157 The Associated Press. "$17.1 Million Awarded in Malpractice Suit." April 19, 2005.

157 The Associated Press. "Judge Awards Parents of Disabled Child $60.9 Million." November 25, 2005.

158 Congressional Budget Office. "Limiting Tort Liability for Medical Malpractice." January 8, 2004. http://cbo.gov/showdoc.cfm?index=4968&sequence=0 (July 6, 2006).

158   Guntheroth, Warren G. "Physician Says No on I-330 and I-336." *Seattle Post-Intelligencer,* November 3, 2005.

158   Galloway, Angela. "Nurses Oppose Initiatives." *Seattle Post-Intelligencer,* October 19, 2005.

160   Anderson, Rick. "Self-diagnosis." *Seattle Weekly,* June 16–22, 2004.

161   *Seattle Post-Intelligencer* staff and news services. "Doctor Convicted in UW Billing Fraud Loses Bid To End Probation." May 10, 2005.

162   Harris, Gardiner. "Big Drug Maker To Plead Guilty in Medicaid Case." *The New York Times,* July 16, 2004.

162   Harris, Gardiner. "Feds Probe 'Payoffs' By Drug Company." *The New York Times,* June 27, 2004.

163   Abelson, Reed and Glater, Jonathan D. "Texas Jury Rules Against the Maker of Fen-Phen, a Diet Drug." *The New York Times,* April 28, 2004.

165   McDonough, Siobhan. "Charity Heads' Salaries Soar Above Inflation Rate, Study Says." The Associated Press, September 20, 2004.

165   Fonda, Daren. "Time 100: The People Who Shape Our World: Jim Sinegal." *Time* Magazine, April 30, 2006.

166   Jackson, Derrick Z. "Snow's Take on Economy Is Unreal." *The Boston Globe,* April 25, 2006.

166   The Associated Press. "House Lawmakers Accept $3,300 Pay Hike." June 13, 2006.

166   Espo, David. "Senate Rejects Bid to Raise Minimum Wage." The Associated Press, June 21, 2006.

167   Solomon, John. "Experiment Volunteers Kept in Dark by Scientists." The Associated Press, January 4, 2005.

168   Colliver, Victoria. "Excessive Medical Expenses: Study Finds That Half of Health Care Dollars Are Wasted." *San Francisco Chronicle,* February 9, 2005.

169   Pear, Robert. "Scam Costs Insurers Millions." *The New York Times,* March 12, 2005.

170   Timmerman, Luke, and Heath, David. "Drug Researchers Leak Secrets to Wall St." *Seattle Times,* August 7, 2005.

175   Milgrom, Peter. "UW Says No to Dental Help for Native Alaskans." *Seattle Post-Intelligencer,* June 29, 2006.

176   Roosevelt, Margot. "Nursing a Grudge." CNN.com, February 28, 2005. http://edition.cnn.com/2005/ALLPOLITICS/02/28/californianurses.tm (November 12, 2006).

177   The Associated Press. "Schwarzenegger Drops Legal Fight Over Hospital Staffing." November 11, 2005.

177   Nossiter, Adam and Dewan, Sheila. "Katrina Doctor, Nurses Accused of Homicide." *The New York Times,* July 19, 2006.

178   Sommerfeld, Julia and Berens, Michael. "Biggest Number of Offenders Are 'Registered Counselors.'" *Seattle Times,* April 24, 2006.

181   Cool, Lisa Collier. "The Preventable Cancer." *Good Housekeeping,* October 1998.

182   Boyles, Salynn. "Fiber Not Protective for Colon Cancer." WebMD Medical News, 2006. http://www.webmd.com/content/article/116/112118.htm (November 19, 2006).

184   Butler, Rhett A. "People Live the Longest in Japan, Monaco, San Marino." April 16, 2006. http://news.mongabay.com/2006/0414-who5.html (July 7, 2006).

188   Freyer, Felice J. "Supreme Court Rules Against Doctor-assisted Suicides for the Terminally Ill." *The Providence Journal,* June 27, 1997.

188   Death With Dignity National Center. "The Oregon Death with Dignity Law." 2006. http://www.deathwithdignity.org/historyfacts (July 7, 2006).

191   Goldberg, Alan B. and Ritter, Bill. "Costco CEO Finds Pro-worker Means Profitability." ABC News, December 3, 2005.

191   D'Arista, Jane. "The U.S. International Investment Position at Year-end 2000." *Capital Flows Monitor,* Financial Markets Center, September 14, 2001.

194   *Seattle Post-Intelligencer* News Services. "Study Shows Obesity Risks May Have Been Overstated." *Seattle Post-Intelligencer,* April 20, 2005.

194   The Center for Consumer Freedom. "Obesity Hype." 2006. http://www.consumerfreedom.com/issuepage.cfm/topic/37 (August 8, 2006).

195   Deveau, Scott. "They'd Trade Year of Life for Thinner Waist." *The Toronto Globe and Mail,* May 18, 2006.

197   Panos, Maesimund B. and Heimlich, Jane. *Homeopathic Medicine At Home.* New York: Tarcher, 1981.

200   Staton, Ron. "Growing Number of Hawaiians Practicing Native Healing Traditions." The Associated Press, August 18, 2005.

200   The Global Academy Institute for Integrative Medicine. 2001. http://www.theglobalacademy.org/int_medicine.asp (November 12, 2006).

202   Bowman, Lee. "Americans Are Forever Going to the Doctor's." Scripps Howard News Service, June 24, 2006.

204   Lewis, Mike, Galloway, Angela, and Castro, Hector. "Killer's Motive Remains Elusive." *Seattle Post-Intelligencer,* March 27, 2006.

204   Castro, Hector. "Killer's Taunt: 'There's Plenty For Everyone.'" *Seattle Post-Intelligencer,* March 28, 2006.

206   Kirby, Paul. "Bonelli Gets 32 Years in Prison for Mall Shooting." Dailyfreeman.com, May 20, 2006. http://www.dailyfreeman.com/site/news.cfm?BRD=1769&dept_id=74969&newsid=16667523&PAG=461&rfi=9 (July 8, 2006).

208   Tanner, Lindsey. "16 Million Americans May Have Anger Ailment." The Associated Press, June 6, 2006.

209   Sherman, Mark. "Violent Crime Shows Increase in 2005." The Associated Press, June 13, 2006.

211   Gillson, Sharon. "Stretta Procedure." About.com, 2006. http://heartburn.about.com/cs/articles/a/stretta.htm (September 8, 2006).

212   Bowman, Lee. "Study Compares Acid Reflux Treatments." Scripps Howard News Service, December 15, 2005.

214   Henderson, Mark. "Drug Companies 'Inventing' Diseases to Boost Their Profits'." *The Times,* April 11, 2006.

217   Hulse, Carl. "GOP Offers Salve for Pain at Pump." *The New York Times,* April 28, 2006.

217   Pope, Charles. "Cantwell Bid to Cut Foreign Oil Imports Dies in Senate." *Seattle Post-Intelligencer,* June 17, 2005.

217   Foss, Brad. "Nation's Petroleum Reserve Nearly Full." The Associated Press, June 8, 2005.

217   Hebert, H. Josef. "EPA Paper May Link Gas Additive With Cancer." The Associated Press, July 22, 2005.

218   Egelko, Bob. "How Bush Sidesteps Intent of Congress: Instead of Vetoing Bills, He Officially Disregards Portions With Which He Doesn't Agree." *San Francisco Chronicle,* May 7, 2006.

218   Heneroty, Kate. "Bush Signs Anti-Torture Legislation, Patriot Act Extension." *Jurist Legal News and Research,* December 31, 2005.

219   National Public Radio. "Citizen Soldiers to be Reduced in Iraq, Afghanistan." February 7, 2006. http://www.npr.org/templates/story/story.php?storyId=5194760 (November 12, 2006).

219   Savage, Charlie. "Bar Group Will Review Bush's Legal Challenges." *The Boston Globe,* June 4, 2006.

219   Pear, Robert. "Medicaid Cuts Will Hurt Poor." *The New York Times,* January 30, 2006.

219   Hunt, Terence. "Bush Defends Exxon's Record Profit." The Associated Press, February 2, 2006.

219   Romero, Simon, and Andrews, Edmund L. "At Exxon Mobil, a Record Profit But No Fanfare." *The New York Times,* January 31, 2006.

220   Lewis, Mike. "Exxon still owes for Valdez spill." *The Seattle Post-Intelligencer*, March 13, 2006.

228   Woodward, Curt. "Gregoire Signs Tougher DUI Law." *Seattle Post-Intelligencer,* March 16, 2006.

230   Allen, Jamie. "Nuclear attack: Now Anything Seems Possible." CNN.com, November 9, 2001. http://archives.cnn.com/2001/US/11/08/rec.nuclear.attack/index.html (November 12, 2006).

230   Preston, Richard. *The Demon in the Freezer: a True Story.* New York: Random House, 2002.

230   The Associated Press. "Greenhouse Gases Hit High in 2004." March 14, 2006.

232   Hollon, Dr. Matthew. "Direct-to-Consumer Advertising: A Haphazard Approach to Health Promotion." *Journal of the American Medical Association,* 2005; 293: 2030-2033.

235   Connolly, Ceci. "Bush Budget Would Cut Popular Health Programs." *The Washington Post,* February 14, 2006.

235   Harlow, John. "Angry Cruise Defends Scientology Bar on Drugs." *The Sunday Times,* June 26, 2005.

235   Evalu8.org. "Scientologist Says Psychiatric Drugs Are Unnecessary, Prompting Calls From Worried Patients on Antidepressants." July 1, 2005. http://evalu8.org/staticpage?page=review& siteid=9375 (July 8, 2006).

237   Thomas, Helen. "Law Legalizes Shameful Treatment." *Seattle Post-Intelligencer,* October 20, 2006.

237   Holland, Gina. "High Court Trims Whistleblower Rights." The Associated Press, May 30, 2006.

238   Neergaard, Lauran. "FDA Women's Health Chief Quits." The Associated Press, September 1, 2005.

238   Davidow, Julie. "FDA Has Lost Its Way, Says Former Official." *Seattle Post-Intelligencer,* February 11, 2006.

238   Neergaard, Lauran. "FDA Chief Abruptly Quits; Bush Names Acting Chief." The Associated Press, September 24, 2005.

239   Harris, Gardiner. "FDA Dismisses Medical Benefit from Marijuana." *The New York Times,* April 21, 2006.

239   Joy, Janet E., Watson, Jr., Stanley J., and Benson, Jr., John A. *Marijuana and Medicine: Assessing the Science Base.* Washington, D.C.: Institute of Medicine, National Academy of Sciences, 1999.

239   Environmental Integrity Project. "Report: EPA Taking 75% Fewer Polluters to Court, Major Polluter Cases Down 90%." October 12, 2004. http://www.environmentalintegrity.org/ pubs/101204_EIP_news_release_FINAL3.doc (July 8, 2006).

242   Heilprin, John. "Environmental Reviews Waived in Push for Oil." The Associated Press, October 19, 2005.

243   Stiffler, Lisa. "Puget Sound a Toxic Stew, Scientists Say." *Seattle Post-Intelligencer,* April 6, 2006.

243   Janofsky, Michael. "EPA to Bar Data From Pesticide Studies Involving Children and Pregnant Women." *The New York Times,* September 7, 2005.

243   Doyle, Michael. "Pesticide Tests May Use Pregnant Women, Kids." McClatchy Newspapers, January 24, 2006.

244   Heilprin, John. "Pesticides Reach Most Rivers." The Associated Press, March 4, 2006.

244   Jaroff, Leon. "Erin Brockovich's Junk Science." *Time* Magazine, July 8, 2006.

245   Whipple, Chris G. "Can Nuclear Waste Be Stored at Yucca Mountain?" *Scientific American,* June 1996.

245   Dininny, Shannon. "Hanford Plant Cost Rises to $11.55 Billion." *Seattle Post-Intelligencer,* June 22, 2006.

245   Heilprin, John. "Ex-chiefs at EPA Assail Bush on Global Warming." The Associated Press, January 19, 2006.

246   Chase, Randall. "Teflon Chemical a Likely Carcinogen." The Associated Press, January 31, 2006.

246   Werner, Erica. "DOE: Suspect Yucca Mountain Work Is Sound, But Will Be Redone." The Associated Press, February 18, 2006.

247   Wagner, Thomas. "Britain Sees a Climate Crisis; Tony Blair Taps Al Gore To Help Cut Greenhouse Gas Emissions." The Associated Press, October 31, 2006.

247   Johnson, Mark. "Court Blocks Attempt To Ease Clean Air Rules." The Associated Press, March 18, 2006.

249   Jesse Ventura, interview by Larry King. *Larry King Live.* Cable News Network, September 20.

249   Coile, Zachary. "House Acts To End Some Food Label Warnings." *San Francisco Chronicle,* March 9, 2006.

250   Pear, Robert. "Ex-Rep. Tauzin To Be Lobbyist For Drug Firms." *The New York Times,* December 9, 2004.

252   Gamboa, Suzanne. "Lobbyist Accused of Bilking Tribe." The Associated Press, June 23, 2004.

252   U-S-History.com. "Tammany Hall." 2005. http://www.u-s-history.com/pages/h705.html (July 8, 2006).

253   Shepard, Scott. "Abramoff Guilty Plea Shakes Capitol Hill." Cox News Service, January 4, 2006.

253   The Associated Press. "Abramoff Pleads Guilty To More Federal Charges." January 4, 2006.

253   Stolberg, Sheryl Gay and Phillips, Kate. "Senate Votes for Ban on Gifts and Meals From Lobbyists." *The New York Times,* March 9, 2006.

253   Dishneau, David and Matt Apuzzo. "Lobbyist Abramoff Begins Prison Sentence." The Associated Press, November 15, 2006.

254   Shenon, Philip. "Ney Admits Guilt in Lobby Scandal." *The New York Times,* September 16, 2006.

254   Pope, Charles. "State's Firms Pump Millions Into Federal Lobbbying." *Seattle Post-Intelligencer,* April 9, 2005.

255 Pear, Robert. "Medicare Law Prompts a Rush for Lobbyists." *The New York Times*, August 23, 2005.

256 Pear, Robert. "Health Care Inquiry Cash Misdirected." *The New York Times*, May 16, 2005.

257 Medicare website. "Prescription Drug Coverage: Basic Information." November 16, 2005. http://www.medicare.gov/pdp-basic-information.asp (July 8, 2006).

261 Epstein, Samuel. "Cancer War Should Focus on Prevention." *Seattle Post-Intelligencer*, April 27, 2005.

262 Cybernation.com. 2006. "How To Cleanse Your Body, Obtain Your Ideal Weight, And Have More Energy Than Your Wildest Dreams!" http://www.cybernation.com/livingston/isagenix (November 19, 2006).

263 Marchione, Marilynn. "New Cancer Drugs 'Multitask'." The Associated Press, May 14, 2005.

264 Berenson, Alex. "A Cancer Drug Shows Promise, at a Price That Many Can't Pay." *The New York Times*, February 15, 2006.

264 Miller, Cathryn. "Respond to Drug Costs With Political Action." *Seattle Post-Intelligencer*, June 26, 2006.

264 Neergaard, Lauran. "$100 Million Project To Get to the Root of Cancer." The Associated Press, December 14, 2005.

264 Neergaard, Lauran. "Experts To Create Genetic Map of Cancer." The Associated Press, December 14, 2005.

265 Herbert, Bob. "Illogical Cutbacks on Cancer." *The New York Times*, March 20, 2006.

265 Michael J. Fox Foundation for Parkinson's Research. "Michael J. Fox Testifies Before Congress on Stem Cell Research," September 14, 2000.

266 Neergaard, Lauran. "Treatments Save Lives and Fertility." The Associated Press, May 9, 2006.

269 *Seattle Post-Intelligencer* News Services. "Miners' Shocking End." January 4, 2006.

270 Kauffman, Matthew. "Charities' Costs Sap Aid for Vets." *Hartford Courant*, November 10, 2005.

270 Wiesen, Sloan C. "NCRP Findings Show Reasonable Reform Measure Could Pump Billions Into Charities While Preserving Foundations." National Committee for Responsive Philanthropy (NCRP), June 2, 2003.

270 Forbes website. "American National Red Cross." 2006. http://www.forbes.com/finance/lists/14/2004/LIR.jhtml?passListId=14&passYear=2004&passListType=Misc&datatype=Misc&uniqueId=CH0013 (July 78, 2006).

270 St. Clair, Jeffrey and Bernardo Issel. "A Field Guide to the Environmental Movement." *These Times*, July 28, 2997.

271 Weisman, Jonathan. "HHS Secretary's Fund Gave Little to Charity." *The Washington Post*, July 21, 2006.

276   Modie, Neil and Scott Gutierrez. "Obama Thrills Crowd Like Celebrity." *Seattle Post-Intelligencer,* October 27, 2006.

277   Wikipedia.org. "Lee Boyd Malvo." November 9, 2006. http://en.wikipedia.org/wiki/Lee_Boyd_Malvo (November 13, 2006).

277   *The Michigan Daily.* "Bin Laden Surfaces in New Taped Threats." January 20, 2006.

282   Eber, Gabriel B. et al. "Nonfatal and Fatal Firearm-related Injuries Among Children Aged 14 Years and Younger: United States, 1993–2000." *Pediatrics,* Vol. 113, No. 6, June 2004, pp. 1686–1692.

284   Wikipedia.org. "Lyndon LaRouche U.S. Presidential campaigns." June 27, 2006. http://en.wikipedia.org/wiki/Lyndon_LaRouche_U.S._Presidential_campaigns (November 13, 2006).

284   Wikipedia.org. "Ross Perot." November 12, 2006. http://en.wikipedia.org/wiki/Ross_Perot (November 13, 2006).

290   Kunz, Diane B. "Marshall Plan Commemorative Section: The Marshall Plan Reconsidered: A Complex of Motives." *Foreign Affairs,* May/June 1997.

294   Connor, Steve. "Glaxo Chief: Our Drugs Do Not Work on Most Patients." *The Independent* (UK), December 8, 2003.

II.   WHAT GOES AROUND COMES AROUND

299   Neergaard, Lauran. "Panel Decries U.S. for Killing Plan To Fight Obesity in Kids." The Associated Press, September 14, 2006.

301   Goldberg, Carey. "Even a Little Extra Fat May Shorten Lifespan." *The Boston Globe,* August 23, 2006.

301, 303   Davidow, Julie. "The Obesity Crisis: Americans' Bodies Are Out of Balance." *Seattle Post-Intelligencer,* September 8, 2004.

301   Nesmith, Jeff. "Hunger Gene Also Suppresses Appetite, Scientists Find." Cox News Service, November 13, 2005.

302   Davidow, Julie. "Kids May Be Getting a Media Overdose." *Seattle Post-Intelligencer,* April 4, 2006.

III.   ROMAN EMPERORS OF OLD

333   Dobnik, Verena. "Man Eats 53¾ Hot Dogs in 12 Minutes." The Associated Press, July 4, 2006.

336   Neergaard, Lauran. "Overdose of Tylenol Ingredient Can Kill." The Associated Press, September 20, 2002.

341   Rousseau, Caryn. "Governor Loses 110 Pounds, Beats Colleague in Marathon." The Associated Press, March 7, 2005.

IV.   THE BEST DAMN WORKOUT EVER

349   CNN. "Most Americans Don't Exercise Regularly." CNN.com, April 7, 2002. http://archives. cnn.com/2002/HEALTH/04/07/americans.exercise (November 8, 2006).

371   Castro, Hector. "Redmond Teen's Condition Amazes Doctors." *Seattle Post-Intelligencer,* October 11, 2004.

376   Donald W. Reynolds Department of Geriatrics website. "Faculty: William J. Evans, Ph.D." 2003. http://www.geriatrics.uams.edu/faculty/detail.asp?ID=62 (July 8, 2006)

378   Bowman, Lee. "Caffeine Metabolism Tied to Heart Attacks." Scripps Howard News Service, March 8, 2006.

388   Real-Hypnosis.com. "History of Hypnosis." 2006. http://www.real-hypnosis.com/ historyofhypnosis.html (August 8, 2006).

V.   J'ACCUSE!

401, 402   National Center for Chronic Disease Prevention and Health Promotion. Tobacco Information and Prevention Source website. 2006. http://www.cdc.gov/tobacco (November 19, 2006).

404   Rising, David. "Health Pioneer Richard Doll Dies." The Associated Press, July 25, 2005.

404   Lynch, Barbara S. and Bonnie, Richard J., Editors. *Growing Up Tobacco Free: Preventing Nicotine Addiction in Children and Youths.* Washington, D.C.: Institute of Medicine, National Academy of Sciences, 1994.

405   Castleman, Barry. Senate Hearing, July 31, 2001. http://www.agiweb.org/gap/legis107/ asbestos.html (November 19, 2006)

About the Author

A born-and-bred New Yorker who has traveled extensively, Nickolas Vassili now resides in Seattle, Washington, with his wife of 36 years and his four grown children. The greater part of his professional life has been focused on show business, from performing to production and everything in between. In Nickolas Vassili's second career as a group therapist, he helped create the foundation for most of the group dynamics now used throughout America. He has written articles, plays, and screenplays. In addition, he helped author a book on dentistry and published newspapers in Europe. Nickolas Vassili guided the fortunes of *Children of the Revolution,* a music phenomenon that is the future of contemporary world music. In regard to his credibility as the world's expert on bulimia, N. V. is 70 years old, in perfect health, and in fantastic physical condition. He feels and looks much younger than most men in their 40s and 50s.

www.ingramcontent.com/pod-product-compliance
Lightning Source LLC
Chambersburg PA
CBHW031814170526
45157CB00001B/50